ECG at a Glance

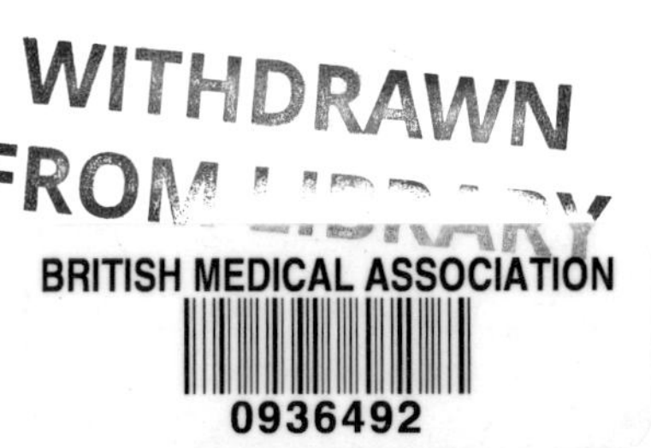

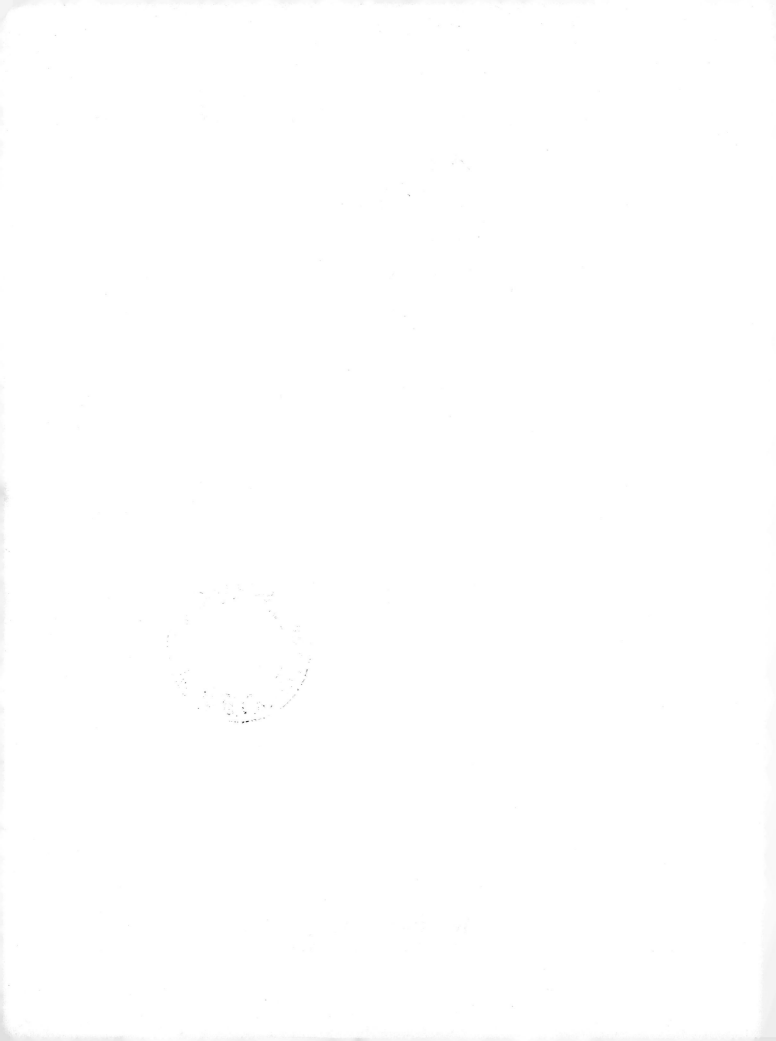

ECG at a Glance

Patrick Davey

Consultant Cardiologist
Northampton General Hospital
Northampton, and
Honorary Senior Lecturer
Department of Cardiovascular Medicine
John Radcliffe Hospital
Oxford

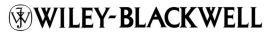

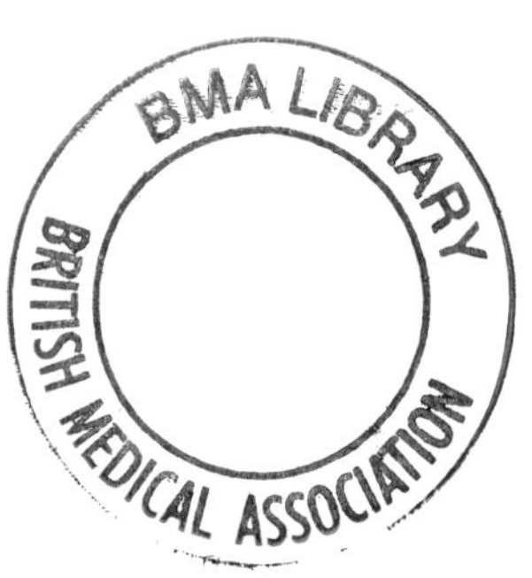

WILEY-BLACKWELL
A John Wiley & Sons, Ltd., Publication

Blackwell Publishing was acquired by John Wiley & Sons in February 2007. Blackwell's publishing program has been merged with Wiley's global Scientific, Technical and Medical business to form Wiley-Blackwell.

Registered office: John Wiley & Sons Ltd, The Atrium, Southern Gate, Chichester, West Sussex, PO19 8SQ, UK

Editorial offices: 9600 Garsington Road, Oxford, OX4 2DQ, UK
The Atrium, Southern Gate, Chichester, West Sussex, PO19 8SQ, UK
111 River Street, Hoboken, NJ 07030-5774, USA

For details of our global editorial offices, for customer services and for information about how to apply for permission to reuse the copyright material in this book please see our website at www.wiley.com/wiley-blackwell

Library of Congress Cataloguing-in-Publication Data
Davey, Patrick,
ECG at a glance / Patrick Davey.
p. ; cm. – (At a glance series)
Includes index.
ISBN 978-0-632-05405-3
1. Electrocardiography – Handbooks, manuals, etc. I. Title. II. Series: At a glance series (Oxford, England) [DNLM: 1. Electrocardiography – Handbooks. WG 39 D248e 2008]
RC683.5.E5D32 2008
616.1′207547–dc22
2007016865

ISBN: 978-0-632-05405-3

A catalogue record for this book is available from the British Library

Set in 9/11.5pt Times by Graphicraft Limited, Hong Kong
Printed in Singapore by Fabulous Printers Pte Ltd

1 2008

Contents

Preface

As you are reading this preface, you wish to learn more about the ECG. Many books will try and persuade you that learning how to interpret the ECG is easy, will require little or no effort, and certainly won't take you long, just a brief read of a short book over a night or two should do it. These views are incorrect. Learning the ECG is difficult, there are many challenges to be overcome, and it will take you a long time before you become competent. As learning takes time and is challenging, ultimately, it is very rewarding.

The basic principle in learning the ECG, as is true for much of medicine, is that you should understand the basics, and then develop this knowledge using individual patients. I hope this book introduces you to the basics, then as it takes you through the many different examples, you can extract the general principles as you go along.

As a guide, I would suggest the following approach to those new to the ECG:

• Start off by reading the first two chapters to give yourself a very basic introduction to the topic. Take a break for a few days, maybe even longer.

• Re-read the first two chapters, then read and understand the four chapters on the basic properties of the normal ECG. Take another break.

• Read the next 11 chapters in Part 2, first briefly revising the four chapters on the normal ECG. As you go along, rehearse in your own mind what you have learnt, and in particular try and understand why things are as they are. Ask yourself questions; use the index to look up the answers.

• These initial sections give you a basic understanding of the ECG; try and embed this knowledge early on.

• Don't overfill yourself too quickly with knowledge from these sections and press on too quickly on to the main body of the book. Whenever you need to, take a break for a few days, or even longer. These initial sections may well take you, gently, a good few weeks to assimilate. Be quite certain that you understand them before you progress onwards to the more clinical sections of the book.

• When you feel ready progress on to the next sections. These six sections are on more advanced areas of the ECG, either a clinical syndrome (e.g. chest pain), a disease process, arrhythmias, complex ECG based investigations, or device therapy. Dip in here in random order as your interest takes you; this is allowed for as there is much repetition in the book, and much cross-referencing. Often the best way to learn is to hang your learning around a case that you have seen. Accordingly, as you see cases on the wards, and in outpatients, look them up in these sections, then follow your curiosity to related chapters.

The mainstay of learning is experience. How many ECGs do you need to read before you are competent? Most national cardiac societies feel about 500 ECGs are needed. Try very hard to read the ECG blind, i.e. before you know what it is meant to show: it is in the intellectual act of you trying to work out what is going on that learning occurs, so you should allow this to happen. Ask more senior colleagues what they think the ECG shows, to confirm or deny your views. The figure of 500 ECGs gives you an estimate of how long it may take you to learn to read the ECG competently. Say you read blind 10 ECGs a week, this will take one year; I think this is an optimistic figure, a more reasonable five ECGs per week gives two years, a more reasonable time period. This means that you will have to 'parallel track' your ECG reading with attachments in many clinical areas, just as you do for your radiological experience. If you do this steadily, you will become most proficient.

Whenever you look at an ECG, ask the following questions:

• 'What does this show?' Examine the ECG systemically (name, date of birth, date and time recorded), then: (1) cardiac rhythm, (2) heart rate, (3) P wave abnormalities, (4) PR interval, (5) QRS duration, axis, whether any Q waves, (6) ST segment, (7) T wave, (8) QT interval. Compare the ECG with a normal one (there are several examples in the book), if possible with an old one from the patient, then summarize how your patient's ECG differs from this. Describe the differences using ECG phraseology, e.g. there is ST elevation leads II, III, and aVF, otherwise the ECG is normal. These are new findings.

• 'What does it mean?' Sometimes one explanation leaps out, e.g. in the above example, an inferior wall ST segment elevation MI.

• 'Consider what the alternative explanations might be?' Most ECGs have a differential diagnosis, for example, might the example above reflect pericarditis?

• 'How can I distinguish these alternatives?' This depends on the situation, in the example above, a cardiac ultrasound.

Try and go through this systematic approach for every ECG you read; this will help you develop an ordered comprehensive approach. In due course you will develop legitimate short cuts, but do so only when you are confident in ECG interpretation.

Though this process of gathering experience takes time, it also provides the fun. Did I get it right? Yes – be pleased, indeed, very pleased. This feeling should drive you onwards. No - try and learn why. This is the frustrating part of learning, though often the most instructive – we learn most from our mistakes, make sure you do.

I would like to wish you good luck, and I hope you enjoy learning about the ECG, it is endlessly fascinating.

Patrick Davey
2008

Acknowledgements

The author and publisher have made every effort to contact copyright holders of previously published figures and tables to obtain their permission to reproduce copyright material. However, if any have been inadvertently overlooked, the publisher will be pleased to make the necessary arrangements at the first opportunity.

Fig. 18.3(b): Collinson, J *et al.* (2000) Clinical outcomes, risk stratification and practice patterns of unstable angina and myocardial infarction without ST elevation: Prospective Registry of Acute Ischaemic Syndromes in the UK (PRAIS-UK). *European Heart Journal*, **21**, 1450–1457, by permission of Oxford University Press.

Fig. 18.3(c): Diderholm, E *et al.* (2002) ST depression in ECG at entry indicates severe coronary lesions and large benefits of an early invasive treatment strategy in unstable coronary artery disease. The FRISC II ECG substudy. *European Heart Journal*, **23**, 41–49, by permission of Oxford University Press.

Table 31.2(b): Morrow, DA *et al.* (2000) TIMI risk score for ST-elevation myocardial infarction: a convenient, bedside clinical score for risk assessment at presentation. *Circulation*, **102**, 2031–2037, by permission of Lippincott Williams & Wilkins.

Fig. 36.3: Brichner, EM *et al.* (2000) Congenital heart disease in adults. *New England Journal of Medicine*, **342**, 256–263, 334–342. Copyright © 2000 Massachusetts Medical Society.

Fig. 42.2: Blomstrom-Lundqvist *et al.* (2003) ACC/AHA/ESC guidelines for management of SVA. *Journal of American College of Cardiology*, **42** (8), 1493–1531, by permission of Elsevier.

Fig. 44.1: Konings, KT *et al.* (1994) High-density mapping of electrically induced atrial fibrillation in humans. *Circulation*, **89**, 1665–1680, by permission of Lippincott Williams & Wilkins.

Fig. 46.1: Ganz, L (1995) Supraventricular tachycardia. *New England Journal of Medicine*, **332** (3), 162. Copyright © 1995 Massachusetts Medical Society.

Table 63.1: Brignole, M *et al.* (2000) New classification of haemodynamics of vasovagal syncope: Beyond the VASIS classification; analysis of the pre-syncopal phase of the tilt test without and with nitroglycerin challenge. *Europace*, **2**, 66–76, by permission of Oxford University Press.

Fig. 64.2: Malik, M *et al.* (1996) Heart rate variability: standards of measurement, physiological interpretation and clinical use. *European Heart Journal*, **17**, 354–381, by permission of Oxford University Press.

Fig. 65.1: Jarcho, M. (2006) Biventricular pacing. *New England Journal of Medicine*, **355**, 288–94. Copyright © 2006 Massachusetts Medical Society.

1 Introduction to the ECG

Fig.1.1

(a)

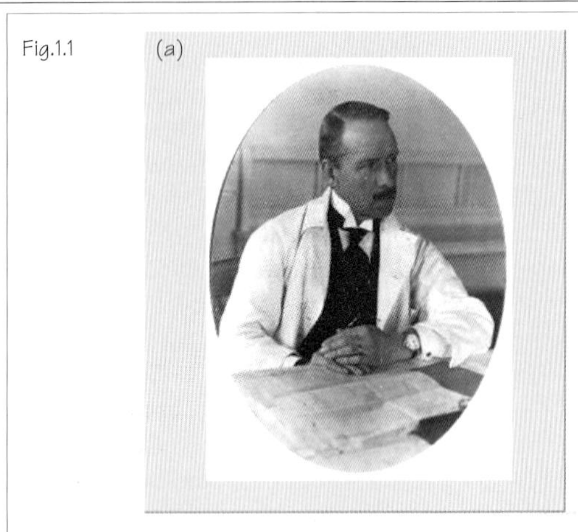

(b)

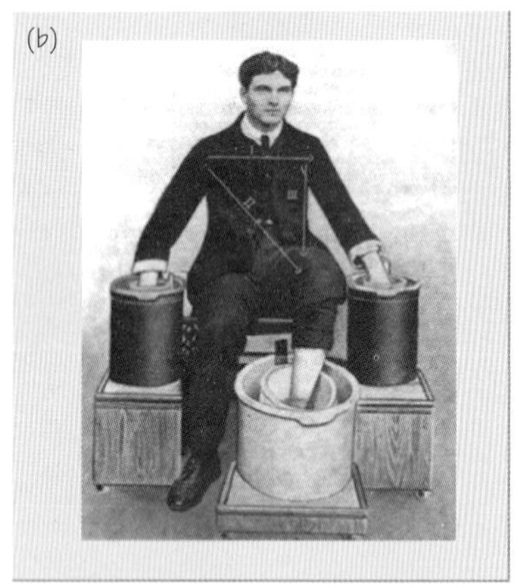

(c)

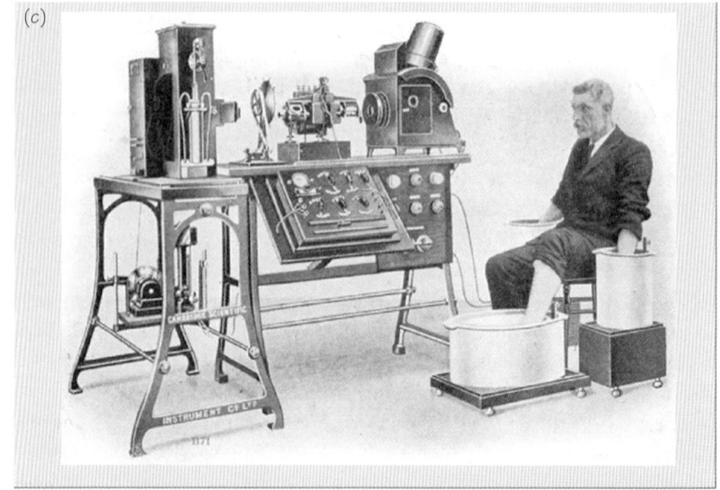
INSTRUMENT CO LTD

(d)

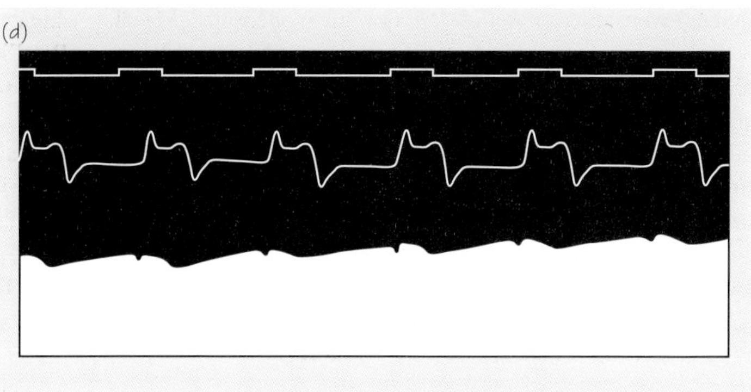

Fig.1.2

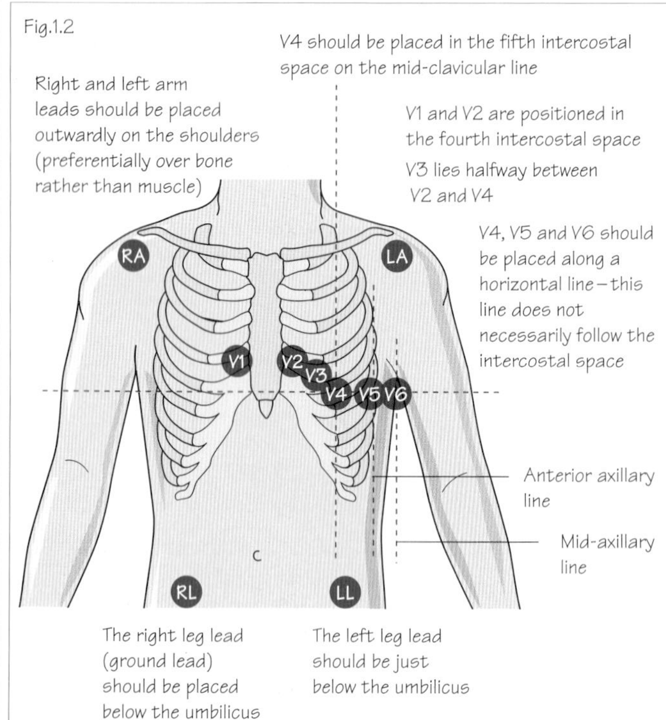
V4 should be placed in the fifth intercostal space on the mid-clavicular line
Right and left arm leads should be placed outwardly on the shoulders (preferentially over bone rather than muscle)
V1 and V2 are positioned in the fourth intercostal space
V3 lies halfway between V2 and V4
V4, V5 and V6 should be placed along a horizontal line – this line does not necessarily follow the intercostal space
RA
LA
V1
V2
V3
V4
V5
V6
Anterior axillary line
Mid-axillary line
RL
LL
The right leg lead (ground lead) should be placed below the umbilicus
The left leg lead should be just below the umbilicus

Fig.1.3

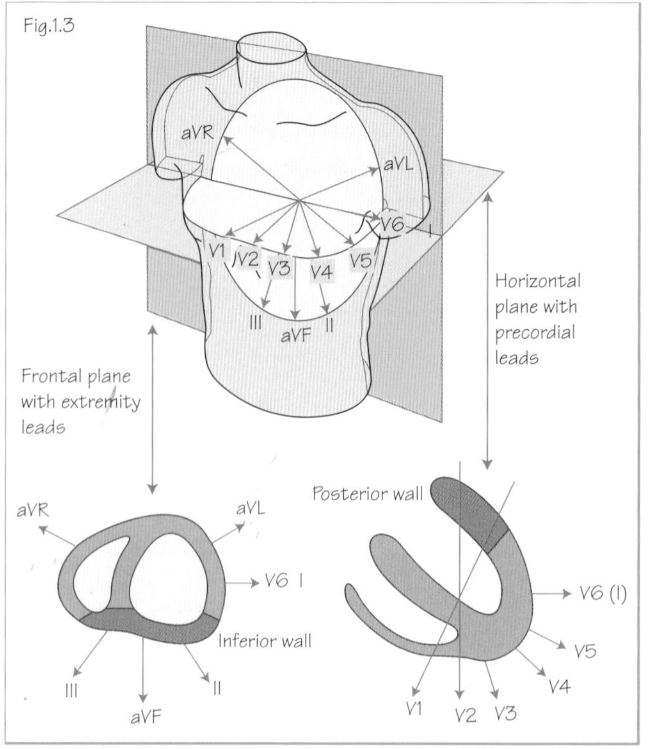
aVR
aVL
V1
V2
V3
V4
V5
V6
III
aVF
II
Horizontal plane with precordial leads
Frontal plane with extremity leads
aVR
aVL
V6 I
Inferior wall
III
aVF
II
Posterior wall
V6 (I)
V5
V4
V1
V2
V3

The electrocardiogram (ECG) is a wonderful tool, cheap, widely available, and incredibly useful. It informs diagnosis, guides and assesses the response to therapy and provides vital data on prognosis. In epidemiological use it gives great insights, e.g. it informs us that 30% of myocardial infarctions (MIs) are clinically silent, and that hypertensive heart disease when associated with certain ECG changes has a high mortality. The ECG informs us not only in acquired heart disease but also in genetic disease, e.g. hereditary long QT or Brugada syndrome. The diagnostic role extends beyond cardiac disease to pulmonary emboli, electrolyte imbalance, rheumatic disease, fitness level, liver disease, diabetes, starvation, etc. It is probably the most useful investigative tool in the whole of medicine.

A brief history of the ECG

The development of the ECG started in the mid 19th century with ideas concerning the role of electricity in the heart, then with the development of increasingly sensitive ways to measure this electricity. The early ECG machines were vast and required a water-cooled jacket! Technological advances in the early 20th century saw recording devices become increasingly small and by 1928 weighed 'only' 50 lbs (22 kg), described as being 'portable'. Weight and size reduction continued and current devices weigh only a few pounds. The modern 12 leads of the ECG were formalized in 1942, with:

- the addition of the three augmented limb leads (aVR, aVL and aVF) of Emanuel Goldberger; to the
- pre-existing three standard leads (I, II, III) so fully explored by the 'greats' of the ECG, Einthoven, Lewis, Mackenzie, and Wilson; and the
- six chest leads (V for voltage 1–6, the technical aspects being formalized in 1938 by the American Heart Association and the British Cardiac Society).

Subsequent years saw an explosion in ECG-based research, and > 150 000 articles on the ECG have now been published!

The ECG in arrhythmias

The early use of the ECG was in arrhythmias, with the classic finding of Wenckebach in 1899 (Wenckebach block), of John Hay in Liverpool in 1905 (Mobitz type II block) and Arthur Cushny, a London professor, in 1907 on atrial fibrillation, an arrhythmia subsequently greatly investigated by Thomas Lewis (University College Hospital, London). Lewis obtained an ECG from a horse with atrial fibrillation and confirmed the diagnosis by examining the atria when the horse was slaughtered! Einthoven made vital contributions and earned the Nobel prize in 1924, the same year that Mobitz published his seminal ECG findings in second degree heart block. The surface ECG findings in many cardiac arrhythmias were elucidated in the mid 20th century, leading inexonerably to greater understanding and better treatment. Catheters allowing the recording of intracardiac ECG signals became available in the mid-century, leading logically to protocols to stimulate the heart to provoke arrhythmias (the electrophysiological study). These intracardiac recordings led to major progress in the diagnosis and treatment of arrhythmias. The external ambulatory recorder, developed by the Montana physician Holter in the 1950s led to discoveries in arrhythmias, circadian rhythm, and cardiac autonomic function (heart rate variability). Technology allowed the development of implantable ECG recorders (the Reveal device), and defined the role of the tilt-table test and carotid sinus massage. Advances continue, e.g. the discovery of the genetic pro-arrhythmic disease by the Brugada brothers in 1992.

The ECG and arrhythmia device therapy

Pacing therapy for slow heart beats had been known of for many years before external devices (bulky and unreliable) became available in 1952. The real breakthrough came in 1958 with the first implantable pacemaker. Subsequent years saw increasing miniaturization, longer battery life, sensing functions and full programmability. Though the knowledge that large direct current applied across the heart could terminate ventricular fibrillation was known from the work of Prevost and Batelli, professors at Geneva, from 1899, it was not until 1947 that Beck, in Cleveland was able to successfully demonstrate defibrillation from ventricular fibrillation (VF) during heart surgery. This led to successful closed chest cardioversion in 1956, and by the 1960s external defibrillators were routinely saving many lives. A logical development was the internal defibrillator, widely available by the mid 1990s. Even more recent is cardiac resynchronization therapy, useful in treating heart failure.

The ECG and coronary disease

The early 19th century saw the discovery of the classic changes of 'full-thickness' myocardial infarction and angina. It was realized early on that many patients with coronary disease had normal resting ECGs. Using exercise to provoke angina, and then record an ECG became widely accepted by the middle third of the century and in 1963 Bruce proposed his classic exercise test. The ability to diagnose coronary disease became widespread, underpinning both the need for and the development of coronary angiography and revascularization. In the 1980s the role of thrombolytic therapy in ST segment elevation but not non-ST segment MI was understood. The role of the ECG in risk stratifying MI continues to evolve, with multiple ECG-based risk scores now available.

Fig. 1.1 (a) Willem Einthoven, in the early 1990s. (b) Early ECG recording required the arms and legs to be placed in saline buckets. (c) An early ECG machine. (d) One of the first ECGs recorded by Augustus Waller (top trace = time, middle trace = chest wall motion, bottom strip = the ECG).

Fig. 1.2 ECG lead placement for an exercise ECG – in a resting ECG the leads to the legs are attached to electrodes just above the ankles. The ECG can be extended further beyond V6, to include leads V7–9, which extend posteriorly on the left chest. The leads can also be extended further rightward beyond lead V1, as 'right-sided chest leads'.

Fig. 1.3 The direction from which the basic 12-leads of the ECG examine the heart.

2 Strengths and weaknesses of the ECG

Fig.2.1

	Patients with the disease	Patients free of the disease	
Diagnostic test positive	A [True +ve]	B [False +ve]	Positive predictive accuracy = Predictive value of a positive test = Post-test likelihood of disease with a positive diagnostic test = A/A+B
Diagnostic test negative	C [False –ve]	D [True –ve]	Negative predictive accuracy = Predictive value of a negative test = Post-test likelihood of no disease with a negative diagnostic test = D/C+D
	Sensitivity = A/A+C	Specificity = D/B+D	Prevalence = pre-diagnostic test likelihood of disease = [A+C]/[A+B+C+D]

Fig.2.2

ECG highly reliable		ECG modestly reliable			ECG highly unreliable
STEMI - diagnosis	STEMI – patent artery following thrombolytic therapy	Non-STEMI	ECG in diagnosing the cause of chest pain in the emergency room (all comers)	ECG in diagnosing the cause of troponin negative chest pain in the ER	ECG in the diagnosis of thoracic aortic dissection
	Exercise ECG for prognosis in chronic stable angina	Exercise ECG for diagnosing IHD in chronic stable angina		Resting ECG for diagnosing IHD in chronic stable angina	
	ECG in confirming the presence of an old STEMI			ECG in confirming the presence of an old non-STEMI	
Arrhythmias (during an episode)	Diagnosis of WPW syndrome between episodes of arrhythmias			Propensity to arrhythmias (outside an arrhythmic episode)	
Presence of ventricular fibrillation			Identification of a group at very low risk of sudden cardiac death post-MI (narrow QRS/no late potentials/high HRV)	Prediction of sudden cardiac death post-MI	Prediction of future sudden cardiac death in the broad population
Internal loop device in the diagnosis of palpitations	Memo device in diagnosing palpitations		External loop recorder in diagnosing palpitations occurring > once/week	24-h ECG in the diagnosis of frequent palpitations	Resting ECG in diagnosing palpitations between events
Internal loop recorder (Reveal® device) in the diagnosis of syncope		External loop recorder in the diagnosis of frequent (≥ 1/week) syncope		Tilt-table test/carotid sinus massage in the diagnosis of syncope	24-h ECG in the diagnosis of syncope
Presence of acquired long QT syndrome	Presence of hereditary long QT syndrome HLQTS	Presence of Brugada syndrome	Prediction of future arrhythmias in those with HLQTS	Prediction of future arrhythmias in those with acquired long QT syndrome	Prediction of arrhythmias occurring in those with Brugada syndrome
	ECG in determining regression of LV hypertrophy	ECG in diagnosing hypertensive heart disease		ECG in predicting future events in those with hypertension	ECG in the diagnosis of hypertension
	Diagnosis of hypertrophic obstructive cardiomyopathy	Diagnosis of acquired LVH		Diagnosis of RV hypertrophy/ ECG in estimating pulmonary artery pressure	
		Left atrial enlargement		Right atrial enlargement	
	Exclusion of heart failure (normal ECG)	Prediction of benefit from multi-site ventricular pacing in heart failure		Presence of heart failure	
	ECG in supporting a clinical diagnosis of aortic stenosis			Diagnosis of the presence of an atrial septal defect	Diagnosis of patent foramen ovale
Diagnosis of the presence of complex cyanotic congenital heart disease (RVH)				Diagnosis of the exact nature of complex cyanotic heart disease	
ECG in the diagnosis of ↑ or ↓ K^+ related arrhythmias		ECG in increasing suspicion of ↑T4 (sinus tachycardia/ atrial fibrillation)	ECG in diagnosing moderate hypo/hyperkalaemia	ECG in increasing suspicion of ↓T4 (bradycardia, long QT interval, ↓ QRS size)	ECG in the diagnosis of isolated ↑ or ↓ in Ca^{2+} or Mg^{2+}

The ECG is a powerful tool, useful diagnostically and therapeutically in suspected cardiac disease, in non-cardiac problems, e.g. non-accidental poisoning, metabolic disturbance, etc, and in monitoring the heart rate of sick patients. ECGs are so widespread that physicians should understand its strengths *and weaknesses*.

Diagnostic role of the ECG

You should be aware of what proportion of those with a diagnosis have a diagnostic ECG, what proportion do not, and what proportion of people with a diagnostic ECG do not have that diagnosis (Fig. 2.1). If you do not have a good idea about these figures, then you do not know whether the ECG has ruled in or out the disease in question and regardless of what it shows, the ECG will have been unhelpful. Usually the problem with the ECG is not so much what it shows (e.g. flat T waves, right bundle branch block, etc) as to the pathological interpretation of these findings. If the finding/interpretation is unique, then the ECG is useful, if there are multiple interpretations then the ECG is less helpful.

Highly diagnostically reliable ECGs

As a generalization, the grosser or more unusual ECG changes are, the more likely there is only one explanation and so the more useful is the ECG. The following conditions have unique ECGs, gross changes, and often only one interpretation:

- ST elevation myocardial infarction (MI) (STEMI), only rarely confused with physiological or pericarditis-related ST elevation.
- Major ST depression during a stress test, in someone at risk of ischaemic heart disease (IHD), fairly reliably indicates coronary disease.
- Arrhythmias are reliably diagnosed on their ECG appearances.
- Wolff–Parkinson–White (WPW) syndrome, 'classic' Brugada/hereditary long QT syndrome (HLQTS).

Moderately diagnostically reliable ECGs

There are often relatively few interpretations to the ECG in:

- Many cases of non-ST segment elevation MI, the ECG is reasonably reliable, e.g. 'proximal left anterior descending (LAD)' pattern or marked 'dynamic' changes.
- Marked left ventricular hypertrophy (LVH) – the grosser the changes, the more reliable is the ECG diagnosis, and the less likely is LVH not to be present. The ECG usually does not reveal the cause of LVH.

Diagnostically less useful ECGs

Most ECG abnormalities are frequent and/or mild, can result from many diseases and are not useful diagnostically:

- T wave flattening, classically due to hypokalaemia – most patients with such ECGs are not hypokalaemic.
- Arrhythmia predisposition may be suspected from the ECG, but the relationship between suspicious ECG findings and actual arrhythmias is weak:
  (a) Conducting tissue disease (e.g. left bundle branch block [LBBB]/long PR interval) predisposes to heart block – most such patients do not have high-grade atrioventricular (AV) block.
  (b) Acquired long QT interval predisposes to torsade-de-pointes (TDP) ventricular tachycardia: most patients with moderate QT prolongation do not have TDP.

This leads to an important principle: if you suspect an arrhythmia, the only way to confirm the diagnosis is to record that arrhythmia!

Prognostic role of the ECG

The ECG can be modestly helpful prognostically, but is rarely the only factor determining outlook:

- ST elevation acute MI, prognosis relates to:
  (a) Site of infarction: best with inferior, worst with anterior MIs.
  (b) Distribution/extent of ST elevation: the more leads, and the greater the sum total, the worse the outlook.
  (c) Degree of ST segment elevation resolution with thrombolytic therapy: the quicker, the more likely reperfusion therapy has opened the artery, the better the outlook.
  (d) Q waves post-MI, especially if extensive, are associated with larger MIs, worse LV function and outlook.
- Non-ST segment elevation MI. Prognosis relates to many factors including resting ECG changes – worst for ST depression, intermediate for T wave inversion.
- Ambient post-MI arrhythmias have some prognostic importance. Ventricular ectopics are weakly related to sudden cardiac death (SCD), but there is a stronger association between non-sustained ventricular tachycardia and SCD. LV function is much more strongly related to outlook.
- QRS duration: in heart failure those with the broadest QRS complexes have the worst outlook.

Limitations to the ECG

The main problems with the ECG are:

- *That the ECG fails to confirm the suspected diagnosis, when it is present*. For example:
  (a) ST depression is not induced during an exercise tolerance test (ETT) in some patients with severe coronary artery disease (CAD), i.e. they have a high-level negative ETT. If you know this, you will not fall into the trap of ruling out CAD solely on the basis of an ETT.
  (b) Intermittent profound bradyarrhythmias, e.g. high-grade heart block or sinus node arrest can occur in those with a normal resting ECG/normal prolonged ambulatory monitoring. If you know this, you may still implant a pacemaker in such a patient to their benefit.
  (c) A single ECG with a normal QT interval does not exclude the long QT syndrome, as diagnostic changes can be intermittently present.

Relying too heavily on the ECG, without knowing its limitations, will lead to the right diagnosis being dismissed – unless the situation is one where the diagnosis will always be confirmed by the ECG (e.g. arrhythmias, ST segment elevation MI [STEMI] – crucially not an MI, which can present with a normal ECG) you must be aware that a normal ECG rarely rules a condition out.

- *The ECG suggests a diagnosis when the patient is normal*, e.g. in musculoskeletal chest pain, the ECG shows ST elevation, misinterpreted as pericarditis/STEMI, whereas it is physiological without pathological significance.
- *The ECG suggests one diagnosis, whereas another is present*, e.g. in syncope, the ECG shows extensive conducting tissue disease, suggesting bradyarrhythmias due to AV block, but in fact ventricular tachycardia is the diagnosis.

Avoid 'putting all your eggs in one basket' on the basis of the ECG; use it to guide diagnosis rather than relying entirely on it.

Fig. 2.1 The definition of sensitivity, specificity, positive and negative predictive accuracy.

Fig. 2.2 The reliability of the ECG in diagnosis and management.

3 Basis of the ECG

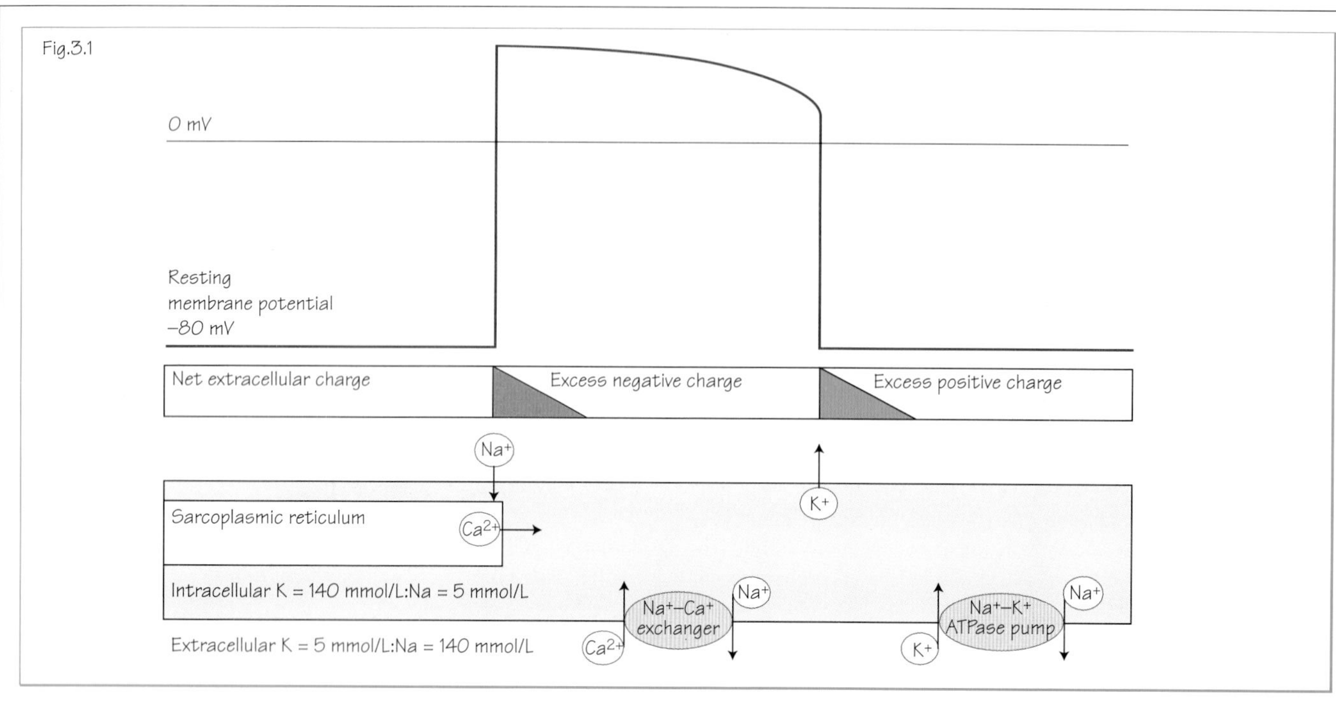
Fig.3.1
0 mV
Resting
membrane potential
−80 mV
Net extracellular charge
Excess negative charge
Excess positive charge
Na+
K+
Sarcoplasmic reticulum
Ca2+
Intracellular K = 140 mmol/L:Na = 5 mmol/L
Extracellular K = 5 mmol/L:Na = 140 mmol/L
Ca2+
Na+–Ca+ exchanger
Na+
K+
Na+–K+ ATPase pump
Na+

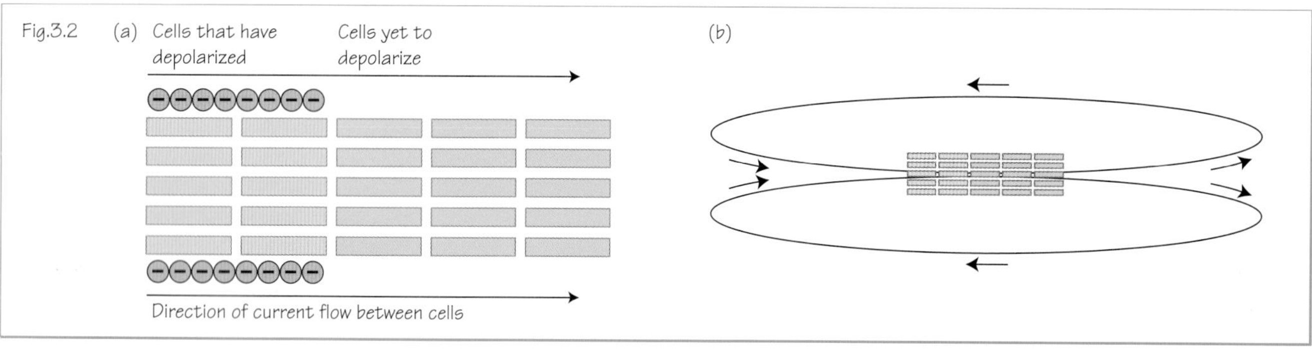
Fig.3.2
(a)
Cells that have depolarized
Cells yet to depolarize
Direction of current flow between cells
(b)

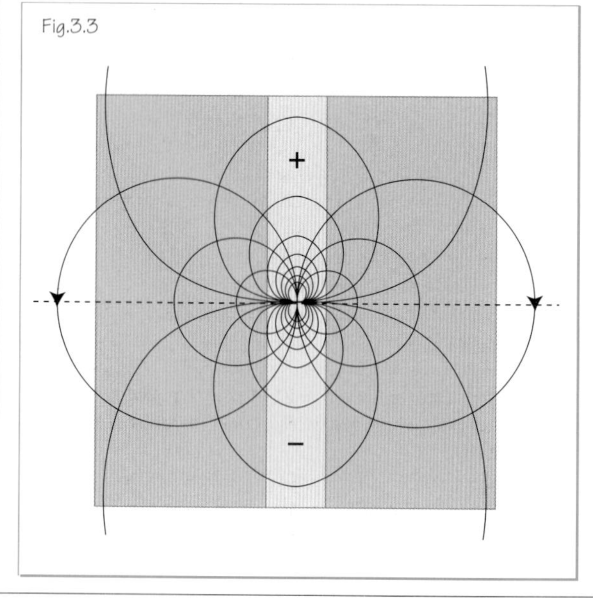
Fig.3.3
+
−

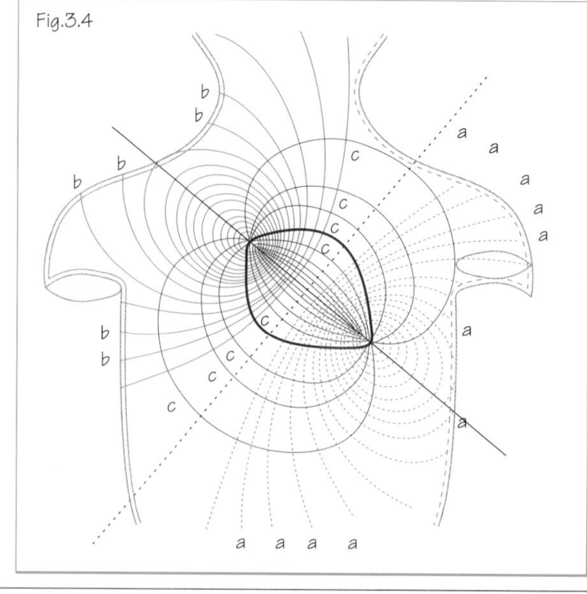
Fig.3.4
a
b
c

The basis of the ECG

The ECG is a clever device designed to detect current flow. The heart generates electricity, which is transmitted to the chest wall, where it can be detected. The ECG records the pattern of spread of electricity in the various phases of the cardiac cycle. Its utility relies on the pattern of spread changing in a characteristic fashion in many diseases. In understanding the ECG, be aware that:

- Electrons carry current, which flows from areas with negative charge to areas with more positive charge; when current moves towards an observing electrode a positive deflection results and vice versa. The ECG only shows a deflection when current is moving in the heart. No current flow means no ECG deflection.
- The basis of current flow around the heart starts off as current flow within individual heart cells, which induce current flow between cells. With depolarization positively charged Na^+ ions move into the cell; with repolarization, positively charged K^+ move out of cells – this leaves excess negative charge outside the cell at the start of the cardiac cycle, excess positive charge outside the cell at the end of the cycle.
- Current flows from areas just depolarized (excess extracellular negative charge) into areas yet to depolarize, then onto an observing electrode. This current flow depolarizes neighbouring cells, firing action potentials, and in sequence fully depolarizing the whole heart. When fully depolarized, the extracellular charge throughout the heart is the same; there is no current flow, and no ECG deflection.
- At the end of the cardiac cycle, individual myocytes repolarize, moving positively charged K^+ ions out of the cells, leaving the outside extracellular space more positive than the extracellular space of those parts of the heart yet to repolarize. Current, as electrons, moves into the repolarized area from the areas of the heart yet to repolarize.
- In summary, the heart does not depolarize or repolarize simultaneously – some areas de/repolarize before other areas, so that in depolarization, current flows into areas about to depolarize, with repolarization, current flows away from areas about to repolarize. This spread of currents give rise to a characteristic sequence of currents flowing over the heart with each heartbeat.
- The utility of the ECG in medicine is that many, but far from all, diseases change this electricity pattern in a characteristic way.
- It is crucial to remember that abnormal ECG reflect deviations in the flow of the current from normal – they may indicate something seriously wrong with the heart, they may not – abnormal ECGs do not always mean the heart is abnormal!

Fig. 3.1 The top part of the figure shows an action potential, with voltage measured by an intracellular electrode; the middle part of the figure shows the net extracellular charge at different times during the action potential; the bottom part of the figure shows ion movement into, out of and within a myocyte during the action potential. The action potential: intracellular $[K^+]$ is 130–140 mmol/L; extracellular K^+ is 4–5 mmol/L. Intracellular $[Na^+]$ is 5 mmol/L, extracellular $[Na^+]$ 140 mmol/L. The resting myocyte membrane is permeable only to K^+; during rest some K^+ moves down its concentration gradient from the inside to the outside of the cell, with its positive charge, leaving negative charge inside the cell. This results in a potential difference between the outside and inside of the cell of –90 mV. The excess extracellular positive charge prevents more positively charged K^+ moving out of the cell. During the upstroke of the action potential (phase 1), the cell membrane becomes impermeable to K^+ and rapidly more permeable to Na^+, which along with its positive charge moves down its concentration gradient into the cell, leaving net negative charge outside the cell, so the interior of the cell becomes positively charged to +30 mV. This positive intracellular voltage triggers the release of Ca^{2+} from its sarcoplasmic reticulum (SR) and other storage sites, initiating myosin contraction. During the plateau phase (phase 2), the cell membrane remains much more permeable to Na^+ than K^+, so the intracellular environment is positively charged. Furthermore, there is also a net flow of Ca^{2+} into the cell, which helps maintains net positive charge in the cell, and myosin contraction. With repolarization the membrane becomes much less permeable to Na^+ than K^+, so K^+ again flows out of the cell (as repolarizing potassium currents), allowing the interior to become negatively charged (phase 3), so restoring the resting status. Ca^{2+} is removed (by SR pumps) from the cytoplasm around this time, terminating myosin contraction. The membrane permeability alters due to the opening and shutting of ion-specific membrane channels (these switch on or off according to the intracellular voltage, spontaneously over time, or in response to hormones and intracellular messengers). Intracellular ionic concentration is maintained by pumps that consume adenosine triphosphate (ATP) (e.g. the Na^+K^+ATP'ase membrane pump).

Fig. 3.2 Current flows between different areas of the heart either when some areas have depolarized and others are still to depolarize or, conversely, when some areas have repolarized and others are still to repolarize. (a) Here depolarized cells are shown with excess negative charge, which flows in the direction of the depolarization wavefront. (b) This shows the current flow loops round the dipole, producing current flow to the side and behind the depolarization wave.

Fig. 3.3 This shows a more complex and so more realistic pattern of current flow than Fig. 3.2b. In the centre is a dipole (labelled as – or + for the polarity at either end), which generates a complex series of looping currents around itself.

Fig. 3.4 The surface correlates of internal current flow, projected onto a torso. The pattern of current flow is complex. There is no current flow towards an observing electrode at right angles to the dipole, and maximal flow directly in front or behind the dipole.

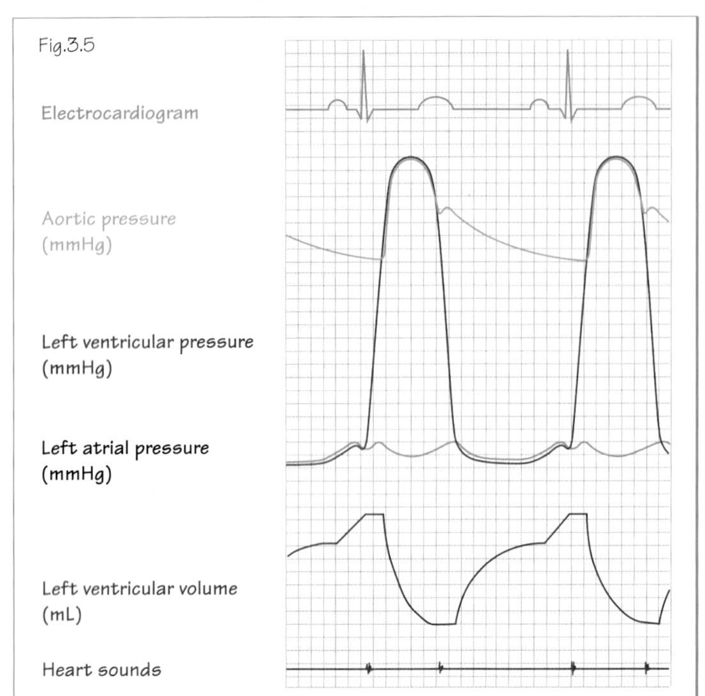
Fig.3.5
Electrocardiogram
Aortic pressure
(mmHg)
Left ventricular pressure
(mmHg)
Left atrial pressure
(mmHg)
Left ventricular volume
(mL)
Heart sounds

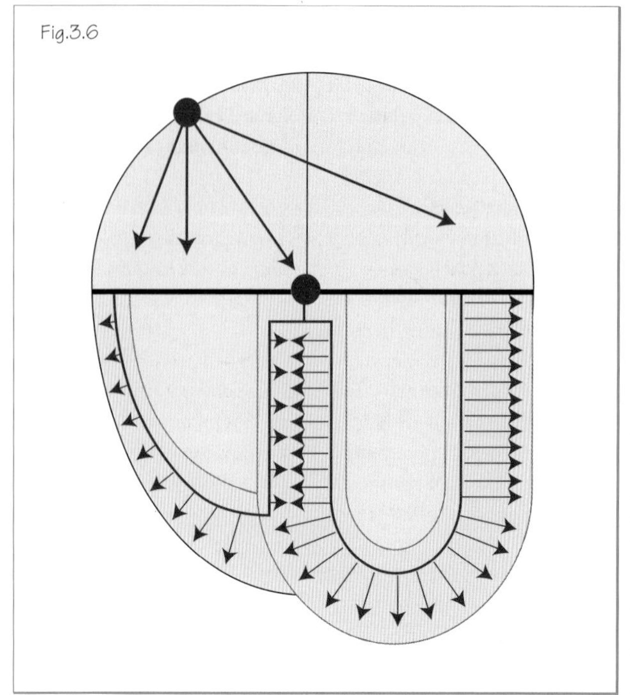
Fig.3.6

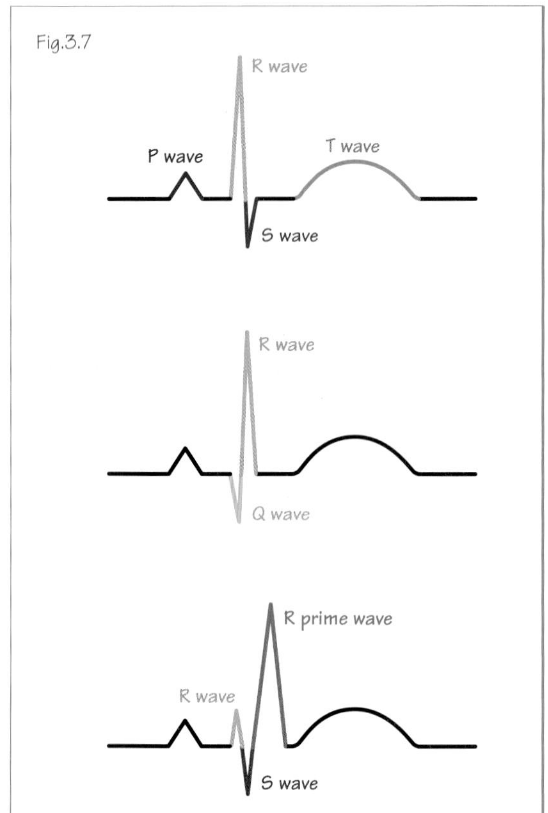
Fig.3.7
R wave
P wave
T wave
S wave
R wave
Q wave
R prime wave
R wave
S wave

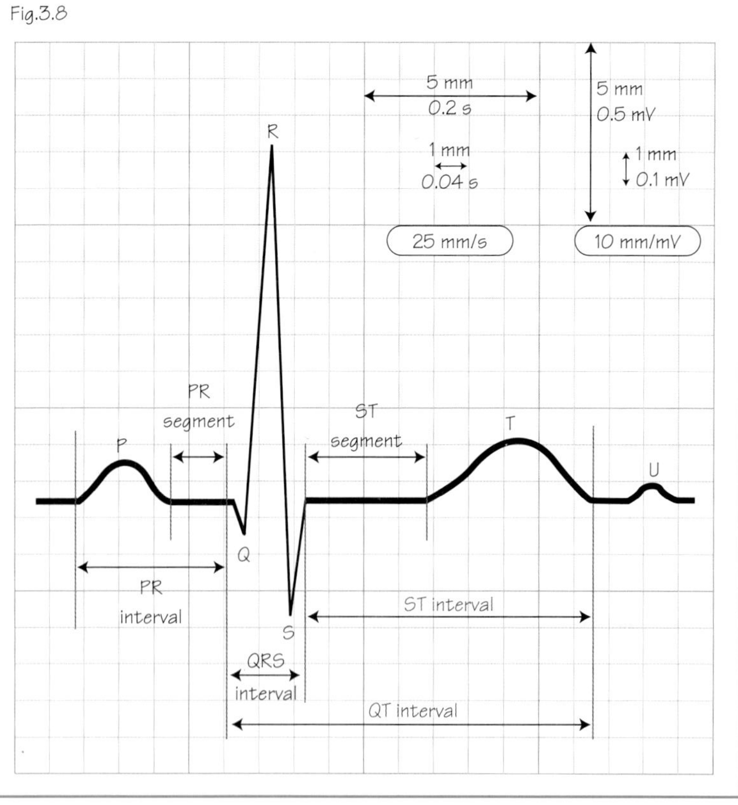
Fig.3.8
5 mm
0.2 s
1 mm
0.04 s
5 mm
0.5 mV
1 mm
0.1 mV
25 mm/s
10 mm/mV
R
P
PR
segment
ST
segment
T
U
Q
S
PR
interval
ST interval
QRS
interval
QT interval

The basic ECG

The ECG is the surface recording of the electricity associated with the cardiac cycle. To understand the ECG you should know: (i) the key components of the cardiac cycle; (ii) when the different parts of the heart depolarize and repolarize; (iii) where the different ECG leads are sited.

The cardiac cycle

1 The heart fills during diastole and contracts during systole.
2 The cardiac cycle begins with electrical activation of the atria, starting at the cardiac pacemaker in the sino-atrial (SA) node, high up in the right atrium.
3 A key property of the heart is that electrical activation (i.e. depolarization of a cell sufficient to fire an action potential) of some heart cells activates adjacent cells (i.e. they become depolarized sufficient for an action potential to fire). So, activation of the SA node initiates a wave of depolarization that spreads over the right atrium and, via the bundle of Bachmann into the left atrium. Electrical atrial activation leads to co-ordinated atrial pumping.
4 The electrical impulse travels downwards into the atrioventricular (AV) node, the only electrical connection between the atria and the ventricles. The AV node delays the electrical impulse, allowing atrial systole to finish before ventricular systole starts.
5 After a short delay (150–200 ms), the electrical impulse crosses the AV node and enters the specialized conducting tissue of the ventricles – the bundle of His, bundle branches and their divisions.
6 The specialized conducting tissue quickly (50–60 ms in health) distributes the electrical impulse throughout the ventricle and into the myocytes, initiating contraction. Though the electrical impulse spreads quickly via the specialized conducting tissue, myocyte-to-myocyte spread of electrical activity is much slower.
7 The specialized conducting tissue is sub-endocardial, so the wave of excitation spreads endocardially to epicardially, and then onto an observing electrode. This accounts for most leads observing the left ventricle having a positive deflection.
8 After depolarization, the action potential of the myocytes has a prolonged plateau phase, during which the ventricular myocytes are contracted, and little current flows.
9 After the plateau phase, repolarization occurs, the intracellular level of calcium falls rapidly and the myocytes relax, starting diastole. Repolarization starts sub-epicardially and spreads sub-endocardially.

Naming of the different waves of the ECG (Fig. 3.7)

- Atrial systole results in the P wave. Atrial repolarization results in a small current flow, not seen, without a named wave.
- Ventricular depolarization is quick and results in the QRS complex:
  (a) A Q wave is defined as an initial negative deflection of the QRS complex.
  (b) An R wave is defined as the first positive deflection of the ventricular complex.
  (c) An S wave is a negative deflection of the QRS complex *following* an R wave – it cannot be the first deflection of the QRS complex.
  (d) An R′ wave (pronounced R prime) is a second positive deflection, i.e. an R wave, followed by an S wave, and then a second R wave.
- During repolarization, current flows result in the T wave, and possibly the U wave.

Siting of the ECG leads

Much work in the early years related to ECG lead positioning and signal processing. It is not necessary to comprehend processing details to understand how the different leads observe the heart (see Figs 1.2 & 1.3). Though an almost infinite array of positions could be used, lead localization is fixed by convention to allow standardization and comparison; non-standard positions (e.g. right ventricle [RV], posterior leads) are used if appropriate.

- The four limb leads are attached to the two arms and legs (**red** = right arm; **yellow** = left arm; **green** = left leg; **black** = right leg): using these leads, positions I, II, III, aVR, AVL and aVF are derived.
- The six chest leads are attached as follows:
  V1 **Red**: fourth intercostal space, right sternal border.
  V2 **Yellow**: fourth intercostal space, left sternal border.
  V3 **Green**: midway between V2 and V4.
  V4 **Brown**: fifth intercostal space, left mid-clavicular line.
  V5 **Black**: level with V4, left anterior axillary line.
  V6 **Violet**: level with V4, left mid-axillary line.

Paper speed and sensitivity

The ECG is usually recorded at a paper speed of 50 mm/s. Each large square is 1 cm long, records 200 ms of activity and is divided into five smaller ones of 40 ms duration. *Always check the paper speed of the recording*. The sensitivity is usually 10 mm/mV. The size of the deflection on the paper relates to the sensitivity setting, if it is increased (e.g. 20 mm/mV) then complexes are larger, and vice versa. At the end of each ECG modern machines insert a square wave pulse of 1 mV for 200 ms; confirming the settings.

Fig. 3.5 The basic elements of the cardiac cycle.
Fig. 3.6 Sequence of depolarization of the heart. The impulse starts at the sino-atrial (SA) node, then activates the atria, both right (downwards and rightwards) and left (via the bundle of Bachmann). The impulse then reaches the atrioventricular (AV) node, is delayed briefly before passing into the bundle branches and more distal Purkinje fibres.

Fig. 3.7 Naming of the different ECG waves. P wave reflects atrial activation, T wave ventricular repolarization. Whether the T wave is positive (i.e. above the line) or negative (below the line) it is always called the T wave. The waves of the depolarization complex (QRS complex) are defined in the text.
Fig. 3.8 The basic ECG nomenclature, demonstrating the basic ECG, recorded at a standard paper speed of 50 mm/s, and sensitivity of 10 mm/mV, and showing the timing of the normal ECG.

4 The normal P wave

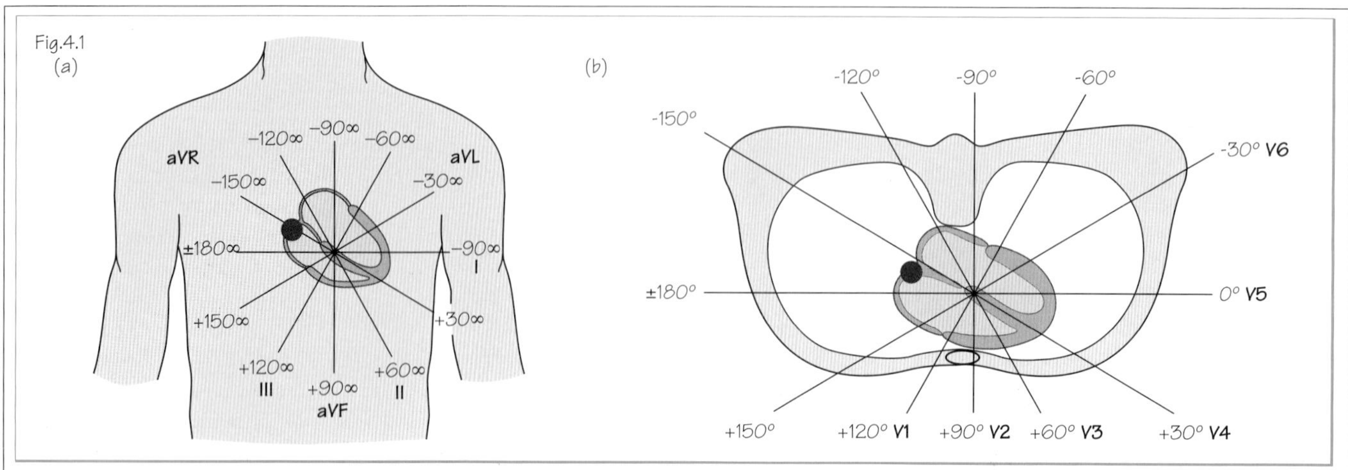

Fig.4.1
(a)
aVR
aVL
−120∞
−90∞
−60∞
−150∞
−30∞
±180∞
−90∞
I
+150∞
+30∞
+120∞
III
+90∞
aVF
+60∞
II
(b)
-120°
-90°
-60°
-150°
-30° V6
±180°
0° V5
+150°
+120° V1
+90° V2
+60° V3
+30° V4

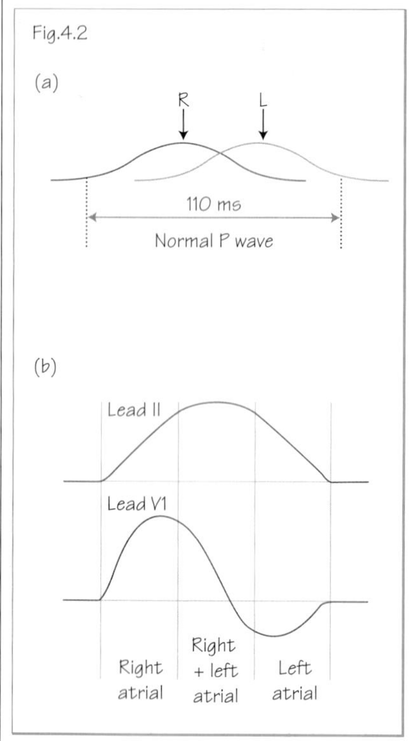

Fig.4.2
(a)
R
L
110 ms
Normal P wave
(b)
Lead II
Lead V1
Right atrial
Right + left atrial
Left atrial

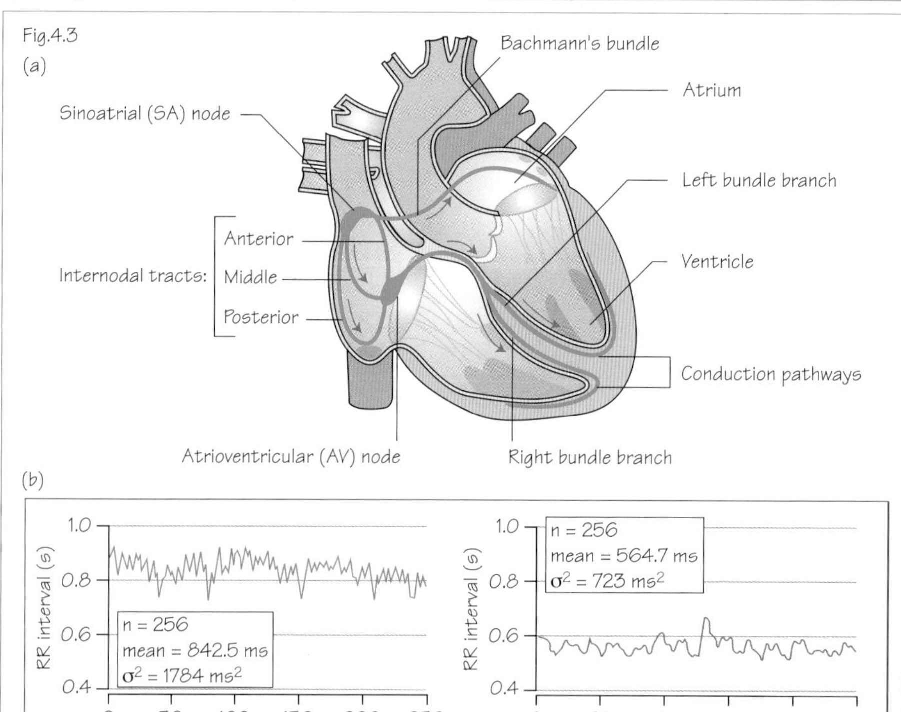

Fig.4.3
(a)
Bachmann's bundle
Atrium
Sinoatrial (SA) node
Left bundle branch
Internodal tracts:
Anterior
Middle
Posterior
Ventricle
Conduction pathways
Atrioventricular (AV) node
Right bundle branch
(b)
RR interval (s)
n = 256
mean = 842.5 ms
σ2 = 1784 ms2
n = 256
mean = 564.7 ms
σ2 = 723 ms2
Beats

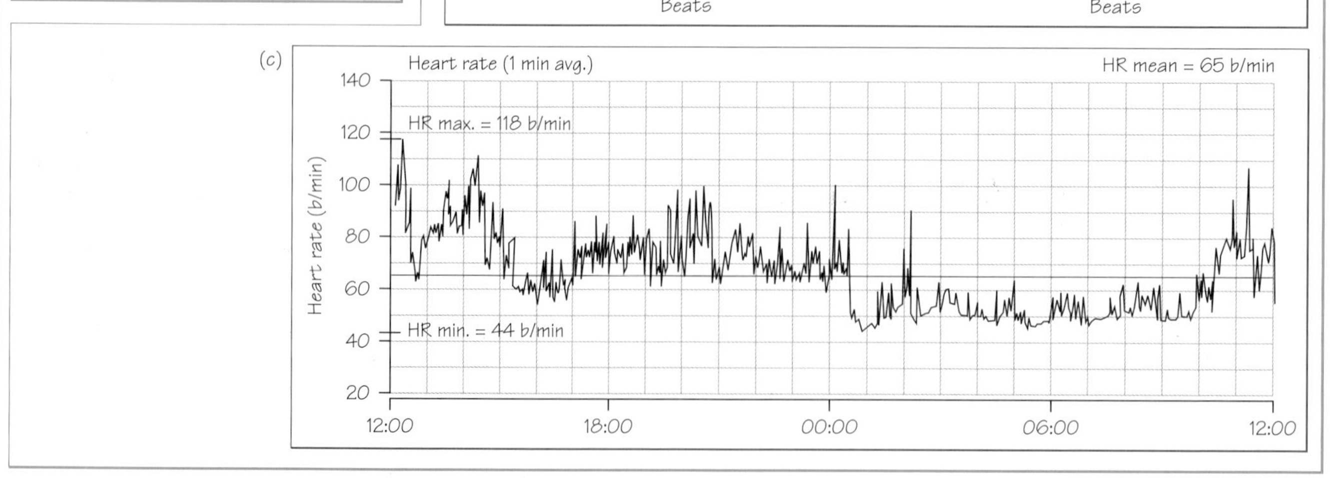

(c)
Heart rate (1 min avg.)
HR mean = 65 b/min
HR max. = 118 b/min
HR min. = 44 b/min
Heart rate (b/min)
12:00
18:00
00:00
06:00
12:00

The P wave reflects the electrical activation of the atria, and allows one to:

• Have some idea of where atrial depolarization started and whether the atria are enlarged, as P wave shape relates to where depolarization starts and the route it takes.

• Assess many properties of the sinus node, including heart rate variability, as the P wave reflects sinus node function.

The key points are:

• The best leads to look at the P wave are those directly in or away from the path of atrial depolarization, i.e. lead II and lead V1 (Fig. 4.1a,b).

• The direction of travel of the depolarizing wave through both atria determines the exact shape of the P wave.

• Depolarization starts at the sinus node (Fig. 4.2a,b), then travels directly into the right atria and, via specialized conducting tissue known as the bundle of Bachmann, into the left atria. The time taken for electricity to travel down the bundle of Bachmann means that left atrial depolarization starts a little while after right atrial depolarization, and accordingly goes on for a little while after right atrial depolarization has finished (Fig. 4.3a–c).

The duration of the P wave reflects how long atrial depolarization lasts. The duration is increased if the wave of electricity travels slower than normal (e.g. some cardiomyopathies), or if the wave travels at the normal speed but the atria is enlarged (see Chapter 7). In the former the P wave size is usually diminished, whereas in the latter the P wave is often of a good or better size.

The size of the P wave reflects both the volume of electrically active tissue and the insulation between the atria and the observing electrode. If the atria have more/larger myocytes, then the size of the P wave increases; conversely if the number/size of myocytes decreases, or there is more insulation between the heart and the ECG electrode (e.g. pericardial effusion, obesity) then the P wave size diminishes.

Sinus node function

The P wave rate reflects sinus node activity, which is more complex than imagined. The easiest way to assess sinus node function is from a 24-h ECG (Fig. 4.3c) and, though it is possible to look at PP intervals, it is more usual to look at RR intervals (predicated on assuming the PR interval is fixed, or changes only slowly). Important measures of sinus node function include:

• Heart rate which responds to activity (e.g. slows during sleep, increases during exercise), psychological influences and disease.

• Heart rate variability. Heart rate fluctuates over very short time periods (seconds and minutes) in response to autonomic influences. These heart rate fluctuations do not change the average heart rate, but do change the instantaneous heart rate. The sympathetic nervous system is believed to alter heart rate with a periodicity of about 0.1 Hz, and the vagus with a periodicity of about 0.25 Hz.

Fig. 4.1 The position of the atria in the chest in the frontal and horizontal planes, illustrating why leads II and V1 are best for examining the P wave. From the frontal plane (a) it can be seen, as depolarization starts superiorly and spreads inferiorly, that the wave of depolarization, and hence the current flow, is largely directed towards lead II, completely so for the right atrium, largely so for the left atrium. From the horizontal view (b) it can be seen that as the sinus node lies high up in the right atria, and to its back, the wave of right atrial depolarization passes directly towards lead V1. However, the wave of left atrial depolarization passes largely away from lead V1. It is easy to see why in left atrial enlargement the late depolarization phase of the P wave is prolonged and negative in lead V1.

Fig. 4.2 (a) Timing and size of the contribution of right and left atria to the shape of the P wave. Right atrial depolarization occurs first, and occupies the first two-thirds of the P wave; left atrial depolarization onset is delayed by about one-third of the duration of the P wave, and then occupies the remaining two-thirds. In health, both contribute equally to the size of the P wave. Thus the first and last thirds of atrial depolarization are exclusively the domain of the right and left atria. Both atria contribute to the middle third of the P wave and hence in health the overall P wave is largest in the middle of the P wave. (b) P wave shape in leads II and V1; both left and right atrial depolarization are directed towards lead II. Right atrial depolarization is directed towards lead V1, though left atrial depolarization is largely away, accounting for the appearance of a late but small negative P wave deflection in lead V1.

Fig. 4.3 (a) Atrial depolarization, which starts at the sinus node, spreads down internodal and interatrial ('bundle of Bachmann') pathways, respectively allowing for right and left atrial depolarization. The impulse then proceeds into the atrioventricular [AV] node and the rest of the heart. (b) Heart rate variability. Two traces of RR interval (essentially the same as PP interval) plotted out against beat number (i.e. instantaneous heart rate). Left lying, right tilted up. Vagal tone, higher when lying, increases high-frequency heart rate variability (σ^2, measured in milliseconds squared), seen as instantaneous increases/decreases in RR interval (sharp 'spikes' on the tachogram). Standing increases sympathetic tone, increasing heart rate (i.e. lessening RR interval) as vagal tone is withdrawn, lessening the high-frequency changes seen when lying (n = number of beats assessed, μ = average RR interval). (c) Trace of heart rate (HR) plotted out against time from a normal 24-h ECG; normal heart rate variability, with a clear decrease in heart rate at night when asleep.

5 The normal QRS complex

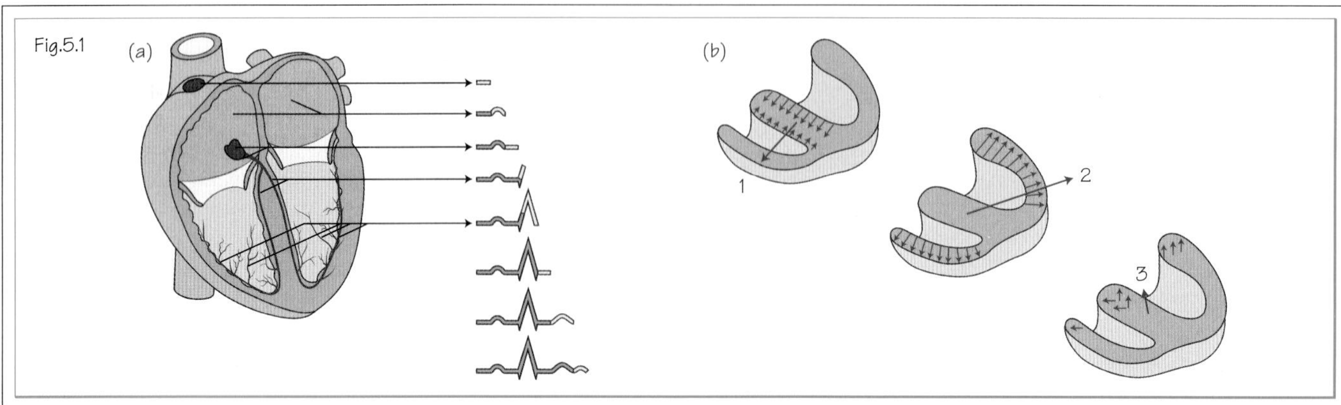

Fig.5.1
(a)
(b)
1
2
3

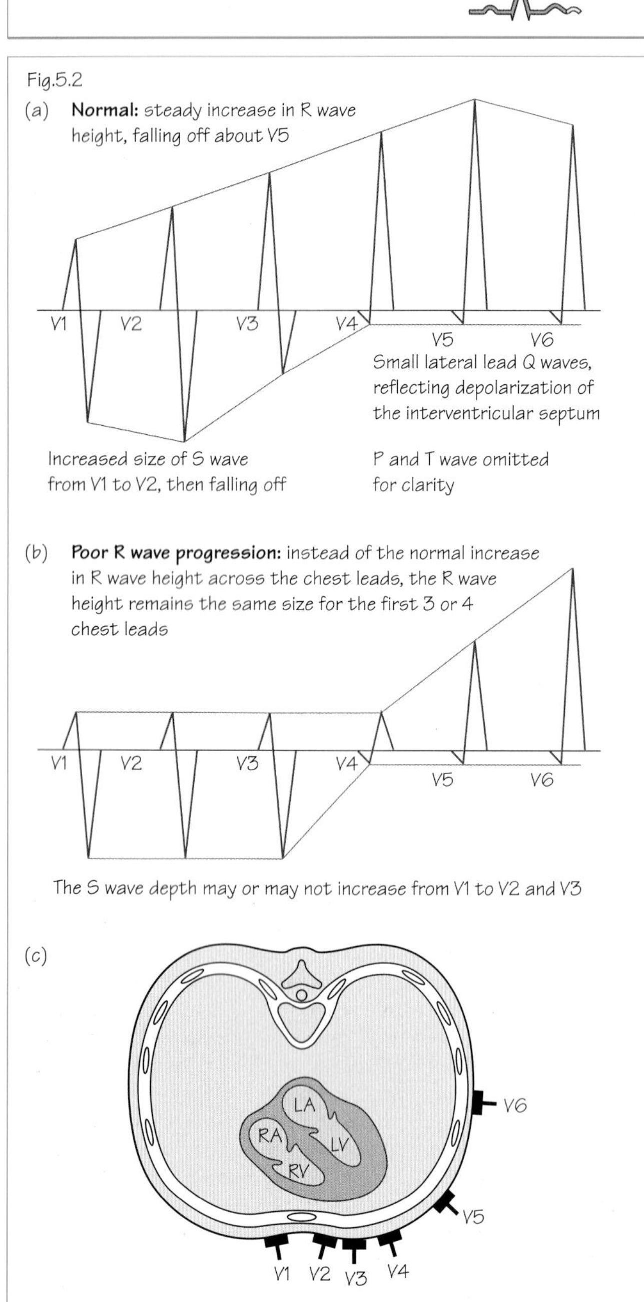

Fig.5.2
(a) **Normal:** steady increase in R wave height, falling off about V5
V1
V2
V3
V4
V5
V6
Small lateral lead Q waves, reflecting depolarization of the interventricular septum
Increased size of S wave from V1 to V2, then falling off
P and T wave omitted for clarity
(b) **Poor R wave progression:** instead of the normal increase in R wave height across the chest leads, the R wave height remains the same size for the first 3 or 4 chest leads
V1
V2
V3
V4
V5
V6
The S wave depth may or may not increase from V1 to V2 and V3
(c)
LA
RA
LV
RV
V6
V5
V1 V2 V3 V4

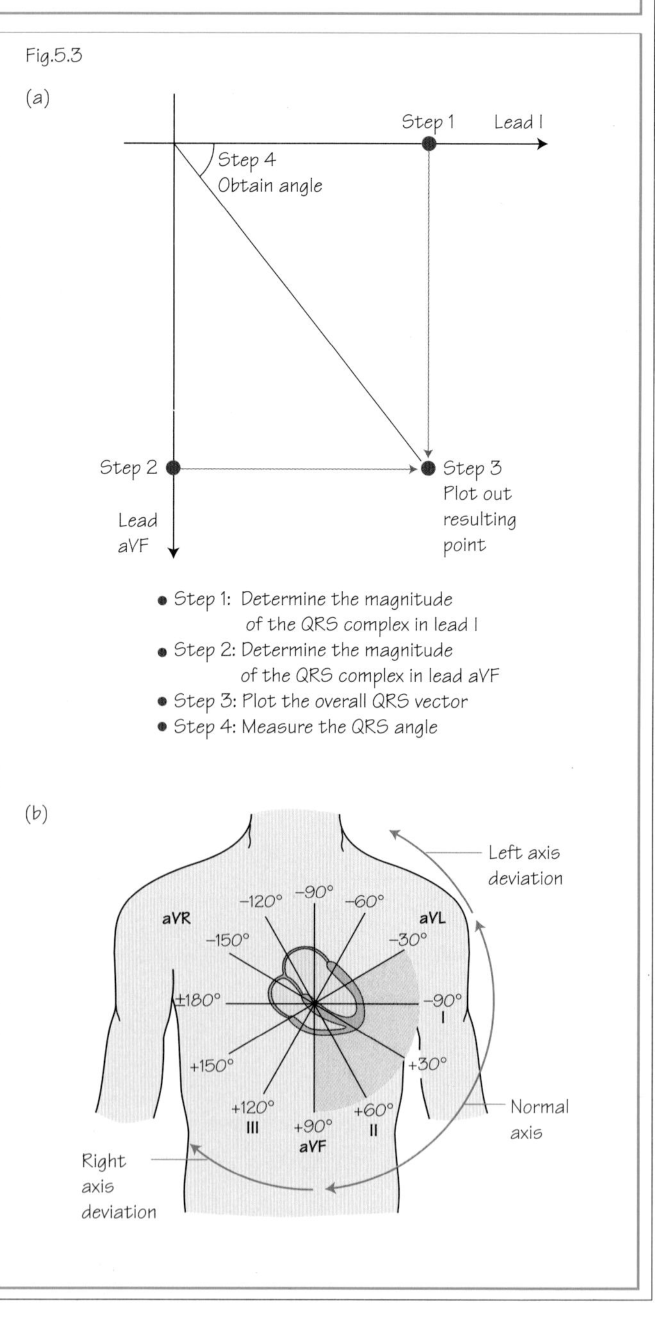

Fig.5.3
(a)
Step 1
Lead I
Step 4
Obtain angle
Step 2
Lead aVF
Step 3
Plot out resulting point
• Step 1: Determine the magnitude of the QRS complex in lead I
• Step 2: Determine the magnitude of the QRS complex in lead aVF
• Step 3: Plot the overall QRS vector
• Step 4: Measure the QRS angle
(b)
Left axis deviation
aVR
aVL
−120°
−90°
−60°
−150°
−30°
±180°
−90°
I
+150°
+30°
+120°
III
+90°
aVF
+60°
II
Normal axis
Right axis deviation

The QRS complex represents ventricular depolarization. The path of depolarization (Fig. 5.1a–c) is from the atria into:

• **The atrioventricular (AV) node**, which slows down the depolarization wave to ensure that atrial contraction is over before ventricular contraction starts.

• Then into the **bundle of His**.

• Then into the **left side of the septum**, with the current then passing both down the septum, and from the left to the right side of the septum (so accounting for the small 'septal' Q waves in left-sided ECG leads).

• Then via the Purkinje cells into the **sub-endocardium of the ventricles**, and through the myocardium towards the epicardium, so producing a co-ordinated contraction that results in the greatest cardiac output for the least energy.

This pattern of depolarization (Fig. 5.1a–c) gives rise to the different shape of the QRS complex in the different leads (Fig. 5.2a–c).

• In the left-sided leads there is often a small Q wave, reflecting septal depolarization (which is directed left → right, i.e. away from the left-sided leads), followed by a large R wave as the bulk of the left ventricle (LV) depolarizes towards the left sided electrodes.

• In the right-sided leads there is a small R wave, followed by a large S wave, as the later QRS complex is dominated by depolarization of the large bulk of the LV rather than the small right ventricle (RV); the LV depolarization wave moves away from the right-sided leads, leading to a negative deflection (the S wave) in these leads.

• There are no large Q waves in the normal ECG (i.e. all Q waves are physiological, being ≤ 2 mm depth, < 1 small square in duration or ≤ 25% of the R wave), as current passes from the endocardium to the epicardium, i.e. always initially towards an observing electrode. The exception to this is lead aVR, which looks 'through' the AV valve 'into' the ventricle, so observing current flow away from it, resulting in a large Q wave.

Important properties of the QRS complex include:

• The upstroke of the QRS complex is very steep, reflecting the fact that the specialized conducting tissue of the ventricle (the His–Purkinje system) distributes the electrical impulse throughout the sub-endocardial ventricular tissue very quickly, allowing myocyte depolarization to be initiated nearly simultaneously.

• The duration of the normal QRS is short, certainly < 120 ms, though more often < 100 ms.

• The overall **vector of depolarization** (Fig. 5.3a,b), termed 'the QRS axis' is determined by plotting the largest R wave in two leads (often lead I and aVF) against each other (Fig. 5.3a,b). A 'quick' way to determine whether the axis is normal is to look at leads I and II; if both QRS complexes are positive, the axis is normal. Left axis deviation results in a negative deflection in lead II and III (positive in lead I). Right axis deviation results in a negative QRS in lead I; lead II is usually positive but may be negative; lead III is positive.

• The **size of the QRS complex** is determined by: (a) the size of the patient (fatter patients have smaller complexes); (b) the ventricular muscle mass – the lead directly opposite the largest mass of ventricular tissue has the largest QRS complex; (c) the age of the patient (older patients have smaller QRS complexes for any given muscle mass).

Fig. 5.1 (a) The specialized conducting tissue of the heart allows the depolarization wave to quickly pass throughout the heart. (b) The sequence of ventricular depolarization. 1. Initially the septum depolarizes, with the bulk of the movement being left to right, accounting for the vector of depolarization being mainly left to right. 2. Subsequently the free walls of both ventricles depolarize. The depolarization vector is dominated by the depolarization of the left ventricle (LV) (which is much larger than the right ventricle [RV]), and is therefore directed towards the left. 3. Finally the terminal portions of the septum, RV and LV depolarize, giving a small superiorly directed vector.

Fig. 5.2 (a) The size of the normal QRS complex in the chest leads. The R wave increases initially as one progresses from lead V1 to V6, while the S wave decreases till a maximum R wave is reached (usually around lead V4). The maximum R wave size is in the lead overlying the largest bulk of the left ventricle. The R wave of the QRS complex then declines slightly in size. The transition point is where the R wave height = the S wave depth, and is usually around lead V3. Its physiological significance is that this is along a line extending down the interventricular septum; (b) shows this in the typical heart. The transition point may be moved either earlier (i.e. towards V1), termed 'clockwise rotation', or towards lead V6, termed 'anti-clockwise' rotation. If the R wave height in the anterior leads does not increase steadily, the term 'poor anterior R wave progression' is applied (c). This can be due to obesity (which results in counter-clockwise rotation of the heart), or to damage to the front of the heart (e.g. an old anterior wall myocardial infarction [MI]). LA, left atrium; LV, left ventricle; RA, right atrium; RV, right ventricle.

Fig. 5.3 (a) Determination of the QRS axis. The maximum R wave in the QRS complex is obtained from two leads (in this example leads I and aVF) at right angles to each other, and plotted out: the resulting angle is measured and termed the QRS axis. (b) Normal and abnormal QRS axis.

6 The T and U waves

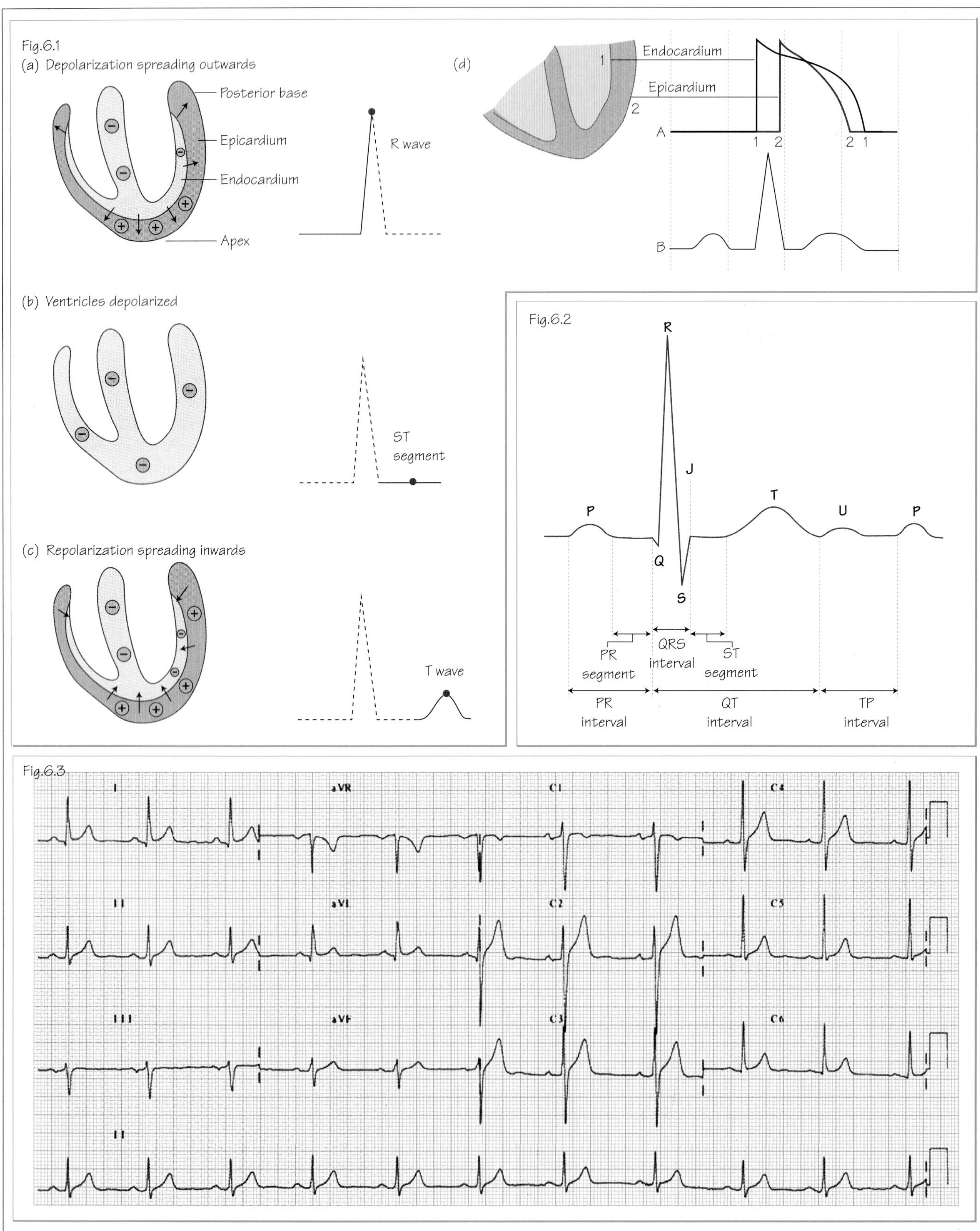

Fig.6.1
(a) Depolarization spreading outwards
Posterior base
Epicardium
Endocardium
Apex
R wave
(b) Ventricles depolarized
ST segment
(c) Repolarization spreading inwards
T wave
(d)
Endocardium
Epicardium
1
2
A
1 2
2 1
B
Fig.6.2
R
J
T
P
U
P
Q
S
PR segment
QRS interval
ST segment
PR interval
QT interval
TP interval
Fig.6.3
I
aVR
C1
C4
II
aVL
C2
C5
III
aVF
C3
C6
II

The T wave reflects current movement during repolarization. In understanding the T wave, note that:

- The direction of *depolarization* is endocardial to epicardial (from inside the heart to the outside), as the first tissue to depolarize is closest to the specialized conducting tissue (the Purkinje cells), which lies just under the endocardium (Fig. 6.1a–c). Depolarization moves positively charged ions into the cell, leaving excess negative charge (electrons) outside the cells, which flow into areas with more positive charge, i.e. areas yet to depolarize (and then on to an observing electrode). Current flow during depolarization is therefore endocardially to epicardially, resulting in an R wave.
- As the action potentials of epicardial cells are shorter than those of endocardial cells these cells, despite being activated later, repolarize earlier, i.e. epicardial cells repolarize first, followed by endocardial cells (Fig. 6.1a–c). Thus, though the direction of repolarization is epicardial to endocardial, in the opposite direction to depolarization, the current flow associated with this is endocardial to epicardial. This current flow moves towards an observing electrode causing a positive deflection, the T wave.
- The key principle is thus established that in health where there is an R wave, there is an upright T (Fig. 6.3). This translates as *the T wave axis* (calculated in the same way as the QRS axis – Chapter 5) *should be within 60° of the QRS axis*.
- Where the R wave is equivocal or absent, the T wave polarity is equivocal or variable; e.g. lead aVL in many people.
- The inferior leads (especially lead III, aVF) often show variable T wave polarity, as the bulk of other parts of the heart balance out any local inferior wall repolarizing current flow. In addition, posture affects the inferior lead T waves – hence during an exercise test an ECG should initially be recorded in the lying, then the standing position.
- aVR (which looks through the atrioventricular [AV] valves at the endocardial surface of the heart) has a deep Q wave and so an inverted T wave.
- In lead V1 (where the bulk of the posterior wall balances out currents from the septum) there is usually only a very small, sometimes absent, R wave, and so usually the V1 T wave is inverted.

From the above it is clear that if one sees a QRS complex with a good R wave, but a flat or inverted T wave, then that ECG is abnormal. In determining the cause, it is actually not very helpful trying to understand the underlying pathophysiology, though from what has been said it is clear that the sequence of repolarization must be altered, with either there being no endo–epicardial differences (flat T waves) or the sequence being reversed with repolarization occurring from the endocardium to the epicardium (inverted T waves). For causes see Chapters 15, 16 and 17.

U waves are positive deflections occurring after the T wave, sometimes merging with it (Fig. 6.1a–c). The origin of the U wave is speculative. Some regard it as reflecting repolarization of papillary muscles. Prominent U waves are normal in youth (< 35–40 years) but are rare in those more elderly. In disease they can occur (but are not inevitable) in hypokalaemia, left ventricular hypertrophy, those on class I anti-arrhythmic drugs, mitral valve prolapse. Bizarre U waves may occur in the extraordinarily rare hereditary long QT syndrome.

Fig. 6.1 (a–c) Sequence of depolarization and repolarization. The diagram shows the specialized conducting tissue of the heart. The depolarization sequence starts at the sinus node, then proceeds through the atria to the atrioventricular (AV) node, then into the specialized conducting system, which in the ventricles is situated sub-endocardially. Thus depolarization proceeds in an inward → outward direction. Repolarization proceeds in the opposite direction to depolarization (outward → inward), but as the current associated with repolarization moves in the opposite direction to the one associated with depolarization (see text), an observing electrode will see a positive deflection both for depolarization (the R wave) in most leads, and for repolarization (the T wave). (d) Sequence of endocardial and epicardial depolarization and repolarization. The endocardium depolarizes first, whereas the epicardium repolarizes first. Endocardial/epicardial differences account for the positivity of the T wave in health (see text).

Fig. 6.2 The U wave. This ECG shows the position of the U wave. Their origin is uncertain, and there maybe a number of physiological explanations. Most people do not show U waves. When present, they may be normal (e.g. the young), or, if associated with flat T waves, may indicate hypokalaemia. If the ECG shows a long QT interval, they may indicate hereditary long QT syndrome. They also occur in other pathologies.

Fig. 6.3 Normal 12-lead ECG. This ECG is used to illustrate the normal T wave. Note that wherever there is a well-developed R wave, the T wave is clearly upright. Where there is a poor R wave, the T wave is equivocal (e.g. lead III, V1), and in lead aVR, where there is no R wave, rather there being a well developed Q wave, the T wave is inverted.

7 Abnormalities in the shape of the P wave – left and right atrial enlargement

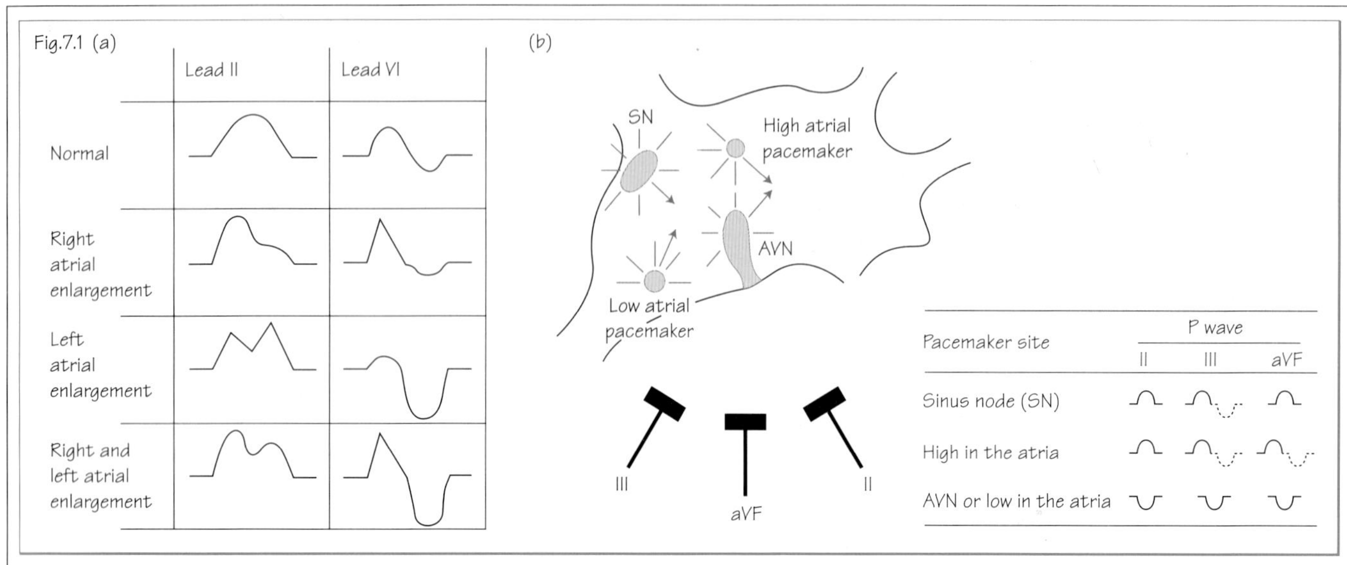

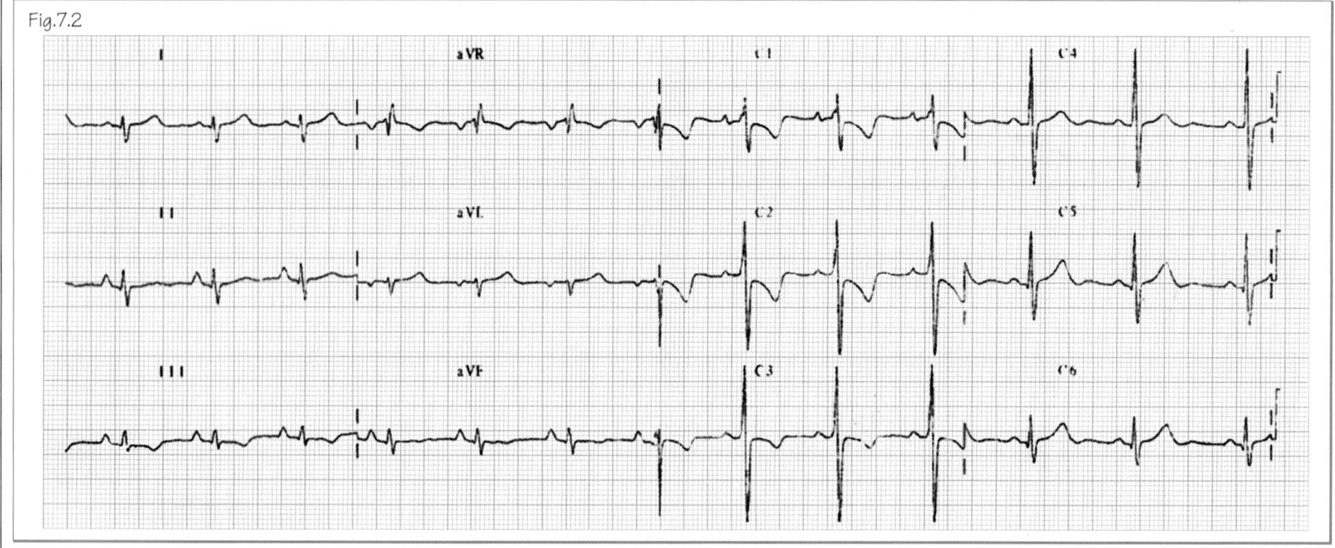

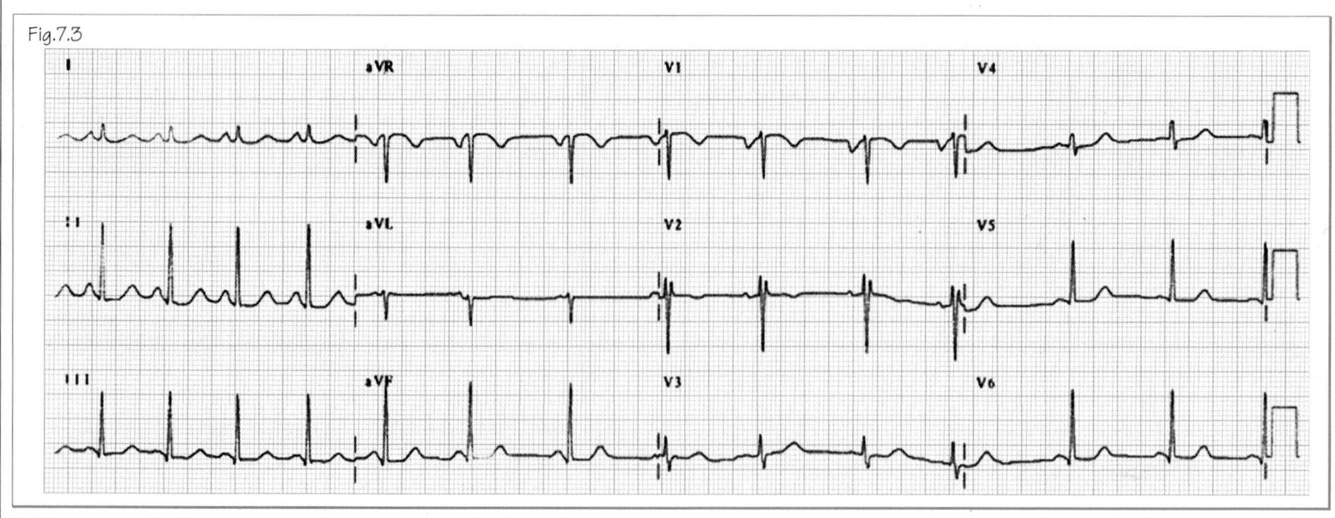

The P wave shape is altered in atrial enlargement (though the relationship between ECG and cardiac ultrasound findings is not close) and arrhythmias. The normal P wave is the sum of the right and left atrial depolarization vectors (Fig. 7.1a,b) and is best examined in lead II and V1:

• Lead II reflects both atria (right atrial [RA] depolarization proceeds towards lead II, left atrial [LA] depolarization is mainly directed to lead II). As the sinus node activates the RA first, the initial part of the P wave reflects RA depolarization, the mid-part both, and the latter part LA depolarization.

• Lead V1 mainly reflects LA depolarization, which moves directly away from lead V1. Right atrial depolarization makes only a small, initial, contribution to the P wave in lead V1.

Right atrial enlargement (Fig. 7.2 and see Fig. 35.1)

The ECG is not reliable in diagnosing RA enlargement. When the RA is enlarged depolarization takes longer (more distance to travel) and involves greater current flows (depolarizing atrial myocytes let in more ions, increasing current flow). The vector directed towards lead II is:

• Larger, so the P wave in lead II becomes taller, usually ≥ 0.15 mV.

• Longer, not usually seen, as normal RA depolarization is over well before the end of the P wave.

Lead V1 is affected by RA enlargement, but less so as the vector of RA depolarization is at right angles to this lead. However, there is an increased voltage here in the first two-thirds of the P wave.

Left atrial enlargement (Fig. 7.3 and see Fig. 33.1)

In LA enlargement, the LA depolarization vector is prolonged and increased:

• In lead II there is a long late high voltage positive deflection after the initial RA P wave, resulting in a classic bifid shape (P mitrale, from rheumatic mitral stenosis). P mitrale is a sign of advanced, rather than early, LA enlargement.

• As the vector of LA depolarization proceeds away from lead V1, after a small initial positive deflection arising from the normal right atria, the P wave is dominated by a late negative deflection (Fig. 7.1a,b). This late negative deflection is *a moderately reliable and sensitive marker of LA enlargement*.

Biatrial enlargement

Biatrial enlargement results in a combination of the above signs: a large P wave in lead II, both early and late on, with a late negative deflection in lead V1.

Causes of atrial enlargement

The clinical situation (history/examination) and associated ECG changes allow a diagnosis. Left atrial enlargement is common in:

• Hypertension: look for ECG left ventricular hypertrophy (LVH).

• Aortic and mitral valve lesions: listen for characteristic murmurs.

• Previous myocardial infarction (MI): Q waves or loss of R wave height on a regional basis.

• Cardiomyopathy: non-specifically abnormal ECG or conducting tissue disease.

Right atrial enlargement is often due to chronic obstructive pulmonary disease (COPD)-related pulmonary hypertension and often the QRS axis is swung to the right. Occasionally in severe pulmonary hypertension a dominant R wave in lead V1 is seen.

Ectopic atrial pacemaker

If the pacemaker is situated other than in the sinus node then the P wave shape differs, according to where the pacemaker is sited (Fig. 7.1a,b). Most ectopic pacemakers are variants of normal: sometimes their presence indicates sinus node disease or, for low atrial pacemakers, an atrial septal defect.

Fig. 7.1 (a) Typical findings in right, left and biatrial enlargement. Normally right atrial (RA) depolarization occupies the first two-thirds and left atrial (LA) depolarization the latter two-thirds of the P wave. The left atrium accounts for the small negative terminal deflection in the P wave of lead V1. In RA enlargement, the RA contribution is increased in size, leading to an increased early phase of the P wave. This contribution is positive in both lead II and V1. In LA enlargement, the late phase is increased; this is positive in lead II (leading to the classic bifid appearance of P mitrale – commonly found in rheumatic mitral valve disease), and negative in lead V1 (LA depolarization is mainly away from lead V1). A late negative deflection in lead V1 is a more sensitive sign of LA enlargement than a bifid P wave in lead II. Biatrial enlargement leads to a combination of these signs. (b) Findings in ectopic atrial pacemaker. The pacemaker can move, usually within the RA, often either higher up, or, more typically, much lower down. The ECG leads 'in line' with this movement are the inferior ones, and the pattern of the ECG changes in a predictable manner, as shown. AVN, atrioventricular node; SN, sinus node.

Fig. 7.2 An ECG showing right atrial (RA) enlargement, from a patient with pulmonary hypertension (QRS axis shifted to the right, a dominant R wave in lead V1, repolarization changes [inverted T waves] leads V1–V3 due to right ventricular 'strain'). Compare with a normal ECG (see Fig. 6.3). The abnormal P wave findings are really quite subtle; there is a peaked P wave in lead II (so-called 'gothic' P wave, or P pulmonale). What amplitude of the P wave in lead II constitutes P pulmonale is debatable. The early positive amplitude of the P wave in lead V1 is also increased; an early voltage in lead V1 of ≥ 0.15 mV (i.e. ≥ 1.5 mm) is fairly suggestive. Unfortunately, most patients with RA enlargement do not have these ECG signs, and most patients with these ECG signs do not have RA enlargement.

Fig. 7.3 An ECG showing left atrial (LA) enlargement. Aside from the changes to the P wave, the ECG is otherwise normal. There is a wide (though surprisingly not bifid) P wave seen in lead II, and a large late negative deflection in the P wave in lead V1. This comes from a patient with severe isolated mitral stenosis, with a very large LA.

8 Increased QRS amplitude

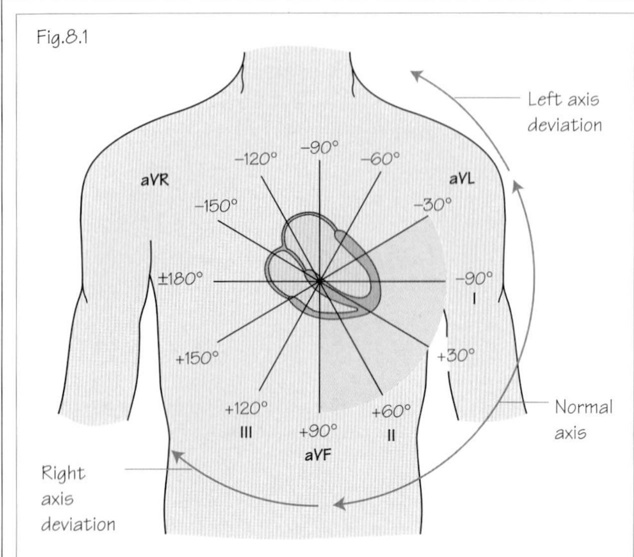

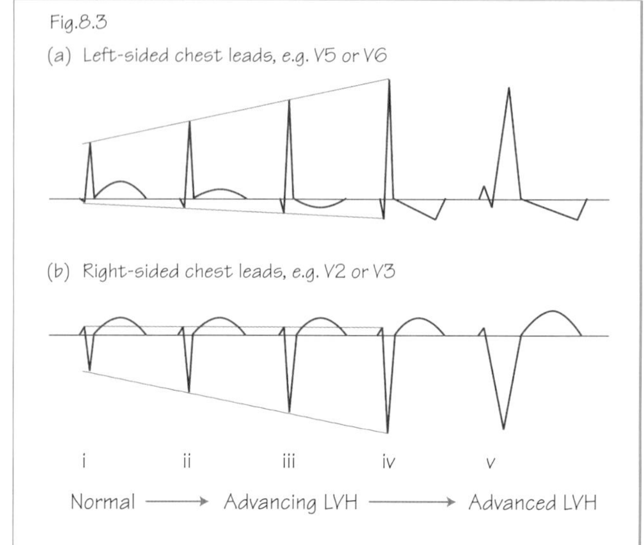

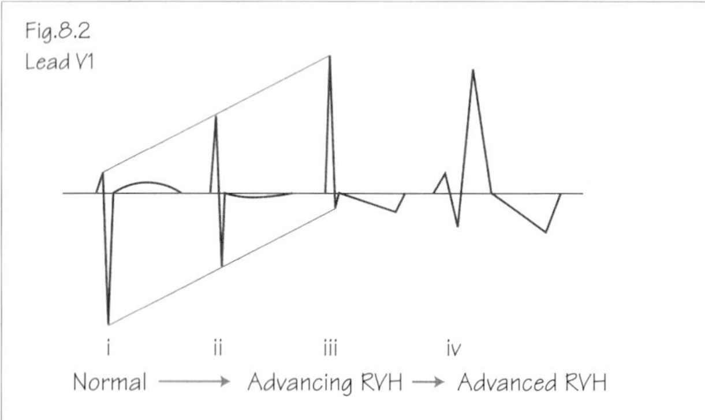

Table 1
Criteria for the ECG diagnosis of right ventricular hypertrophy (RVH).

• Butler–Leggett formula*			
Directions	Anterior (A)	Rightward (R)	Posterior-leftward (PL)
Amplitude	Tallest R or R' in lead V1 or V2	Deepest S in lead V1 or V6	S in lead V1
RVH formula: A + R − PL ≥ 0.70 mV			
• Sokolow–Lyon criteria† – RVH = R wave in lead V1 + S wave in lead V5 or V6 ≥ 1.10 mV			
Adapted with permission from *Butler PM, Leggett SI, Howe CM *et al.* Identification of electrocardiographic criteria for diagnosis of right ventricular hypertrophy due to mitral stenosis. *Am J Cardiol* 1986; **57**: 639–43: and from †Sokolow M, Lyon TP. The ventricular complex in right ventricular hypertrophy as obtained by unipolar precordial and limb leads. *Am Heart J* 1949; **3**: 273–94			

Table 2
Criteria for the ECG diagnosis of left ventricular hypertrophy (LVH).

- Romhilt–Estes criteria
  1. Voltage criterion: R or S in any limb lead ≥ 0.20 mV or S in lead V1 or V2 or R in lead V5 or V6 ≥ 0.30 mV — 3 points
  2. Left ventricular strain: ST segment and T wave in opposite direction to QRS complex
     – without digitalis — 3 points
     – with digitalis — 1 point
  3. Left atrial enlargement: terminal negativity of the P wave in lead V1 > 0.10 mV in depth and 0.04 s in duration — 3 points
  4. Axis shift: left axis deviation of ≥ −30° — 2 points
  5. QRS duration: ≥ 0.09 s — 1 point
  6. Intrinsicoid deflection in lead V5 or V6 ≥ 0.05 s — 1 point

  Total possible score 13 points
  Probable LVH = 4 points; definite LVH = 5 points
- Sokolow–Lyon criteria
  S wave in lead V1 + R wave in lead V5 or V6 > 3.50 mV or R wave in lead V5 or V6 > 2.60 mV
- Cornell sex-specific voltage criteria
  – Women: R wave in lead aVL + S wave in lead V3 > 2.00 mV
  – Men: R wave in lead aVL + S wave in lead V3 > 2.80 mV
- Cornell voltage–QRS duration product criteria
- Gubner–Ungerleider criteria
  – R wave in lead I plus S wave in lead III ≥ 2.5 mV
- Minnesota Code 3-1
  – R wave in lead V5–6 > 2.6 mV or
  – R wave in leads II, III, aVF > 2.0 mV or
  – R wave in lead aVL > 1.2 mV

The size of the QRS complex depends on:

• The number and activity of myocytes. Myocytes may become less numerous with age. Myocytes are more electrically active in youth (< 40 years) and in ventricular hypertrophy.

• The insulation between the heart and the observing electrodes. A pericardial effusion, or obesity, diminishes the amount of electricity reaching the electrodes. The latter is easily diagnosed, the former, either by clinical signs or, rarely, by beat-to-beat variation in the amplitude of the QRS complex (see Chapter 25).

Right ventricular hypertrophy

Right ventricular hypertrophy (RVH) results in greater voltages from the right ventricle (see Fig. 8.2), resulting in:

1 The QRS axis shifts to the right (see Fig. 8.1).

2 Leads looking at the right ventricle show greater positive deflections. In particular, in lead V1 the size of the R wave increases – instead of the normal situation where there is a very small R wave followed by a deep S wave, in RVH the R wave can equal the height of the S wave, or indeed can be much larger than the S wave (called a dominant R wave). The R wave remains narrow (unlike right bundle branch block).

3 In severe RVH there may be T wave changes (see below).

4 The left-sided chest leads are unchanged in RVH (the bulk of the right ventricle, even when hypertrophied, cannot rule out the influence of the large bulk of the left ventricle on the left-sided leads).

5 Signs of right atrial enlargement may be present (see Chapter 7 and Fig. 35.1), with the P wave becoming peaked early on in lead II and V1.

Left ventricular hypertrophy

In left ventricular hypertrophy (LVH), greater voltages are generated by the left ventricle, which results in:

1 The QRS axis shifting to the left.

2 Those leads looking at the left ventricle show an increased deflection, i.e. leads I, II, aVL, and V5 and V6.

3 Conversely, those leads looking away from the left ventricle show increased negative deflections, i.e. there is an increased size of the S waves in leads V2 and V3.

4 There may be signs of left atrial enlargement (bifid P wave in lead II, lead V1 P wave dominated by a late negative deflection).

5 In severe LVH there may be T wave changes (see below).

Despite the above, it is often rather difficult to be unequivocally clear on ECG grounds as to whether ventricular hypertrophy is present. Various 'rules' have been proposed (Tables 8.1 & 8.2). However, those 'rules' which make hypertrophy certain, miss most cases and those 'rules' that capture most hypertrophy also capture many non-hypertrophy cases (i.e. high specificity rules have low sensitivity, and high sensitivity rules have low specificity – see Chapter 2). There are no ideal rules; those using the ECG regularly will adapt the rules in light of their experience.

• In practice, most cases of RVH have fairly unremarkable ECGs – no rules therefore allow one to reliably diagnose RVH, and if this diagnosis is important, other investigations should be used (e.g. echo-derived pulmonary artery pressure).

• For LVH, many ECG readers use:

(a) The size of the R wave in lead aVL ≥ 11 mm, a specific but not sensitive finding.

(b) S in V2/3 + R in V5/6 ≥ 45 mm (in the young) or ≥ 40 mm (in those ≥ 40–45 years), a sensitive but not specific finding.

Repolarization changes in ventricular hypertrophy

In severe hypertrophy, the sequence of *repolarization* in the mass of hypertrophied tissue alters, from the normal epicardial to endocardial sequence to the reverse, i.e. endocardial to epicardial spread. This is because the action potential is differentially prolonged in the endocardium and becomes longer than the epicardial APD. As the direction of the current flow associated with repolarization changes, so the direction of the T wave changes over the largest bulk of hypertrophied tissue, from upright to negative, usually in a 'reverse-tick' pattern. In severe LVH, T wave inversion is found in leads I, II, aVL, (sometimes V4), V5, V6, and in RVH in leads V1, V2 and sometimes (rarely) V3. These repolarization changes were previously called 'strain'; they indicate more severe hypertrophy, usually more advanced underlying heart disease (e.g. aortic valve disease) and usually a worse prognosis (especially in hypertensive heart disease). Sometimes, they are the only signs of hypertrophy, as the voltage criteria may not be met. Repolarization changes are sometimes useful in confirming the diagnosis of LVH.

Fig. 8.1 Homunculus demonstrating the normal QRS axis, left and right axis deviation.

Fig. 8.2; Table 1 The ECG signs of right ventricular hypertrophy (RVH). The impact of RVH is on the QRS axis (which shifts to the right (a) and the right-sided chest leads (b)); there is no impact on the left-sided chest leads. As RVH advances, the size of the R wave in lead V1 gradually increases (ii), becoming dominant (iii). In advanced RVH, in addition to a 'dominant' R wave in lead V1, the T waves in the right-sided chest leads flattens and then inverts ('strain', or 'repolarization changes'). Finally, right bundle branch block occurs (iv).

Fig. 8.3; Table 2 ECG consequences of advancing left ventricular hypertrophy (LVH). (a) As LVH progresses, increasing left axis deviation occurs, the height of the R wave in the left-sided leads increases (often with increasing size of the initial small Q wave in leads V5 and V6, due to increased voltages generated by left to right depolarization of the larger interventricular septum). The T wave in the lateral leads first flattens (ii), then inverts (see iv) ('strain' or 'repolarization changes'). (b) In the right-sided leads, the S wave deepens, but there is no impact on the ST–T wave. In advanced LVH left bundle branch block often occurs (v). RVH, right ventricular hypertrophy.

9 Q waves and loss of R wave height

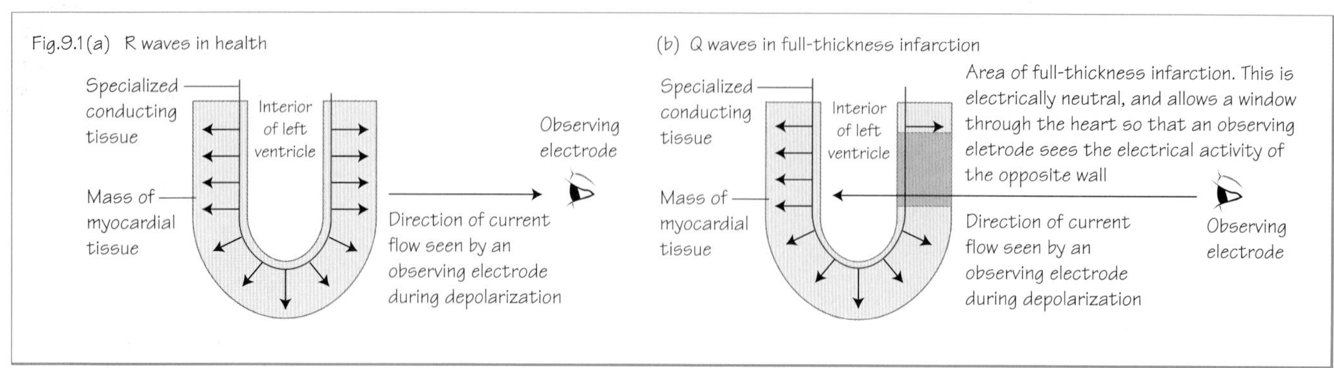

Fig.9.1 (a) R waves in health (b) Q waves in full-thickness infarction

Fig.9.2
(a)

(b)

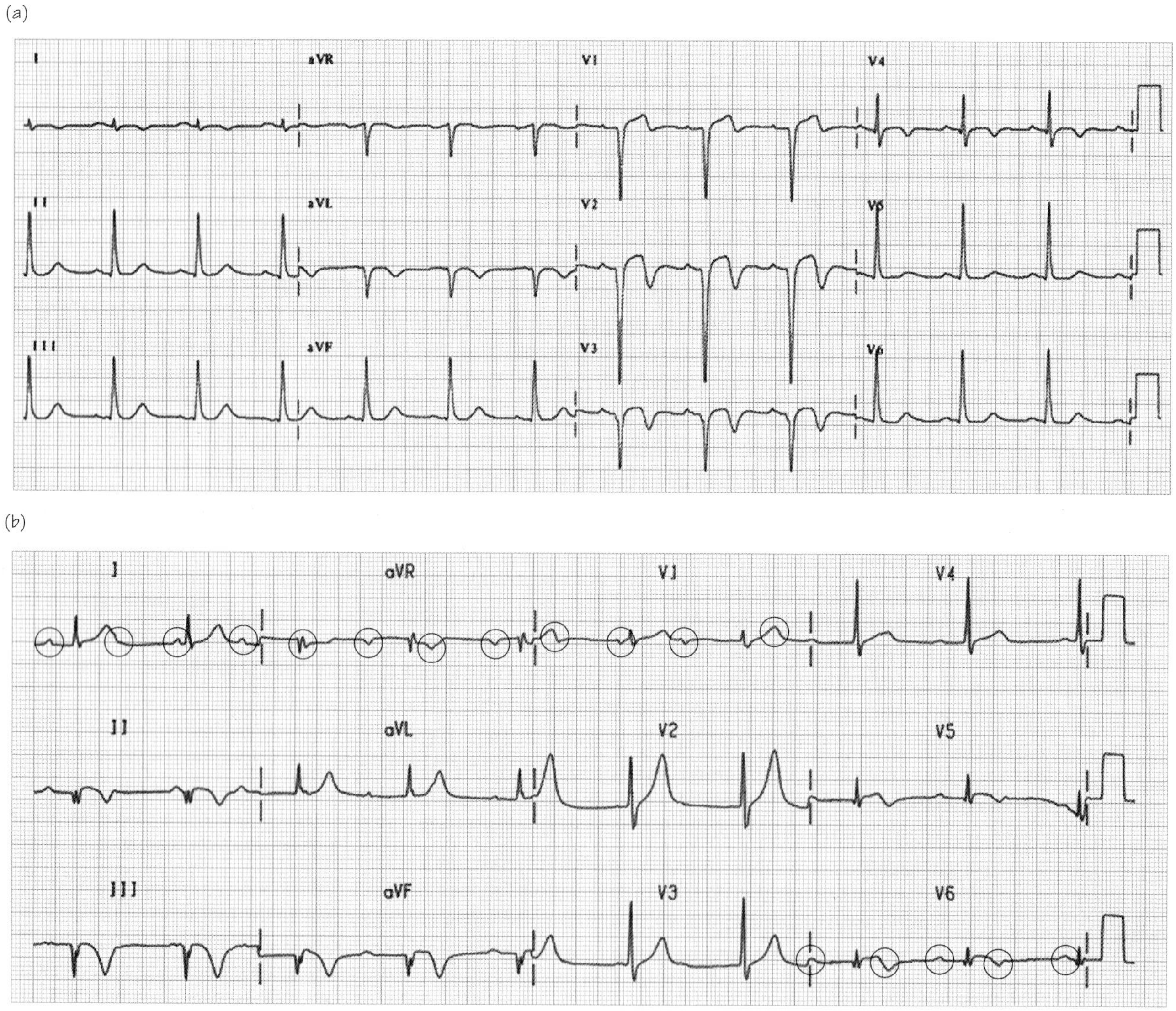

Pathological Q waves are a key finding as they indicate significant cardiac damage. They must be distinguished from physiological Q waves, which occur in:

- The left-sided chest leads, where they reflect left-to-right septal depolarization. They are small ≤ 2.5 mV and brief < 40 ms.
- Lead aVR, which looks through the atrioventricular (AV) valve at the endocardial surface of the heart.

Pathological Q waves do not fulfil the criteria for being physiological and indicate an 'electrical window' in the part of the heart directly facing the electrode, which allows currents from the opposite wall to influence the electrode in an unopposed fashion (Fig. 9.1a,b). As depolarization proceeds from the endocardium to the epicardium, the electrode looking directly into the heart through this electrical window sees a Q wave rather than an R wave. Pathological Q waves indicate:

- An old transmural myocardial infarct; the Q wave distribution reflecting which artery has occluded (Table 9.1).
- Less commonly another pathology, such as left ventricular hypertrophy (LVH) (increased Q waves in the left-sided leads in association with large R waves), or occasionally hypertrophic cardiomyopathy (large Q waves, in the inferior leads, without substantial R waves).
- A rare cause of Q waves is myocarditis or dilated cardiomyopathy.

Damage insufficient to cause Q waves, but sufficient to result in the death of some cells in the heart (i.e. sufficient numbers survive so that some electrical activity continues), leads to a decrease in size of the R waves, without Q wave formation. Pathologically small R waves can be difficult to diagnose unambiguously, as there is so much variation in normal R wave height (healthy thin young patients have large R waves, healthy elderly obese individuals small ones). With experience readers develop a good instinct about what is normal for a particular individual. Pathological loss of R wave height usually follows the regional distribution of coronary arteries. If this affects the anterior wall, it is termed poor anterior R wave progression (see Fig. 5.2). Though this can be caused by rotation of the heart due to obesity, if there is T wave inversion in any of leads V2–V6 then the probability of anterior wall damage is greatly increased.

Table 9.1 Distribution of Q waves related to site of coronary artery occlusion.

Classification, according to site of Q waves	Leads demonstrating Q waves	Likely site of occlusion*
Standard		
Anterior	V1 to 4	LAD
Posterior	Dominant R wave in lead V1, i.e. R wave > S wave	Cx
Inferior	II, III, aVF	RCA, sometimes Cx
Lateral	V5/6	Variable; distal RCA, side-branch of Cx
Combinations		
Antero-lateral	I, aVL, V1 to 6	Large LAD
Infero-lateral	II, III, aVF, V5/6	Large RCA
Infero-posterior	II, III, aVF, dominant R wave lead V1	Large RCA or Cx
Infero-postero-lateral	II, III, aVF, dominant R wave lead V1, V5/6	Very large RCA/Cx

* There are many other possible sites of occlusion for the patterns described, these are the most likely.
Cx, circumflex coronary artery; LAD, left anterior descending coronary artery; RCA, right coronary artery: large vessel means both long and occlusion more proximally.

Fig. 9.1 The mechanism underlying pathological Q waves. The normal situation is shown if (a) where an observing electrode sees the wave of depolarization passing towards it, so producing an R wave. An observing electrode directly over an area of full-thickness myocardial infarction (or indeed scar tissue from any pathology) does not see the normal endocardial to epicardial spread of excitation (which normally results in an R wave). Rather, the electrode sees into the cardiac cavity, and so the spread of depolarization of the opposite wall, which moves away from the electrode, rather than towards it, causing a Q wave (b). The distribution of the Q waves reflects which coronary artery has occluded (see Table 9.1).

Fig. 9.2 ECGs showing Q waves. (a) Anterior wall myocardial infarct; sinus rhythm, P wave is unremarkable. Pathological Q waves in leads V1–3, really quite deep, with biphasic T waves, i.e. initially up and then down. This is a sign that the myocardial infarction (MI) causing the septal Q waves is recent, i.e. ≤ 1–7 days or so. After a few weeks the T waves become fully upright, so resuming their normal polarity. The T wave abnormality does extend more laterally, certainly into lead V4, and, albeit rather subtly, into leads V5 and V6. (b) Infero-lateral-posterior MI. This ECG is complex, with many abnormalities. Though the QRS rate is reasonable, being about 60 bpm, giving the impression that the rhythm is sinus; in fact it is not. The rhythm is complete heart block, as there is no consistent relationship between the atrial (P waves circled) and the ventricular activity. There are inferior lead (II, III, and aVF) Q waves, and the lateral leads (V5 and V6) are not nearly as tall as they should be (compare with (a) above); this is because there has also been a lateral lead infarct, resulting in the loss of much myocardium, and thus a loss of R wave height. Furthermore, lead V1 is abnormal; the main part of the QRS complex should go downwards (i.e. there should be a deep S wave). However, instead, the R wave is much larger than the S wave, a 'so-called dominant (lead V1) R wave', as there has also been a posterior wall MI (see Fig. 13.2). The deep inferior lead T wave inversion suggests that the MI is very recent, within the past few days (old MIs have upright 'T's). The extent of Q waves, loss of R wave height, and posterior MI signs suggests that the MI is very large, has affected the inferior, lateral and posterior part of the left ventricle, and is likely to be due to the occlusion of a very large right or circumflex coronary artery. Left ventricle (LV) function is likely to be poor.

10 QRS axis deviation

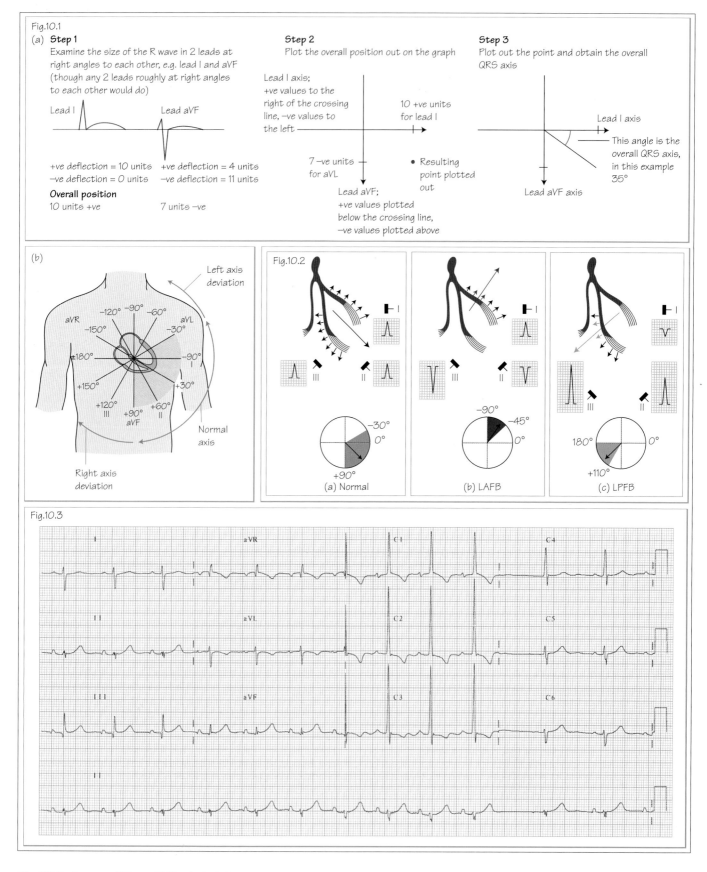

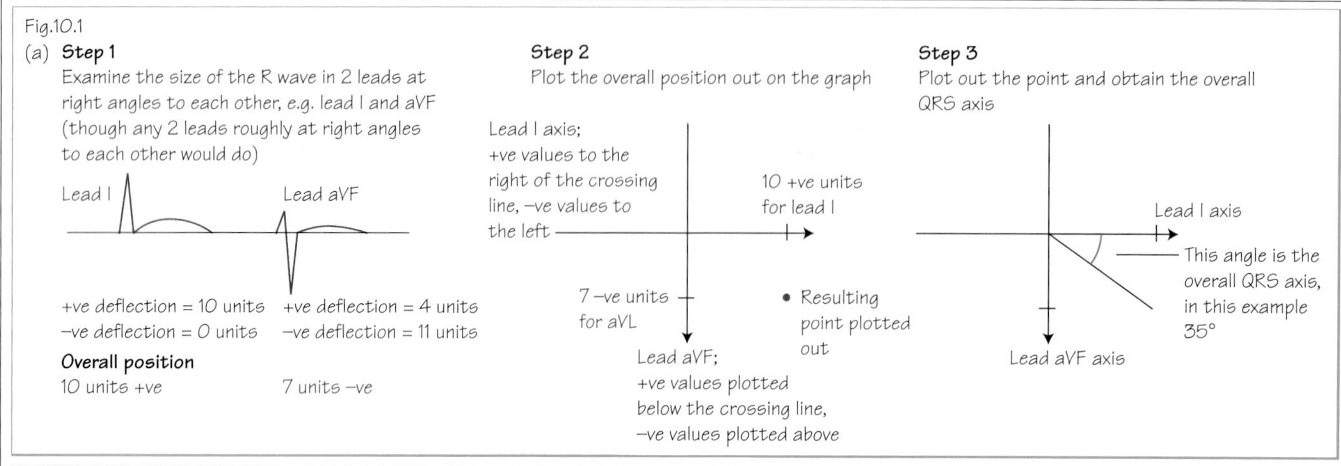
Fig.10.1
(a) Step 1
Examine the size of the R wave in 2 leads at right angles to each other, e.g. lead I and aVF (though any 2 leads roughly at right angles to each other would do)
Lead I
Lead aVF
+ve deflection = 10 units
–ve deflection = 0 units
+ve deflection = 4 units
–ve deflection = 11 units
Overall position
10 units +ve
7 units –ve
Step 2
Plot the overall position out on the graph
Lead I axis;
+ve values to the right of the crossing line, –ve values to the left
10 +ve units for lead I
7 –ve units for aVL
Resulting point plotted out
Lead aVF;
+ve values plotted below the crossing line,
–ve values plotted above
Step 3
Plot out the point and obtain the overall QRS axis
Lead I axis
This angle is the overall QRS axis, in this example 35°
Lead aVF axis

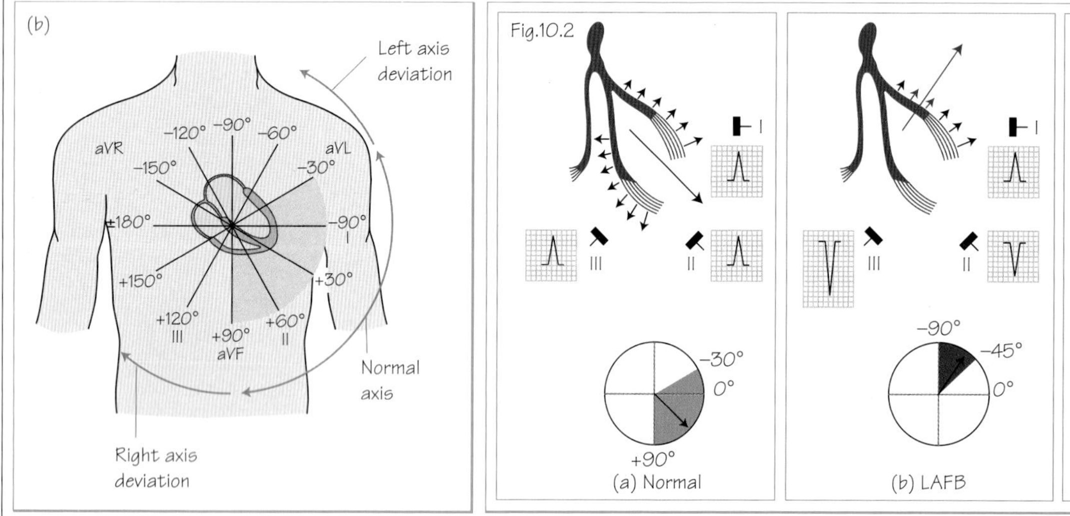
(b)
Left axis deviation
aVR
–120°
–90°
–60°
aVL
–150°
–30°
±180°
–90°
I
+150°
+30°
+120°
III
+90°
aVF
+60°
II
Normal axis
Right axis deviation
Fig.10.2
I
III
II
–30°
0°
+90°
(a) Normal
–90°
–45°
0°
(b) LAFB
180°
0°
+110°
(c) LPFB

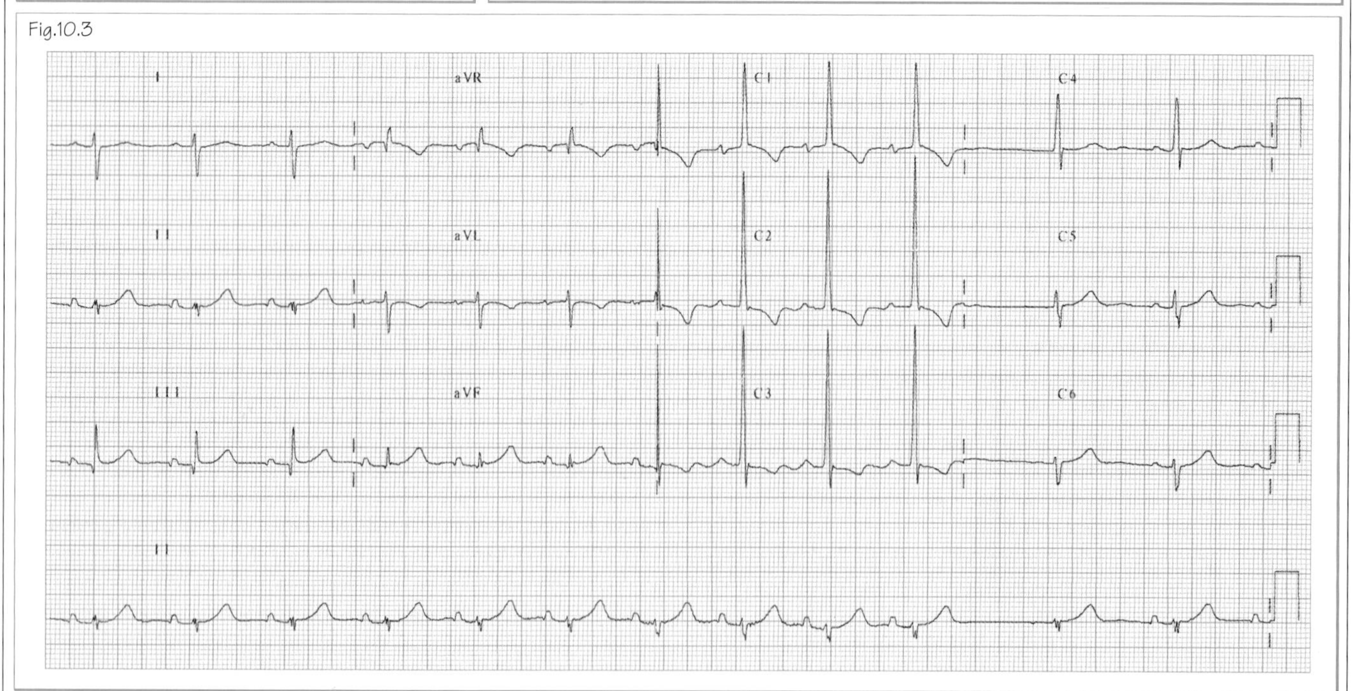
Fig.10.3
I
aVR
C1
C4
II
aVL
C2
C5
III
aVF
C3
C6
II

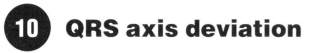

The wave of depolarization spreads over the ventricles in a co-ordinated fashion, and it is possible to determine its direction of travel, the QRS axis, both for a particular moment in time (instantaneous QRS vector) and overall for the whole of the depolarization phase (overall QRS axis). How and why is this done?

Determination of the QRS axis

The wave of depolarization crossing the ventricles has the properties of a vector, that is, it possesses both direction and speed:

• The instantaneous vector can be determined from knowledge of the instantaneous QRS amplitude in each of three ECG leads at right angles to each other (orthogonal leads, traditionally X, Y and Z leads). The instantaneous vector produces a plot of the vector of depolarization over the QRS cycle (vectorcardiography). The plots obtained are complex, used infrequently and most cardiologists are inexperienced in their interpretation. They usually add little to the data in the standard 12-lead ECG.

• The overall frontal (i.e. obtained from the standard frontal leads) vector of the overall QRS complex can easily be obtained (Fig. 10.1a,b).

Meaning of the overall QRS axis

The overall QRS vector shows the direction of depolarization of the bulk of the ventricular mass. As such, it is mainly directed towards the main muscle mass being depolarized, i.e. in health, towards the left ventricle. It is useful as it changes in a characteristic fashion in disease.

Left axis deviation

There are two common interpretations:

1 More left ventricular muscle to depolarize, i.e. left ventricular hypertrophy (LVH) is present, which usually also causes prominent left-sided R waves and deep right-sided S waves. Occasionally LVH occurs with just an axis shift and no increase in QRS amplitude. Once suspected this diagnosis is best confirmed by cardiac ultrasound.

2 Left ventricular depolarization is delayed as the conducting tissue is damaged. The left anterior fascicle of the left bundle branch supplies much of the anterior part of the left ventricle. If this is damaged, the left anterior part of the left ventricle depolarizes late, which then predominates the depolarization vector, resulting in left axis deviation (Fig. 10.2a–c).

Right axis deviation

There are two common interpretations:

1 More right ventricular muscle mass, i.e. right ventricular hypertrophy is present (Fig. 10.3).

2 The posterior lying bulk of the left ventricle is depolarized late, due to disease in its conducting tissue, the posterior fascicle of the left bundle (Fig. 10.2a–c). Other conducting tissue disease may also be present, e.g. long PR interval, right bundle branch block.

Catches in measuring the QRS axis

The QRS axis can really only be measured accurately from the 12-lead ECG if there are no Q waves; large Q waves (e.g. inferiorly) prevent any firm conclusion being reached.

Fig. 10.1 (a) How to determine the overall QRS axis. **Step 1**: Determine the overall (R–S) wave amplitude in two leads at right angles to each other (here leads I and aVF are used, as these correspond to the X and Y axis on a standard graph. Any combination of leads can be used, though those at right angles to each other are preferred). **Step 2**: plot these points out on the appropriate graph. **Step 3**: Determine the overall QRS axis. A very rough rule is that the direction of the QRS axis is in the direction of the standard lead with the largest R wave. A rough rule is that if leads I and II have overall +ve QRS complexes, and lead III overall –ve, then the axis is normal. If either lead I or lead II is negative, then either there is left axis (lead I +ve, lead II and III –ve) or right axis deviation (lead I –ve, lead II +ve or –ve, lead III +ve). (b) Normal and abnormal QRS axis. The figure shows the heart, frontal leads, and the direction of observation. Normal QRS axis is outlined between –30° and +90°. Left axis deviation is ≥ –30, right axis deviation is ≥ +90.

Fig. 10.2 Mechanism of axis deviation in partial left bundle damage. (a) Normal: current passes down the specialized conducting tissue, with the left ventricle dominating the axis, as this is much larger than the right ventricle. The left bundle is divided into two branches, the anterior hemi-fascicle, and the much larger posterior hemi-fascicle, which respectively supply the antero-superior and postero-inferior part of the left ventricle. When the anterior hemi-fascicle is blocked (b), this part of the heart is activated late, so resulting in left axis deviation. Likewise, when the larger left posterior hemi-fascicle is blocked (c), the part of the heart normally supplied by this conducting tissue is activated late, resulting in right axis deviation. A convenient way to remember which axis deviation results from which hemi-fascicular block is to remember that **l**eft **a**nterior hemi-fascicular block causes **l**eft **a**xis deviation. LAFB, left anterior fascicular block; LPFB, left posterior fascicular block.

Fig. 10.3 Right axis deviation in right ventricular hypertrophy (RVH). The sequence of ECG changes with increasingly severe RVH is: (i) the earliest sign is right axis deviation; (ii) next the R wave in lead V1 increases in size; (iii) finally, right bundle branch block occurs. This ECG shows gross RVH. The features include: (a) some prominence to the P wave in lead II, suggestive (not diagnostic) of right atrial enlargement; (b) QRS axis shifted to the right (negative QRS in lead I and II, +ve QRS in lead III; the computer calculation of the axis is 151°); (c) dominant R wave in lead V1, highly prominent R waves in leads V2 and V3; (d) an unusual feature is the small R waves in the left lateral chest leads – common in patients with RVH due to congenital heart disease (as here) but not in other causes of RVH.

11 Long PR interval and QRS broadening

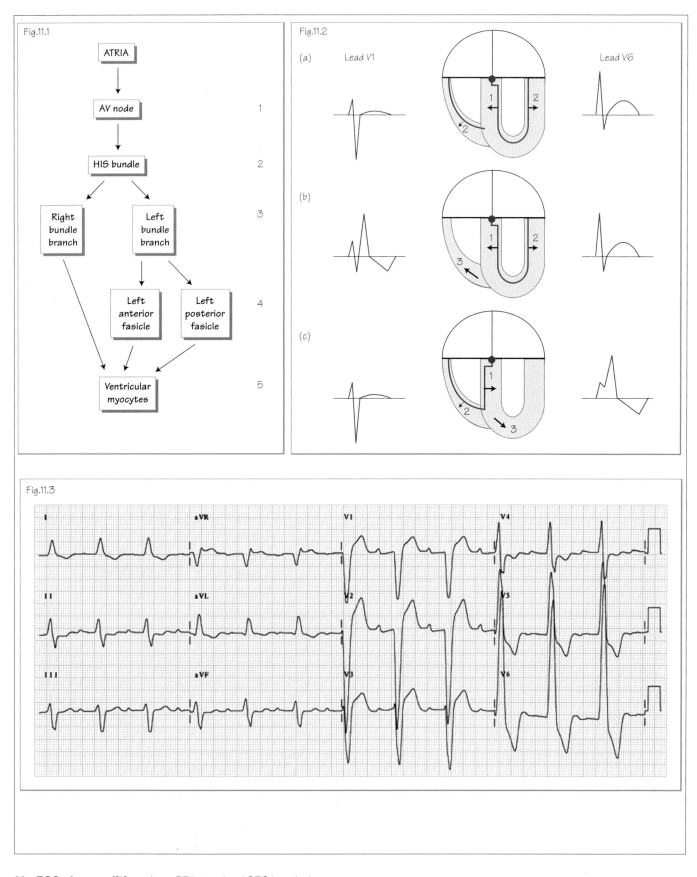

Fig.11.1

ATRIA

AV node 1

HIS bundle 2

Right bundle branch

Left bundle branch 3

Left anterior fasicle

Left posterior fasicle 4

Ventricular myocytes 5

Fig.11.2

(a) Lead V1 Lead V6

1 2

2

(b)

1 2

3

(c)

1

2

3

Fig.11.3

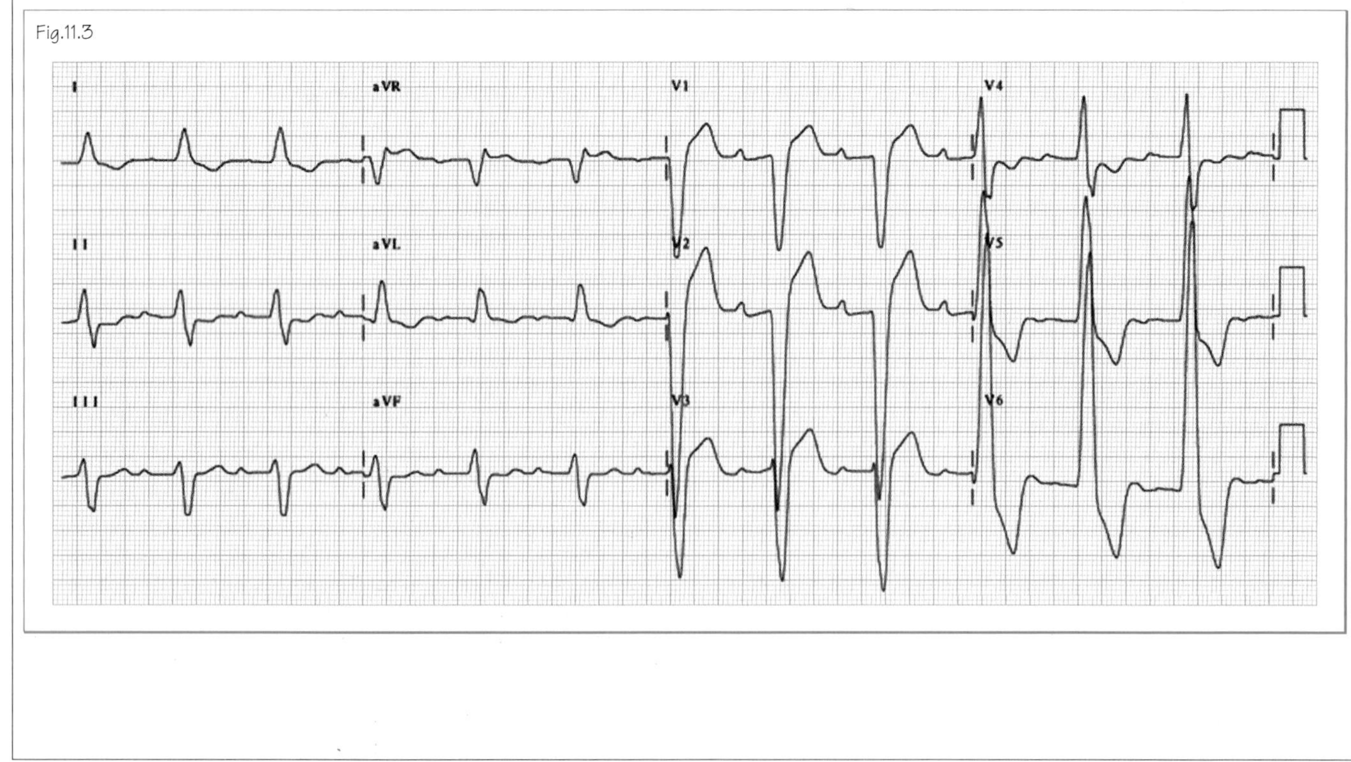

The normal wave of depolarization passes from the sinus node into the atrioventricular (AV) node, the bundle of His, the right and left bundles and their various branches then into myocardial cells (Fig. 11.1). Disruption at any point between the sinus node and the bundle of His can prolong the PR interval; disruption below this broadens the QRS complex resulting in bundle branch block. When bundle branch block occurs, the electricity passes through the myocardium, not using the specialized conducting tissue cells. This is much slower than normal, and results in a broad QRS complex (Fig. 11.2a–c).

PR interval prolongation

The PR interval is the time between the start of the P wave and the first QRS deflection. The normal PR interval is lengthened by high vagal tone/low sympathetic tone (sleep, etc.) and low heart rates, and shortened by exercise and high heart rates. These influences need to be factored into deciding whether the PR interval is prolonged. In most people at rest the PR interval is ≤ 200 ms. PR interval prolongation can result from disease of the AV node, the bundle of His, or both bundle branches (Fig. 11.1). It is not possible to determine from the 12-lead ECG why PR interval prolongation has occurred; if this is important then invasive measurement may be indicated (see Chapter 55).

Bundle branch block

The duration of the QRS complex reflects the duration of ventricular depolarization. It is prolonged if the speed of travel of the depolarizing wave is decreased, if the heart size/muscle mass is increased or, as is often the case, both apply, i.e. electricity passes more slowly over a larger distance.

Right bundle branch block (RBBB) causes the right ventricle to be activated late, so right-sided leads see unopposed activity late on resulting in a late deflection in lead V1 (Fig. 11.2a–c). Full block of the left bundle gives rise to delayed and slowed activation of the left ventricle, so broadening the QRS complex in the left-sided leads (Fig. 11.2a–c). Partial blockage of the left bundle results in axis deviation without QRS broadening (see Fig. 10.2):

- Left axis deviation, for damaged anterior branch (delayed activation of the left lateral left ventricle).
- Right axis deviation, for damaged left posterior fascicle (delayed activation of the posterior left ventricle, which lies to the right of the lateral ventricle).

Bi- and tri-fascicular block

Bi-fascicular block is the term used when any two of the following occur:

- PR interval prolongation (Fig. 11.3).
- RBBB.
- Right or left axis deviation (left posterior/anterior hemi-fascicular block).

Tri-fascicular block is applied to: PR interval prolongation + RBBB + right/left axis deviation. It indicates extensive conducting tissue disease that frequently progresses to second or third degree heart block. The term block is a misnomer, as tri-fascicular block implies complete heart block – conduction delay is perhaps a better term. Be aware that though syncope in patients with extensive conducting tissue disease is likely to be due to bradyarrhythmias due to high-grade AV block (e.g. second or third degree block) in those with impaired left ventricular function, especially if due to coronary artery disease, it is possible that syncope may be due to ventricular tachycardia, and this may need to be actively excluded (e.g. by ventricular stimulation study, see Chapter 65).

Fig. 11.1 Damage to the conducting tissue at 1 or 2 leads to prolongation of the PR interval; damage to the left or the right bundle at 3 leads to a broad QRS complex with a normal PR interval. If both the right and left bundles are damaged, then the PR interval can be prolonged. Damage at 4 leads to axis deviation, with a normal PR interval. If there is extensive damage to the myocardium (5), e.g. cardiomyopathic processes, then the QRS complex is broadened. AV, atrioventricular.

Fig. 11.2 ECG changes in bundle branch block. (a) Normal: the septum depolarizes L → R first, both ventricles then depolarize simultaneously (endocardially to epicardially) resulting in a narrow complex QRS complex. (b) Right bundle branch block (RBBB): the septum and left ventricle depolarize normally, resulting in relatively normal QRS complexes in leads looking at the left ventricle (e.g. I, II, aVL, V4–6). The right ventricle depolarizes late, resulting in a late positive deflection in lead V1. (c) Left bundle branch block (LBBB) results in the septum being depolarized right to left (rather than the normal left to right), so there are (i) no physiological Q waves in left-sided chest leads; and (ii) delayed activation of the left ventricle, resulting in a large late positive deflection in left ventricle (LV) leads.

Fig. 11.3 Long PR interval. The time from the start of the P wave to the start of the QRS complex in lead V1 is 320 ms (normal PR ≤ 200 ms). This ECG also shows full left bundle branch block (LBBB), with a broad negative QRS in lead V1, very broad and positive in lead V6. Some patients with LBBB show an 'M' pattern in lead V6 (i.e. upwards, then a small downward deflection, then a much greater upwards deflection) – not seen here. This patient has disease affecting more than one part of the conducting system; such extensive conducting tissue disease not infrequently progresses to complete heart block.

12 Delta waves

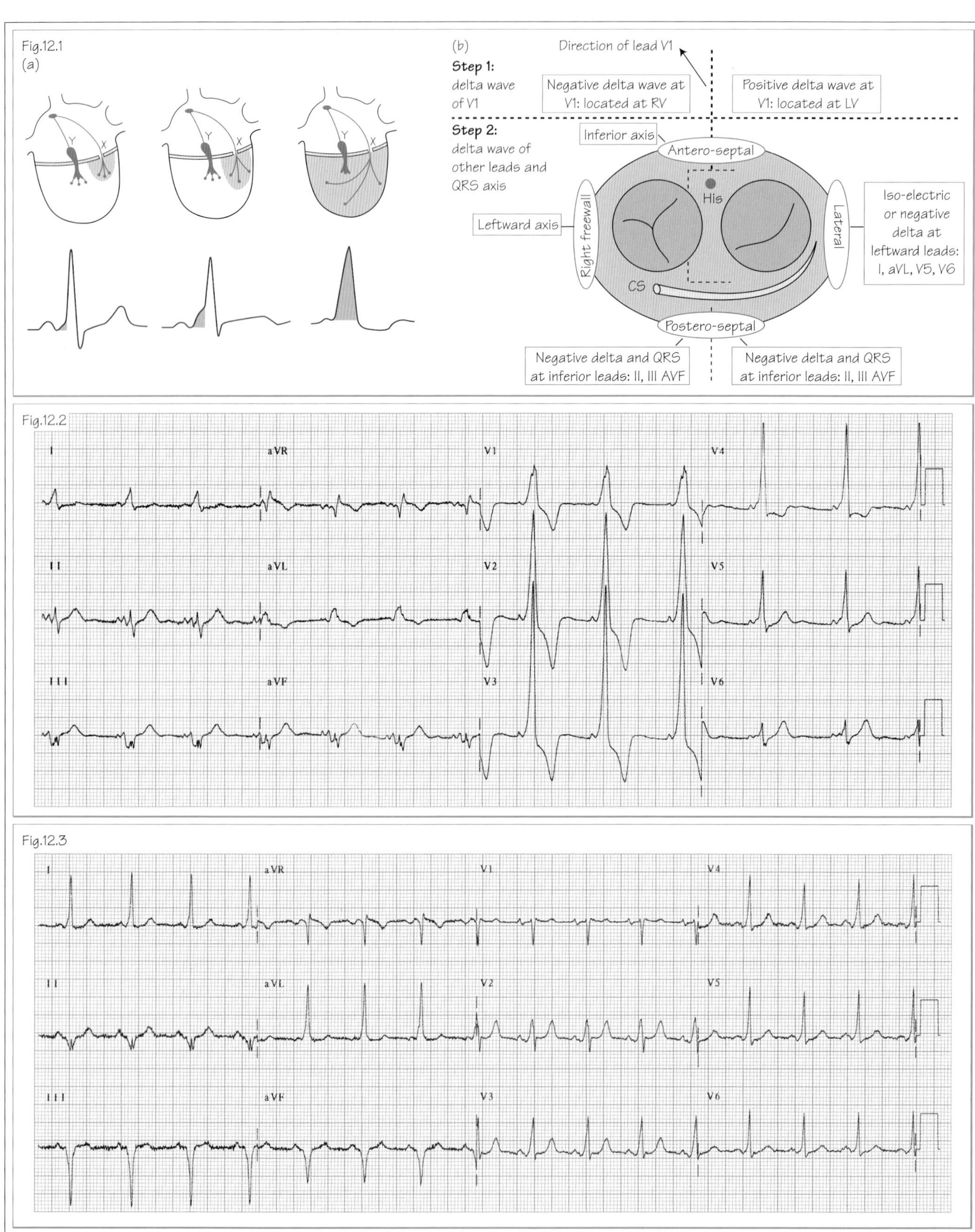

Fig.12.1
(a)
(b)
Direction of lead V1
Step 1:
delta wave of V1
Negative delta wave at V1: located at RV
Positive delta wave at V1: located at LV
Step 2:
delta wave of other leads and QRS axis
Inferior axis
Antero-septal
His
Leftward axis
Right freewall
Lateral
Iso-electric or negative delta at leftward leads: I, aVL, V5, V6
CS
Postero-septal
Negative delta and QRS at inferior leads: II, III AVF
Negative delta and QRS at inferior leads: II, III AVF
Fig.12.2
I
aVR
V1
V4
II
aVL
V2
V5
III
aVF
V3
V6
Fig.12.3
I
aVR
V1
V4
II
aVL
V2
V5
III
aVF
V3
V6

Delta waves are pathognomonic of the Wolff–Parkinson–White (WPW) syndrome, and are due to early ventricular activation from an accessory pathway bypassing the atrioventricular (AV) node.

Mechanism of the delta wave

In health the only electrical connection between the atria and the ventricle is the AV node. In WPW syndrome there is an extra electrical connection between the atria and ventricle (an 'accessory' pathway), down which depolarization passes, bypassing normal AV conduction. Accessory pathways, unlike the normal AV node, do not delay conduction, so depolarization via the pathway reaches the ventricle before the normal current down the AV node. The premature arrival of depolarization in the ventricle causes an early start to the QRS complex, resulting in a short PR interval. Depolarization spreads from its arrival site by cell-to-cell transmission, which is slow, resulting in a 'slurred' upstroke to the QRS complex, the 'delta wave' (Fig. 12.1a,b). The characteristics of the QRS complex in those with a delta wave are: (i) a short PR interval; (ii) the first part of the upstroke is 'slurred'; (iii) the latter part of the QRS is normal, as the QRS complex is a mixture of the depolarization induced by the accessory pathway and by normal AV electrical conduction. The delta wave:

- Is large if the amount of the heart activated prematurely is large and vice versa (Fig. 12.1a,b).
- Polarity (that is, the axis) can be used to determine the location of the accessory pathway (Fig. 12.1a,b). Most cases with a positive deflection in leads V1 have a left atrial to left ventricle pathway; those with a negative deflection in V1 have a right atrial to right ventricular pathway.

Variations of accessory pathways

- Permanently visible accessory pathways, i.e. ECGs taken at different times, all show a delta wave (Figs 12.2 & 12.3). These are the only pathways that lead to sudden cardiac death (SCD) (see below).
- Intermittently visible pathways, where the delta wave comes and goes over time.
- Concealed, the pathway is not visible during sinus rhythm, either as: (i) the pathway is so far from the sinus node that by the time the impulse reaches the pathway ventricular activation, which has occurred via the normal route, is largely over, i.e. there is no/hardly any ventricle left to activate via the pathway; or (ii) the pathway only allows impulse transmission from the ventricles to the atria not from the atria to the ventricle, i.e. one-way conduction. These pathways only allow orthodromic tachycardia and not pre-excited atrial fibrillation, so there is no risk of SCD. They conduct slowly; the clue to their presence is during tachycardia the P wave is a long way from the QRS complex, buried in the ST segment or even the T wave.

Equivocal delta waves

Often it is easy to determine whether or not a delta wave (and so accessory pathway) is present but, on occasions, this can be very difficult. The presence of a delta wave can be confirmed (or denied) by an 'adenosine test'. Adenosine, given by intravenous bolus, temporarily (2–6 s) prevents all conduction through the normal AV node. When an accessory pathway is present the entirety of the ventricle is activated via the pathway, i.e. a very large and obvious delta wave occurs (see Fig. 46.2), when no pathway is present, complete heart block occurs (but only for 2–6 s, so there is no danger of asystole).

Clinical features of the WPW syndrome

An accessory pathway provides a mechanism for tachyarrhythmias (see Chapter 46): (i) orthodromic tachycardia; (ii) antidromic tachycardia; (iii) atrial fibrillation, which occasionally leads to (iv) ventricular fibrillation and sudden cardiac death (SCD). The annual incidence of SCD is 0.15%, i.e. 3% over 20 years, so most patients with WPW syndrome have a normal life expectancy. Sudden cardiac death in WPW syndrome is confined to patients whose pathways have short refractory periods capable of generating very high heart rate during atrial fibrillation (≥ 250 b/min). All patients with WPW syndrome and persistently visible delta waves should have their SCD risk assessed (see Chapter 46) and the pathway ablated if this is high.

Fig. 12.1 (a) Delta wave in Wolff–Parkinson–White (WPW) syndrome. This diagram shows variable activation of the ventricle by current passing through the accessory pathway, leading to variable size of the delta wave (outlined in red on the ECG). The delta wave size reflects how much ventricular tissue is depolarized by the accessory pathway, the more the bigger the delta wave. A large delta wave reflects an accessory pathway very close to the start of the atrial wave of depolarization or a pathway that conducts impulses to the ventricle very quickly (a 'slick' pathway). (b) Localization of the accessory pathway in relation to the atrioventricular (AV) valves. Determine the 'polarity' of the delta wave in lead V1 (i.e. is it upright, i.e. positive, or absent, i.e. negative). Then, keeping as appropriate to the right- or left-hand side of the diagram, use the delta wave in the other leads to determine pathway location.

Fig. 12.2 A gross example of Wolff–Parkinson–White (WPW) syndrome. The PR interval is very short (look at leads V1–6), and the QRS upstroke is very slurred, due to the delta wave. The QRS complex is positive in lead V1, so the pathway is left sided (Fig. 12.1b); the inferior leads show negative QRS complexes inferiorly so this is a left-sided postero-septal pathway.

Fig. 12.3 Wolff–Parkinson–White (WPW) syndrome; much more subtle than in Fig. 12.2. At first glance this looks like an old inferior wall Q wave myocardial infarction (MI) (Q waves in leads II, III and aVF), with left ventricle (LV) hypertrophy (aVL = 15 mm, normal < 11 mm). However, further inspection reveals small and rather subtle delta waves, with a short PR interval, especially in the antero-lateral chest leads (V2–6). This is WPW syndrome with a right-sided pathway (lead V1 complex is negative); the inferior wall MI is not real, the ECG pattern is termed 'pseudo-infarction' and the Q waves disappear when the pathway is ablated.

13 ST elevation

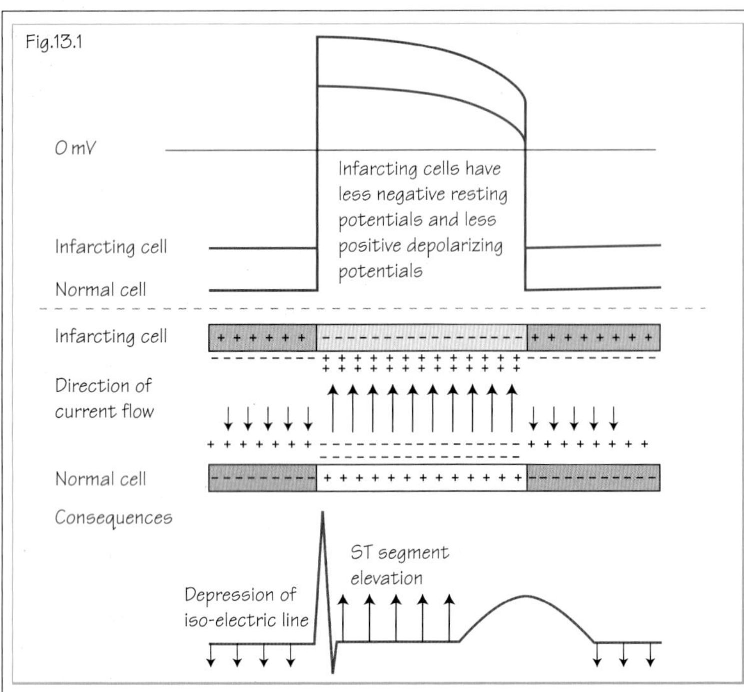

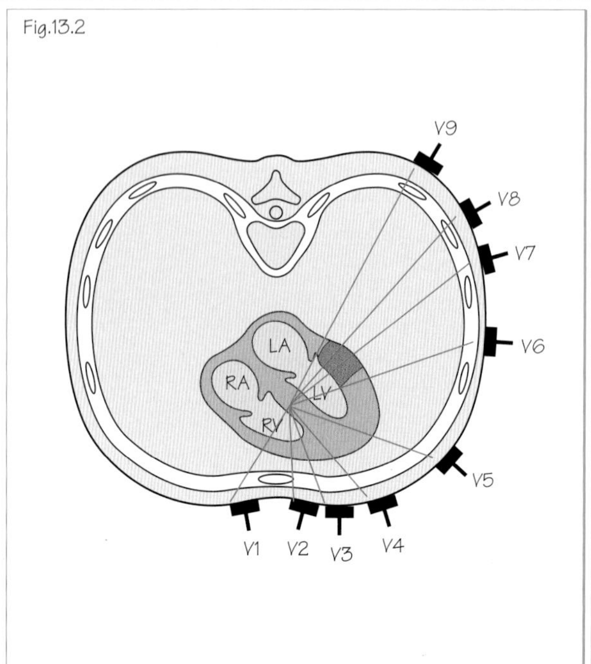

Fig.13.3

(a)

I aVR C1 C4

II aVL C2 C5

III aVF C3 C6

(b)

I aVR V1 V4

II aVL V2 V5

III aVF V3 V6

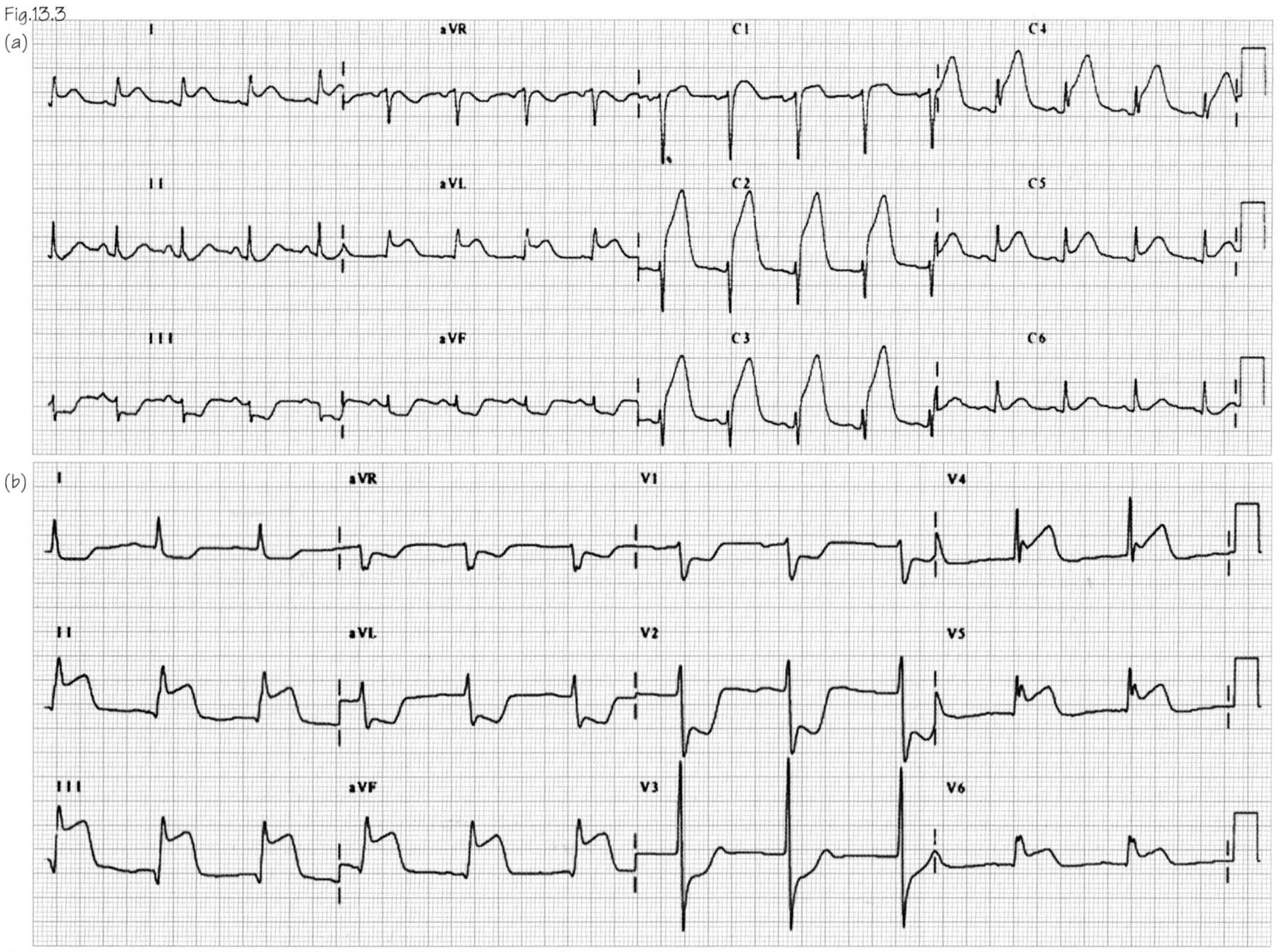

Pathological ST elevation is an important finding, sometimes indicating the presence of a life-threatening myocardial infarct. However, not all ST elevation is pathological, and not all pathological ST elevation is due to infarction. Causes include:

1 'Physiological'.
2 ST segment elevation myocardial infarction (STEMI).
3 Bundle branch block (see Chapters 53 and 54).
4 Pericarditis.
5 Brugada syndrome (see Chapter 39).
6 Other causes, including left ventricular aneurysm, hyperkalaemia and hypothermia.

The important clinical decision usually is to differentiate between one of the first three listed above.

Physiological ST elevation

This is extremely common. There are no cardiac symptoms, ST changes are usually confined to leads V1, V2 and V3; cardiac ultrasound demonstrates no wall motion abnormality. Changes are 'fixed', unlike the evolving changes of STEMI.

ST segment elevation myocardial infarction

In STEMI the sub-epicardial myocardium is more ischaemic than the sub-endocardial tissue. Ischaemic cells let in less positive charge from the extracellular space during depolarization, leading to an excess of external positive charge around damaged cells. Electrons from the less ischaemic areas flow in to neutralize this charge, and onto the observing electrode (Fig. 13.1), causing ST elevation. The iso-electric line is also depressed between depolarizations (Fig. 13.1). It can sometimes be difficult to differentiate ST elevation due to myocardial infarction (MI) from other causes; in STEMI the ST elevation is often 'convex' upwards, whereas in pericarditis the ST elevation is more usually 'concave' upwards. *There are exceptions to this.*

Thirty per cent of MIs have ST elevation; the remaining 70% do not. The importance of differentiating STEMIs from non-STEMIs is that the former benefit from thrombolysis, the latter do not. The leads in which ST elevation occurs reflects the site of infarction, and which coronary artery has blocked (see Table 9.1). The exception to this is posterior wall infarction (circumflex artery occlusion), which causes ST depression in leads V1–3 (Fig. 13.2). Circumflex occlusion is often associated with an inferior wall MI (Fig. 13.3a,b).

ST elevation only persists whilst the infarcting cells are still alive – when they have died (usually after 1–12 h), the ST elevation disappears to be replaced by Q waves (see Chapter 9), T wave inversion (hours–days later), and days–weeks later as the remaining damaged cells are restored to health, re-inversion of the T waves back to a normal polarity.

Pericarditis

In acute pericarditis the mechanism of ST elevation is similar to STEMIs – damaged myocardial cells adjacent to the pericardium let in less positive charge during depolarization, leaving excess external positive charge, neutralized by electrons flowing in from healthy sub-endocardial myocardial cells. The volume of damaged sub-epicardial cells is less in pericarditis than in STEMIs (so there is less external positive charge requiring neutralization), ST elevation is less substantial (> 2 mm ST elevation in pericarditis is rare, though common in STEMIs) and is neutralized more quickly, so lessening ST elevation late on in the plateau phase. Pericarditis-related ST elevation often affects many leads.

Fig. 13.1 Mechanism of ST elevation in myocardial infarction (MI). Highly simplified action potentials of normal and infarcting cells. Infarcting cells between depolarizations have less negative intracellular potentials, so the negative charge that would have been intracellular is now extracellular. This flows away from the damaged sub-epicardial region towards the healthier endocardial area, i.e. away from an observing electrode, so depressing the resting iso-electric line. With each depolarization the damaged cells let in less positive charge than normal during the plateau phase, resulting in excess positive charge in the extracellular space around the sub-epicardial cells, neutralized by electrons flowing in from the sub-endocardial area, which flow on to an observing electrode, causing ST elevation.

Fig. 13.2 Why posterior wall infarction results in anterior lead ST depression. No lead looks directly at the posterior wall of the heart. Leads extended further round the chest (e.g. modified leads V7, V8 and V9) to overlie the posterior wall would show ST elevation in posterior infarction. Posterior leads are not routinely used, so clues must be obtained elsewhere. V1 (and V2, V3) look through the middle of the heart directly at the endocardial surface of the posterior wall. These leads see the ECG signs of infarction, but reversed (as they examine this part of the heart from the inside, not the outside). So, acutely, instead of ST elevation occurring ST depression in seen. The equivalent of a Q wave from a posterior infarct is an R wave in lead V1 (as septal depolarization is now unopposed by the posterior wall). LA, left atrium; LV, left ventricle; RA, right atrium; RV, right ventricle.

Fig. 13.3 ECG showing ST segment elevation myocardial infarction (STEMI). (a) Acute anterolateral STEMI (ST elevation in lead I, aVL, V1–5), with ST depression in lead II (just!), III and aVF. The major deflection of the P wave in lead V1 is a late negative one, indicating left atrial enlargement. This ECG suggests occlusion of the proximal left anterior descending coronary artery, or possibly the left main stem. Prognosis in part relates to the number of leads with ST elevation; the more, the greater the mortality. Seven leads with ST elevation indicate a higher than average mortality. (b) Inferior lead STEMI: ST elevation is seen in the inferior (II, III and aVF) and lateral leads (V4–6). There is evidence of posterior infarction with downward sloping ST depression in leads V1–3. If the ST elevation is greater in II than III, usually it is the right coronary artery that is occluded, whereas if lead III ST elevation is greater than in lead II (as here) usually the circumflex artery is blocked. The lateral and posterior changes suggest a very large and probably dominant circumflex has occluded.

14 ST depression

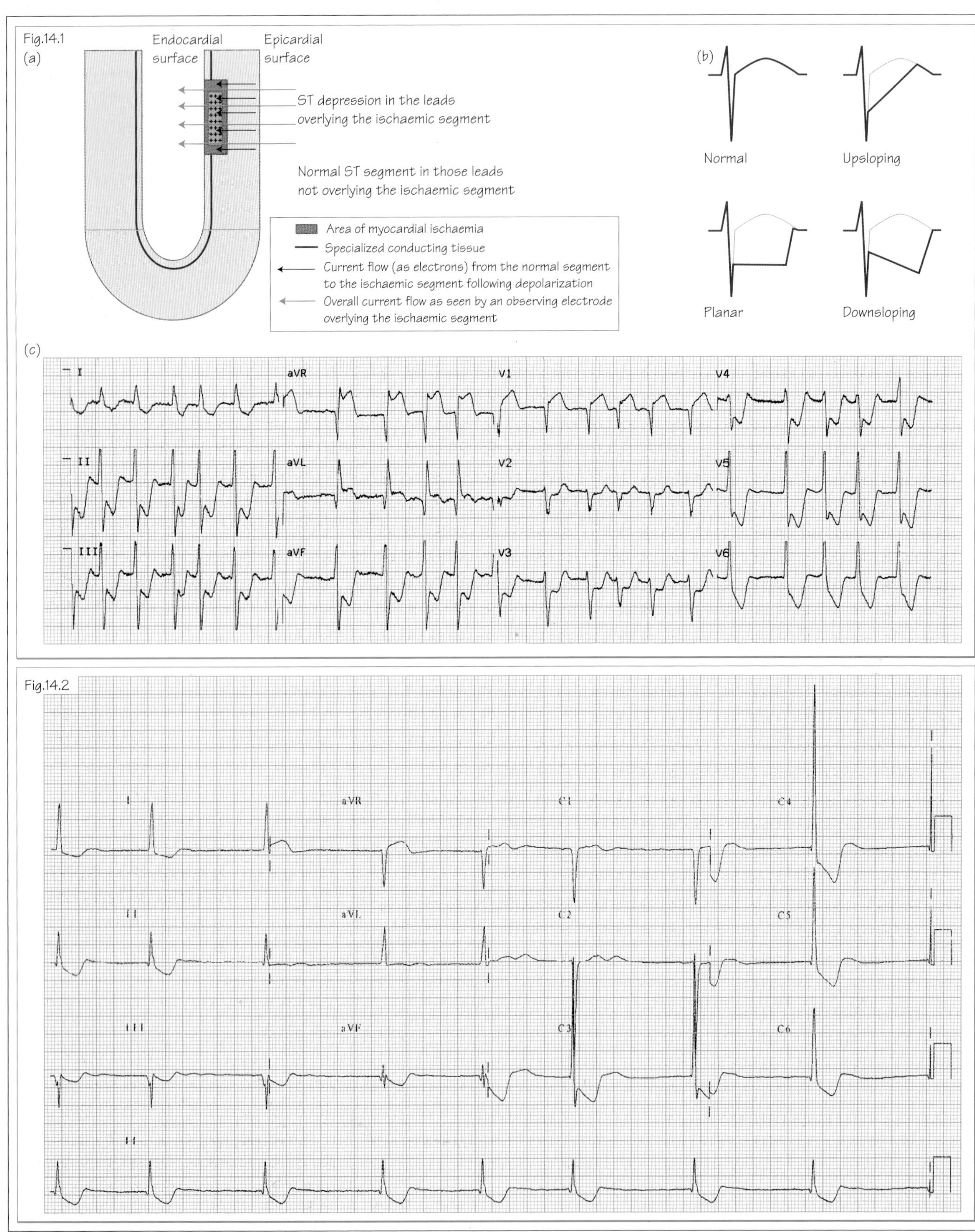

Fig.14.1
(a)
Endocardial surface
Epicardial surface
ST depression in the leads overlying the ischaemic segment
Normal ST segment in those leads not overlying the ischaemic segment
Area of myocardial ischaemia
Specialized conducting tissue
Current flow (as electrons) from the normal segment to the ischaemic segment following depolarization
Overall current flow as seen by an observing electrode overlying the ischaemic segment
(b)
Normal
Upsloping
Planar
Downsloping
(c)
I
aVR
V1
V4
II
aVL
V2
V5
III
aVF
V3
V6
Fig.14.2
I
aVR
C1
C4
II
aVL
C2
C5
III
aVF
C3
C6
II

ST depression is common, and has a large differential diagnosis:
• Ischaemia.
• Left ventricular hypertrophy (LVH).
• Drugs, especially digoxin.
• Myocardial disease.
• Bundle branch block (see Chapters 53 and 54).
• Hyperventilation (see Chapter 38).
• Unknown (usually 'fixed', i.e. does not change over time).

Ischaemic related ST depression

In angina due to epicardial coronary artery disease the sub-endocardium is more ischaemic than the sub-epicardium. Ischaemic cells let in less positive charge than normal during depolarization. This excess positive charge is neutralized in the plateau phase by electrons flowing in from the adjacent healthy sub-epicardial tissue, away from an observing electrode, which in turn causes ST depression (Fig. 14.1a–c). Clues that ST depression is ischaemic in origin include:
• The presence of typical angina during the recording.
• The regional distribution of the ST changes, reflecting the regional distribution of the coronary arteries.
• Dynamic ECG changes, i.e. ST depression comes and goes, unlike ST depression in LVH and digoxin, which are 'fixed', not varying over time.
• In the resting ECG, ST depression due to ishaemic heart disease (IHD) is often either planar or downsloping.
• In the exercise ECG, the exact shape of the ST depression relates to the likelihood of finding coronary artery disease (Fig. 14.1). However, any form of ST depression can be associated with coronary disease (including upsloping ST depression), and indeed a few patients with critical coronary disease have no ST changes during an exercise test.

Left ventricular hypertrophy

Left ventricular hypertrophy typically results in downsloping ST depression in the lateral leads (leads I, aVL, and V5 and V6).
• Left ventricular hypertrophy prolongs epicardial action potentials more than endocardial ones, reversing the normal current flow during repolarization. Endocardial areas repolarize first, so reversing the repolarization wave which now passes endocardially → sub-epicardially, producing T wave inversion.
• The mechanism for the downsloping pattern is unclear, but reflects differential changes induced by LVH in sub-epicardial versus sub-endocardial cellular electrophysiology and collagen deposition.
• The pattern of lead involvement reflects whether leads look at the bulk of the LV muscle mass. If ST depression occurs in leads V3 and 4, a cause other than/additional to acquired LVH should be suspected.
The clue that ST depression is LVH-related is that the voltages of the left-sided QRS complexes are increased, though this is not universal (especially in obese subjects).

Digoxin related ST depression

Digoxin shortens sub-endocardial action potentials more than sub-epicardial ones, leading to 'reverse-tick' (Fig. 14.2) ST depression in the lateral leads, mimicking the distribution of ST changes in LVH. It can be distinguished from LVH-induced ST changes by:
• Knowing that the patient is taking digoxin!
• The absence of increased left-sided QRS voltages (i.e. no LVH). There are, clearly, some exceptions to this, e.g. hypertensive heart disease complicated by atrial fibrillation (AF).
• The presence of AF, a common reason for prescribing digoxin.
Many other drugs, especially in overdose, can cause transient ST changes, both at rest and during exercise.

Myocardial disease associated ST depression

This is not rare. Any primary myocardial pathology can result in ST depression in any combination of leads, i.e. not confined to the lateral leads. Usually the ST depression is 'fixed', i.e. does not change over time. The ST depression is usually rather mild; cardiac ultrasound and angiography are diagnostic. Occasionally persisting ST changes relate to old pericarditis – the pathophysiology is that there is mild (clinically non-relevant) ventricular myocyte damage in the areas adjacent to the pericardium.

Fig. 14.1 (a) The mechanism of ischaemia-related ST depression. During ischaemia due to coronary disease the sub-endocardial cells become ischaemic; they have higher resting membrane potentials and let in less +ve charge during the action potential upstroke, leaving excess external +ve charge. This is neutralized by electrons flowing in from the normal sub-epicardial tissue, causing ST depression in an observing electrode. (b) Different forms of ST depression. On the exercise ECG, the ST depression most strongly associated with ishaemic heart disease (IHD) is downsloping ST depression, followed by planar ST depression, with upsloping ST depression being the least likely to indicate coronary artery disease. It is crucial to realise that upsloping ST depression (and even a completely normal ECG) can be found during exercise in those with coronary disease, even when severe! In acute coronary syndromes, ST depression on the resting ECG is associated with almost as bad an outlook as ST elevation. (c) An ECG showing widespread ST depression, in a patient with unstable angina during chest pain. The rhythm is atrial fibrillation (the patient is not on digoxin), there is mild ST elevation in lead aVL, ST elevation in lead V1 (due to posterior wall ischaemia) and there is gross ST depression in most other leads, especially inferiorly and anterolaterally. The patient had a tight left main stem stenosis and a blocked right coronary artery. The ST changes resolved when angina settled.

Fig. 14.2 An ECG showing 'reverse-tick' lateral lead ST depression due to digoxin. Atrial fibrillation (no visible P waves, so this is either a junctional rhythm, or atrial fibrillation – it is AF, as the QRS rate is so irregular) at a slow heart rate of 45–50 b/min. Prominent voltages in the left-sided chest leads, especially lead V4, suggest left ventricle hypertrophy (LVH). There are very marked 'reverse-tick' ST depression in many leads, especially left-sided ones. There are several interpretations to the ST depression; it might reflect digoxin and/or LVH (which may reflect hypertension, but as it comes so far across the chest leads, may reflect a cardiomyopathy), or the ST depression may reflect ischaemia. In fact this patient had hypertensive heart disease, with digoxin toxicity. When the digoxin was stopped, most of the ST depression went, and the heart rate speeded up.

15 Mild T wave flattening

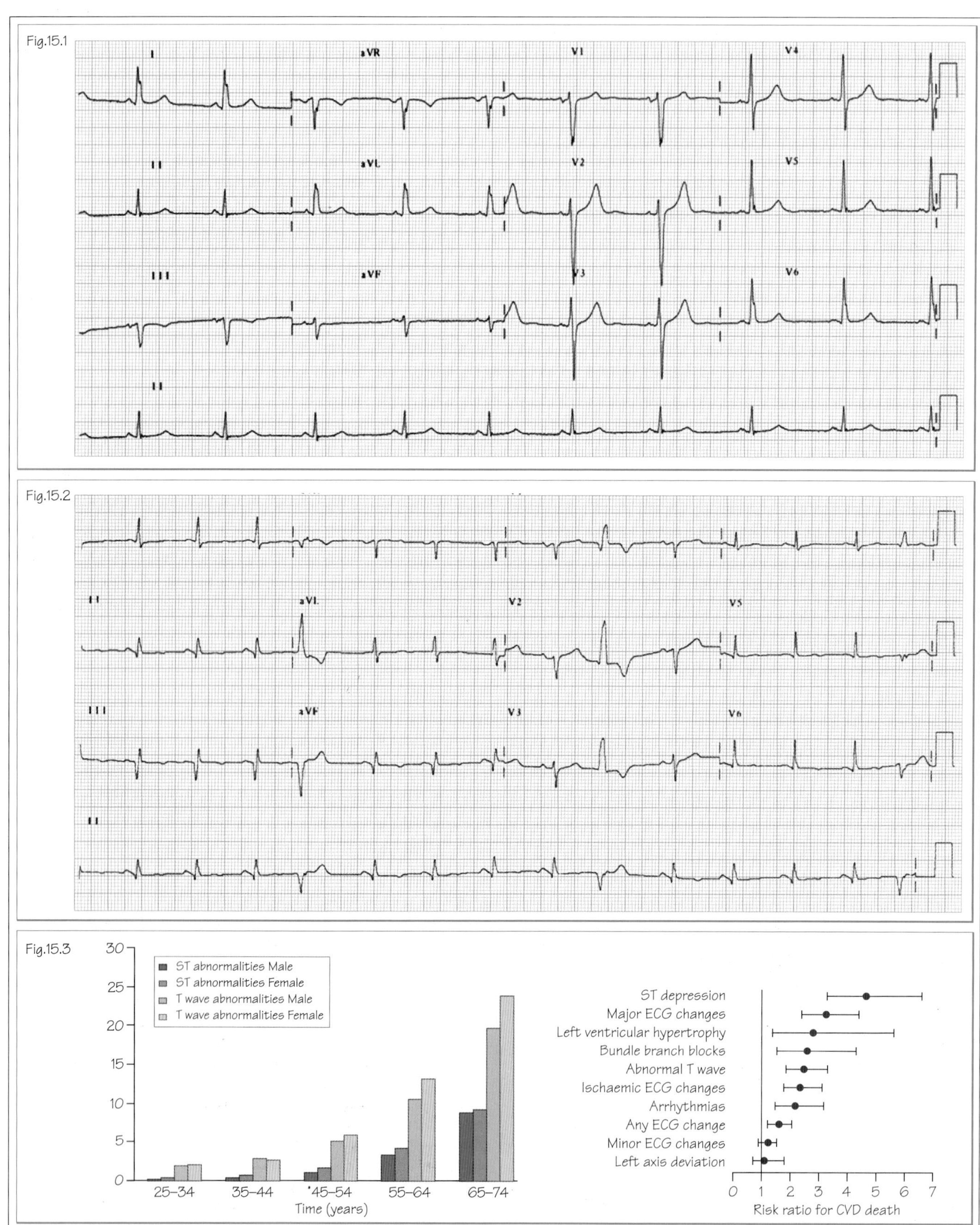

Flattening of the T wave is one of the commonest ECG abnormalities – establishing the underlying diagnosis is a good test both of ECG reading skills and competence as a diagnostician!

The normal T wave (Fig. 15.1):

- Follows the polarity of the QRS complex, i.e. where there is an R wave, the T wave is upright; where there is a Q wave, the T wave is flat or negative (e.g. lead aVR).
- Is usually of substantial size in leads with large R wave (see Chapter 6).

Flat T waves are easily recognised by experienced observers, but are more difficult for the novice, because there is no easy way of diagnosing normality. Generally speaking T waves ≤ 25% of the height of the R wave raise the suspicion of T wave flattening: the smaller they are than this as a proportion of the R wave the greater the suspicion that they are abnormally flat (Fig. 15.2). Flat T waves can mean almost anything! Diagnostic clues come from the clinical situation, as well as the nature of associated ECG changes.

ECG normal aside from mild T wave flattening

- Metabolic changes: low K^+ levels (prominent U waves sometimes occur), and hyperventilation (usually in those obviously anxious, resolving as anxiety goes).
- Drugs, including digoxin.
- Myocardial disease, though often associated with quite abnormal ECGs, can occur with relatively mild ECG abnormalities, including isolated mild T wave flattening. The diagnostic clue is the presence of symptoms and/or signs of heart failure. A cardiac ultrasound is usually diagnostic.
- Coronary disease; the resting ECG often gives very few clues as to the presence of coronary disease, but occasionally (especially in acute coronary syndromes) isolated T wave flattening is seen, usually regional, i.e. confined to the territory of a coronary artery, often fluctuating over time.
- Pericardial disease: previous or current symptoms of pericarditis are rarely found. There are usually no diagnostic tests.
- Unknown, perhaps frustratingly, is the largest category, where these findings occur despite appropriate investigations showing no major structural heart disease. This is particularly so in the elderly.

Associated with other ECG changes

- Prominent left ventricle (LV) voltages – if T wave flattening is confined to the lateral leads, then they are likely to reflect LV hypertrophy. If not, coronary disease should be suspected.
- Q waves: if the T wave flattening is in the same leads as Q waves they have no additional meaning beyond that of the Q waves (a transmural myocardial infarction [MI]). If they are in distant leads they may indicate coronary disease in the non-infarct related artery. As multivessel coronary disease may benefit prognostically from revascularization, distant T wave flattening should lower the threshold for angiography.

Approach to flat T waves

It can be seen from the above list that almost anything can cause flat T waves, including nothing! This means one must have a careful approach to this problem. You should use the finding of flat T waves to consider that there may be either a cardiac problem, or an electrolyte one (most commonly low K^+ levels). However, the ECG in itself is not that helpful, as it neither rules in nor out any disease process. A sensible approach it to: (i) measure electrolytes; (ii) order a cardiac ultrasound; (iii) be guided by the clinical situation in deciding on further investigations (e.g. coronary angiography if symptoms suggest critical coronary disease), or indeed, whether any more tests at all are indicated!

Fig. 15.1 A normal ECG. With regard to the T wave, the important points to note include the following. (i) Wherever the R wave exceeds the S wave, the T wave is very well formed. (ii) Where the S wave exceeds the R wave (e.g. lead III) the T wave is flat. In lead V1, where S is also greater than R in health, the T wave is inverted. This is an important point, as an important but subtle sign of ischaemia from disease of the circumflex coronary artery is an upright T wave in lead V1. (iii) In lead aVR the T wave is always inverted. (iv) The T wave forms a much greater proportion of the R wave height in the septal chest leads (V1–3) than the lateral chest leads (V4–6). (v) The size of the R wave, and hence the polarity of the T wave in lead III can vary with respiration.

Fig. 15.2 An ECG showing flat T waves. This ECG shows multiple abnormalities – there are generally flat T waves throughout all the leads, with only V2 and V3 having anything approaching a normal T wave. There are deep Q waves in lead III and aVF, suggestive of an old inferior wall myocardial infarct, and the QRS complexes in the chest leads are rather small (which could reflect obesity or old infarction in the anterior territory as well). There are frequent ventricular ectopics, seen on the lead II rhythm strip at the bottom to all be the same morphology (i.e. to originate from the same electrophysiological substrate). There are various interpretations of this ECG. In addition to old infarction (inferior Q's, anterior loss of R wave, which may indicate obesity). The T wave flattening is widespread, and may reflect low K^+, widespread coronary artery disease or left ventricular dysfunction from any other cause. The ectopics may reflect low K^+ in the setting of structural heart disease, or the structural heart disease itself.

Fig. 15.3 Incidence and consequence of major and minor ECG abnormalities in epidemiological studies. ST and T wave incidence rises with age, and shows no sex dependence. CVD, cardiovascular disease.

16 Deep T wave inversion

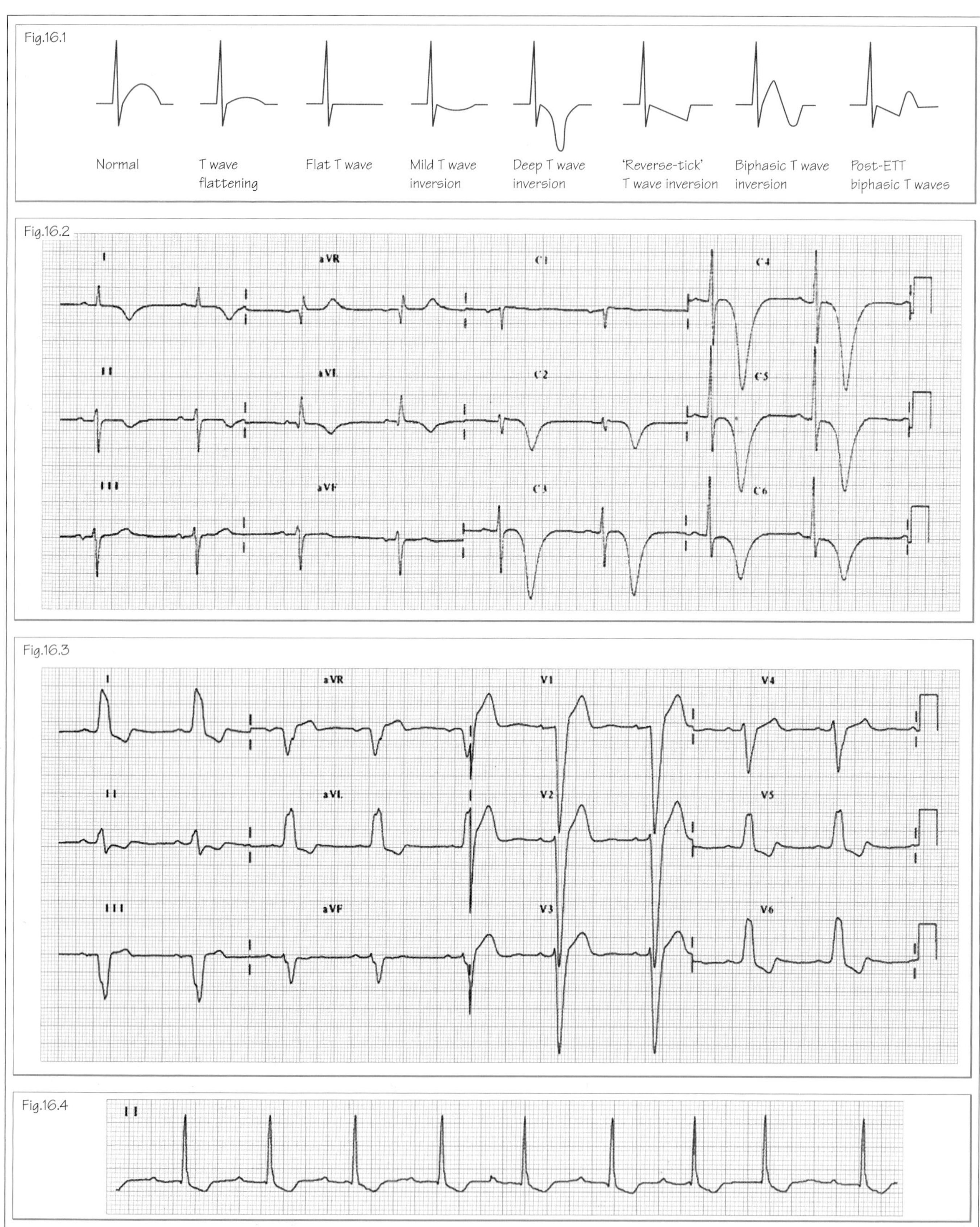

Fig.16.1
Normal
T wave flattening
Flat T wave
Mild T wave inversion
Deep T wave inversion
'Reverse-tick' T wave inversion
Biphasic T wave inversion
Post-ETT biphasic T waves
Fig.16.2
I
aVR
C1
C4
II
aVL
C2
C5
III
aVF
C3
C6
Fig.16.3
I
aVR
V1
V4
II
aVL
V2
V5
III
aVF
V3
V6
Fig.16.4
II

Major T wave inversion is important as it often indicates a major illness.

ECG features of T wave inversion

The normal T waves follow the polarity of the R wave: in health leads with large R waves have upright T's, leads with equivocal R waves have flat T waves, and leads with deep S waves have inverted T's. T wave inversion can only be diagnosed when it occurs in a lead with a large R wave where an upright T wave is expected. If the R wave should be large, but isn't due to disease, then T wave changes are secondary to the process that has affected the R wave. T wave abnormalities include T wave flattening/mild inversion (see Chapter 15); major T wave inversion is discussed here.

Morphology of T wave inversion

- The inverted T wave may be symmetrical, with the down slope and upslope having the same angle, common in coronary disease (Figs 16.1 & 16.2).
- Asymmetrical T wave inversion: the down slope is much shallower than the upslope, resulting in a 'reverse-tick' appearance. Common in left ventricular hypertrophy (LVH), bundle branch block (BBB) (Fig. 16.3), coronary disease and digoxin (Fig. 16.4).
- Biphasic T waves, with the first part going up, and the second part down. This is common in acute coronary syndrome and following a myocardial infarction.
- Biphasic T waves, with the first part going down, and the second part up. This pattern is common in coronary disease in the few minutes after exercise, reported as 'following exercise typical ischaemic repolarization changes occurred.' Its presence increases the probability of coronary disease.

Causes of deep T wave inversion

1 Coronary disease.

2 Bundle branch block; the clue is the wide QRS complex.

3 Left ventricular hypertrophy: the clue is the increased left-sided voltages. The LVH can be acquired, e.g. hypertension related, with T inversion confined to the lateral leads, or generic, e.g. hypertrophic cardiomyopathy (HCM), when much more generalized T wave changes are seen.

4 Others, including drugs, e.g. psychotropics.

ECG clues to the diagnosis of T wave inversion

There are several clues to the diagnosis available from the ECG and the clinical situation:

- Broad QRS; the cause is BBB. In right BBB, T wave inversion occurs in the right-sided leads, and in left BBB, in the left-sided leads (Fig. 15.3).
- Changes confined to the lateral leads (I, II, aVL, V5 and V6) can relate to: (i) LVH (left ventricular voltages are increased, T wave inversion is 'reverse-tick'); (ii) digoxin (patient usually in atrial fibrillation, no ECG LVH) (Fig. 15.4); (iii) ischaemia, especially if the T wave inversion is symmetrical and dynamic (i.e. changes over time).
- Changes in the distribution of a coronary artery. Several patterns are well described: (i) Pan-anterior deep symmetrical T wave inversion is so likely to be due to a high-grade lesion in the proximal left anterior descending (LAD) artery that this ECG is known as an 'LAD-pattern ECG'. This pattern is occasionally seen in other conditions (below). (ii) Deep inferior T wave inversion, sometimes extending laterally to leads V5 and V6 likely due to a tight narrowing in the right coronary artery. (iii) Other patterns, especially if extensive, can be found in hypertrophic cardiomyopathy.
- Non-ishaemic heart disease causes of pan-anterior T wave inversion are usually diagnosed from the clinical situation. (i) Acute sub-arachnoid haemorrhage, this reflects a major catecholamine surge causing coronary vasospasm and sub-endocardial ischaemia/infarction. The more severe the neurological deficit, the more likely ECG abnormalities, troponin release, cardiac dysfunction, pulmonary oedema and death. (ii) Tako-tsubo syndrome (after a Japanese octopus-catching pot), otherwise known as transient left-ventricular apical ballooning syndrome, results in anterior T wave inversion, transient left ventricle dysfunction in an unusual pattern, following severe emotional trauma, usually in women. (iii) Drugs. (iv) Other causes, including HCM.

T wave changes over time

If the T wave changes come and go over brief (hours to days) time periods, they are likely to reflect severe coronary disease. Occasionally this dynamic pattern relates to hyperventilation.

Fig. 16.1 Different forms of T wave abnormalities. T wave flattening, flat, and mild T wave inversion are non-specific findings (see Chapter 15). Deep symmetrical T wave inversion is common in non-ST segment elevation myocardial infarctions (NSTEMIs), with some drugs, and in sub-arachnoid haemorrhage. 'Reverse-tick' T wave inversion is found with digoxin, in bundle branch block (BBB), and ischaemia. Biphasic T waves are common in acute coronary syndrome (ACS); there is a variant where the initial part of the T wave is slopes down (there can also be ST depression), and then the T wave has a late prominent positive deflection.

Fig. 16.2 This ECG shows the classic 'proximal LAD' pattern. The patient is in sinus rhythm. There are good (probably normal sized) R waves throughout the ECG (i.e. there has been no previous myocardial infarction). Antero-laterally (i.e. leads I, II, aVL and V2–6) there is deep symmetrical T wave inversion (i.e. the downslope is the same configuration as the upslope, unlike 'reverse-tick' T wave inversion). This pattern is almost pathognomonic of a high-grade acute (i.e. thrombotic) lesion in the proximal portion of the left anterior descending coronary artery, requiring early revascularization. There are several much rarer causes of this ECG (see text).

Fig. 16.3 T wave inversion in left bundle branch block (LBBB). This ECG shows sinus rhythm, normal PR interval, and a broad QRS complex, with the morphology of LBBB. The lateral leads (I, II, aVL, V5, V6) show abnormal repolarization; whether this is called ST depression, or T wave inversion is semantic. It is universal in LBBB, and indicates that the direction of the repolarizing current is reversed.

Fig. 16.4 ECG with digoxin effect. Sinus rhythm, long PR interval (280 ms), due to digoxin's vagal enhancing effect. Normal QRS complexes. 'Reverse-tick' T wave. Digoxin increases the chance of ST depression occurring during an exercise test, regardless of whether or not coronary disease is present.

17 QT interval and U wave abnormalities

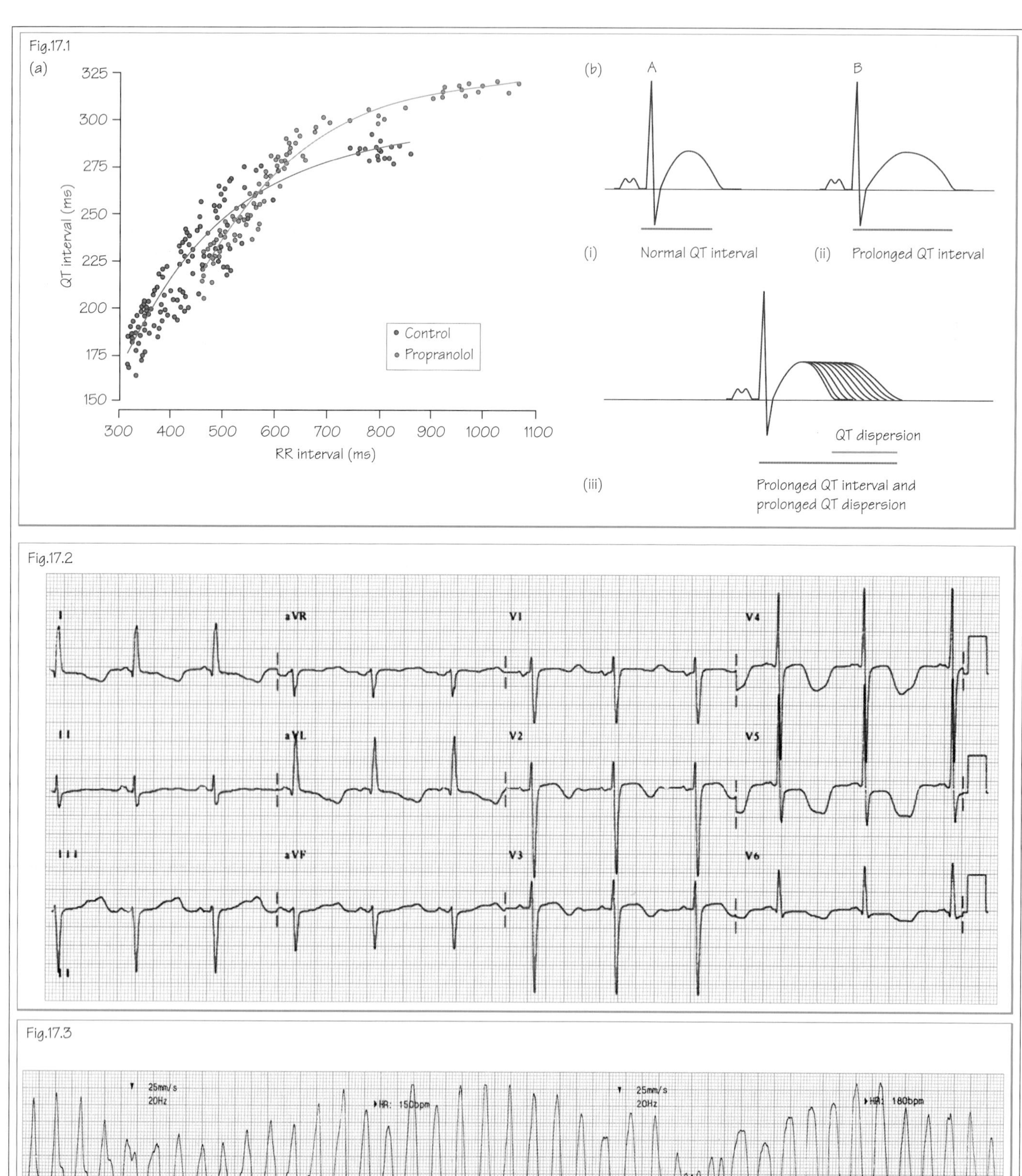

The QT interval reflects the time from the onset of depolarization to the offset of repolarization. It is altered by:

- Heart rate, an exceptionally powerful influence. High heart rates shorten the QT interval. The QT interval–heart rate (QT–HR) relationship changes within an individual over time and between individuals in health, sickness and with drugs, leading to problems in correcting for heart rate, and making scientifically unsound the use of a single formula for such correction (e.g. Bazett's correction: QTc = QT/√(RR interval [QTc = QT interval corrected to its value at 60 b/min, QT = the actual QT interval measured at a particular RR interval]). Ideally, to correct for heart rate, the individuals QT–HR relationship should be determined (e.g. exercise stress test/24-h ECG). If this is impossible, then the best formula to use, as it removes the influence of heart rate on the QT interval, is Fridericia's correction (QTc = QT/^{3}√ (RR interval).
- Autonomic nervous system activity. High vagal tone (and maybe low sympathetic tone) prolongs the QT interval; the opposite shortens the QT interval. Vagal tone has a diurnal rhythm, is high at night so lengthening nocturnal QT interval by ± 20 ms.
- Sex and age have a small influence on the QT interval (women and older subjects have slightly longer QT intervals).
- Physiological genetic differences; twin studies show that the genetic influence on the QT interval is high (50% of inter-individual QT interval variability is genetic).

Pathological influences on the QT interval

- The duration of depolarization (i.e. the QRS complex). Prolonged depolarization (e.g. left bundle branch block) prolongs the QT interval.
- Myocyte action potential duration (APD). If APD is prolonged, the QT interval is prolonged. Action potential duration can be prolonged throughout the heart, causing a long QT interval in all leads, or prolonged regionally, causing increases in QT interval in some but not other leads (Fig. 17.2).

Why the QT interval is important

- Some diseases and many drugs, prolong it, so a long QT interval is a diagnostic clue.
- QT interval prolongation can lead to life-threatening arrhythmias of the torsade-de-pointes (TDP) type ventricular tachycardia variety.

Disease processes prolonging the QT interval

- Left ventricular dysfunction, the commonest cause; prolongation is proportional to the severity of left ventricular dysfunction.
- Critical myocardial ischaemia.
- Drugs; class III anti-arrhythmics (amiodarone and sotalol) universally prolong the QT interval. Non-sedating anti-histamines, macrolide antibiotics, beta-blockers at low heart rates and anti-fungals are amongst a substantial list of drugs that may prolong the QT interval and (other than beta-blockers) lead to TDP and death.
- Metabolic: low K^+ and Mg^{2+}, especially in heart failure.
- Endocrine disease: hypothyroidism, though this is unlikely to result in TDP.
- Nutritional; starvation (e.g. Thai refugees, voluntarily or surgically treated obese patients, anorexia).
- Alcoholism.
- Stroke, especially intracranial haemorrhage.
- Genetic disease, e.g. hereditary long QT syndromes (HLQTS).

Consequences and management

- None – many have no ill effects.
- Torsade-de-pointes ventricular tachycardia, causing syncope and/or sudden cardiac death, treated by immediate cardioversion. Further episodes are prevented by removing relevant drugs, correcting metabolic upset, and pacing (higher heart rates shorten the QT interval). In rare cases isoprenaline is needed. For HLQTS, an implantable cardioverter defibrillator (ICD) may be appropriate.

Fig. 17.1 (a) The influence of heart rate on the QT interval. The inverse relationship between heart rate and QT interval is shown. This data comes from one individual during an exercise test, first when drug free, second when given propranolol. Exercise increases heart rate (shorter RR intervals) and shortens the QT interval. Propranolol shortens the QT interval at high heart rates, but lengthens it at lower heart rates (other beta-blockers have different effects). Note: (i) the strong negative relationship between heart rate and QT interval; and (ii) the QT heart rate relationship differs within an individual over time and with interventions (e.g. propranolol). (b) QT interval, normal (i), uniform prolongation (ii), and prolongation of variable severity in the different leads. (iii). Uniform prolongation is a risk factor for torsade-de-pointes (TDP) type ventricular tachycardia whereas variable prolongation (measured as $QT_{longest\ lead}$–$QT_{shortest\ lead}$, termed QT dispersion) is proposed as a marker of propensity to re-entrant arrhythmias (though the sensitivity/specificity is low, so this marker is not used clinically).

Fig. 17.2 An ECG from a patient with syncope on QT interval prolonging psychotropic medication: sinus rhythm, unremarkable P wave shape, PR interval. The QRS complex is increased (in lead aVL 14 mm, normal ≤ 11 mm; S lead V2 + R lead V5 = 49 mm, normal ≤ 35 in this age group) suggesting left ventricular hypertrophy (LVH). Note the bizarre T waves, inverted anterolaterally, in a very odd pattern, and with a prominent late 'hump' (?U wave) in lead III. The heart rate is 68 b/min, the QT interval 620 ms, with Bazett's correction (see text) 661 ms (normal ≤ 440 ms) and with Fridericia's correction (see text) 646 ms. Syncope was due to torsade-de-pointes (TDP).

Fig. 17.3 A typical example of torsade-de-pointes (TDP; French, 'twisting of the points') type ventricular tachycardia. Fast heart rate, broad QRS complexes, which increase then decrease in size over 10–15 beats. The arrhythmia substantially reduces but usually does not remove cardiac output. Episodes terminate spontaneously (the usual outcome), usually after < 20–30 s, or degenerate into ventricular fibrillation. Typical TDP starts with a short–long–short RR interval sequence, e.g. a premature ventricular ectopic (premature, hence short RR interval), which induces a physiological pause (long RR interval), which results in further QT interval lengthening, and TDP (the first beat occurs early on, so there is a short RR interval). Suppressing any tendency the heart may have towards pauses (using a pacemaker, or isoprenaline), and hence QT prolongation, can suppress TDP.

18 Acute chest pain

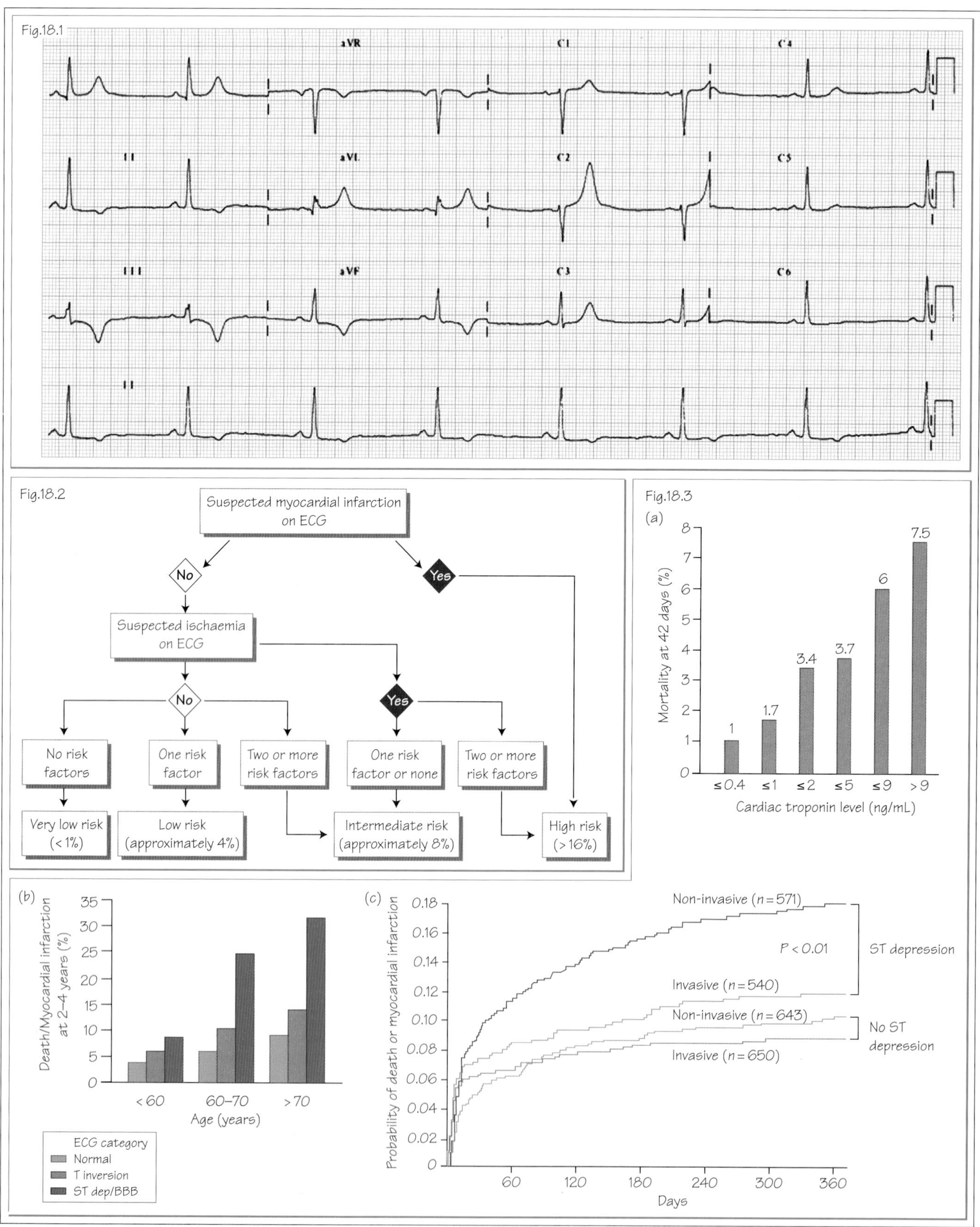

Fig.18.1
aVR
C1
C4
II
aVL
C2
C5
III
aVF
C3
C6
II
Fig.18.2
Suspected myocardial infarction on ECG
No
Yes
Suspected ischaemia on ECG
No
Yes
No risk factors
One risk factor
Two or more risk factors
One risk factor or none
Two or more risk factors
Very low risk (< 1%)
Low risk (approximately 4%)
Intermediate risk (approximately 8%)
High risk (> 16%)
Fig.18.3
(a)
Mortality at 42 days (%)
1
1.7
3.4
3.7
6
7.5
≤0.4
≤1
≤2
≤5
≤9
>9
Cardiac troponin level (ng/mL)
(b)
Death/Myocardial infarction at 2–4 years (%)
< 60
60–70
> 70
Age (years)
ECG category
Normal
T inversion
ST dep/BBB
(c)
Probability of death or myocardial infarction
Non-invasive (n = 571)
P < 0.01
ST depression
Invasive (n = 540)
Non-invasive (n = 643)
No ST depression
Invasive (n = 650)
Days

In managing chest pain one aims to establish the diagnosis and start treatment as soon as possible. *The working diagnosis should be based on the clinical features* (demographics, history, examination) rather than on tests (unless they are categorically diagnostic).

Prognosis in chest pain

Conditions with a high risk of death/serious injury include high-risk acute coronary syndrome (ACS) (non-ST segment elevation myocardial infarctions [NSTEMIs; Fig. 18.1] and ST segment elevation myocardial infarctions [STEMIs]), acute aortic syndromes, pulmonary emboli, chest infection with pleurisy and pneumothorax. Each has specific demographics, histories, physical examination and 'typical' ECGs (see Chapters 20, 29, 30 and 31), which may establish the diagnosis. If not, form a working diagnosis from the clinical features and prove this using advanced tests, while excluding other conditions if they are dangerous and possible. If it is still not possible to reach a clear-cut diagnosis, proceed on the basis of the probability of dangerous chest pain. The ECG can help risk stratification, and the predictors of prognosis in acute chest pain are:

- Normal ECG, associated with a good (not perfect) long-term outcome, as most dangerous chest pain is due to ishaemic heart disease (IHD) and most dangerous manifestations of this are associated with an abnormal resting ECG. There are exceptions as follows. (i) Two to five per cent of myocardial infarctions (MIs) have a normal presentation ECG but the usual MI-related complications (including death). The diagnosis of MI must use the clinical features as well as the ECG – heavy ('crushing'), severe ('the worst ever') retrosternal pain, with sweating, nausea and vomiting. Patients with such symptoms should be observed for ≥ 12 h before reaching a benign diagnosis. (ii) Some high-risk ACS present with a normal ECG, and only later does the ECG becomes abnormal, hence again the need for observation and further ECGs. (iii) Some severe non-cardiac disease presents as chest pain with a normal ECG, e.g. pulmonary emboli (sinus tachycardia is often present) and aortic dissection (ECG often normal). *Do not rule out dangerous conditions on the basis of a normal ECG – always factor in the clinical features.*
- ST elevation or Q waves not known to be old (early relative risk ± 17× increased).
  (a) ST elevation due to MI is a key finding (differentiate from physiological, pericarditis or other causes).
  (b) Old MI, which may leave a legacy of T wave abnormalities, loss of R wave height or pathological Q waves.
- ST depression is a common and important finding and in ACS is associated with as poor an outlook as ST elevation MIs. ST depression/T wave inversion not known to be old increases relative early risk sevenfold. In most ACS associated with ST depression, the ST depression is *dynamic*, i.e. it fluctuates over time, sometimes being present (usually when pain occurs) and sometimes not. Dynamicity is an important feature to look for. ST depression that is 'fixed' (i.e. does not fluctuate over time) may relate to an ACS, but may relate to another cause (e.g. old peri- or myocarditis or an old MI), and it may be that the current episode of chest pain is unrelated to the heart.
- ST/T wave flattening, by far the commonest finding, is usually unhelpful. In young patients it may help diagnostically, but not in the elderly (as mild ECG abnormalities are so common).
- T wave inversion (see above).
- New left bundle branch block (LBBB) is a key finding suggesting new myocardial ischaemia.
- Old LBBB does not help in risk stratification, so use clinical features and troponin.

Sometimes one cannot make a clear-cut diagnosis, and then it can be helpful to ask the question, if this is an ACS, what is the prognosis? The condition can then be managed appropriately according to risk. The risk of harm in ACS relates to:

- Presenting pain similar to that of previous infarction or angina.
- Extent of risk factors: age, hypertension, diabetes, smoking.
- Previous MI/heart failure.
- Systolic blood pressure < 100 mmHg, high heart rate. Crepitations greater than or equal at the base.
- ECG changes (see above).
- Raised biomarkers for myocardial necrosis, especially troponin (Fig. 18.3a–c); C-reactive protein (CRP) and brain natriuretic peptide (BNP) are also relevant.

Fig. 18.1 High-risk acute coronary syndrome (ACS): sinus rhythm, normal P wave, PR interval and QRS complex. The abnormalities are confined to the T waves, with impressive inferior lead (II, III and aVF) T wave inversion symmetrically and T wave flattening laterally (V5/6). Very mild ST elevation in leads I and aVL, i.e. both ST elevation and depression is a very high-risk clinical situation. Severe multivessel coronary disease was found.

Fig. 18.2 Risk classification in patients presenting to the emergency room with acute chest pain considered due to ishaemic heart disease (IHD). Myocardial infarction (MI) was suspected if the ECG showed ST-segment elevation of ≥ 1 mm or pathological Q waves in ≥ 2 leads, findings not known to be old. Ischaemia was suspected if the ECG showed ST-segment depression of ≥ 1 mm T-wave inversion in ≥ 2 leads and if these findings were not known to be old. Risk factors included systolic blood pressure ≤ 110 mmHg, bilateral rales heard above the bases, and known unstable IHD (defined as worsening of previously stable angina, new onset of angina after infarction or after a coronary revascularization procedure, or pain the same as that associated with a prior MI). Basic clinical data is surprisingly good at predicting prognosis.

Fig. 18.3 (a) Troponin level and outcome. There is a strong graded relationship between troponin rise and adverse events. Note: (i) not all patients with a raised troponin are at high risk; and (ii) not all 'troponin-negative' are at low risk. Troponin-negative patients need further risk stratification by pre-discharge exercise stress testing. (b) Age and ECG changes relate to risk in unstable angina, i.e. there should be a lower threshold to admit/invasively investigate the elderly. (c) Interaction between ECG changes, risk and benefit from an invasive policy (i.e. early coronary angiography and percutaneous coronary intervention [PCI]/coronary artery bypass graft [CABG]).

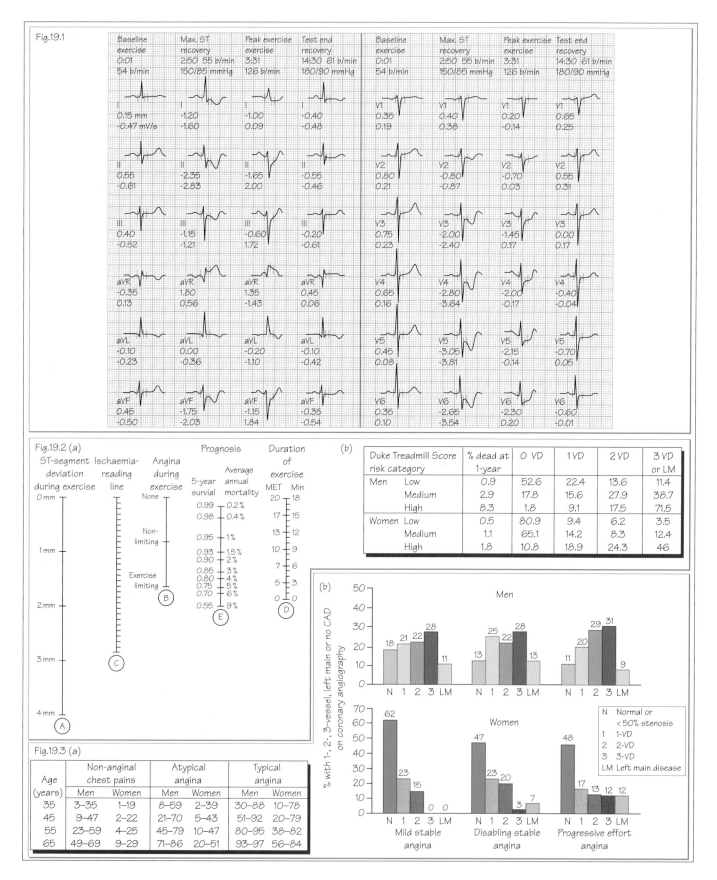

19 Chronic chest pain

Fig.19.1

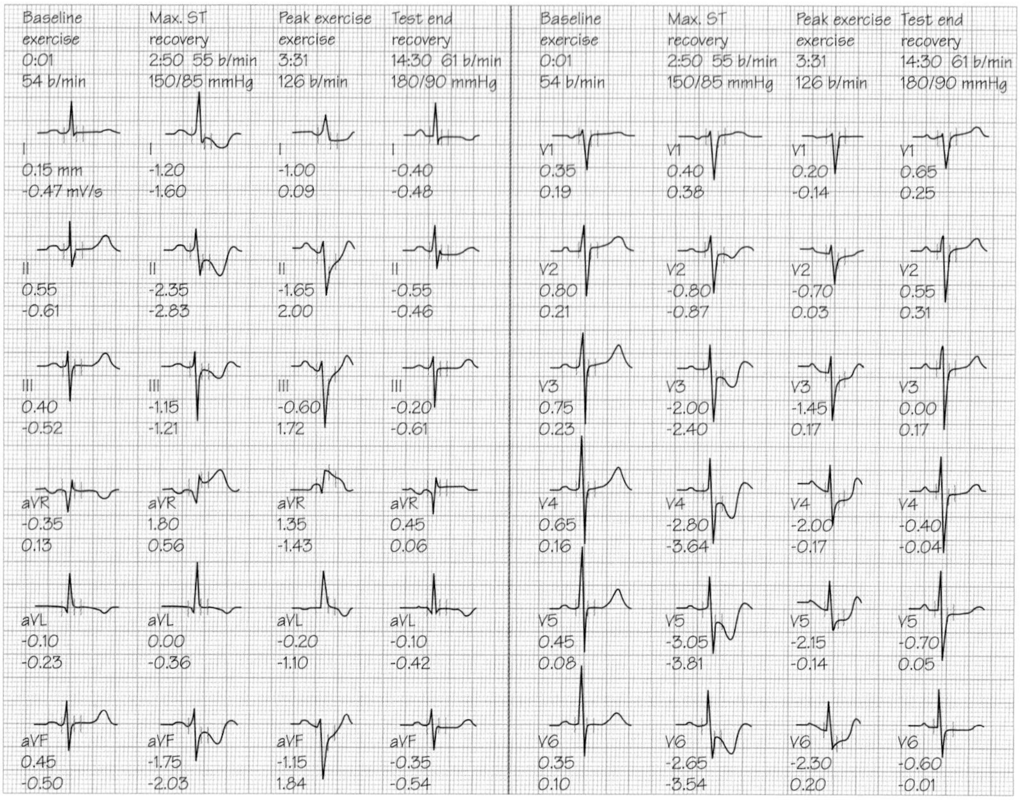

Lead	Baseline exercise 0:01 54 b/min	Max. ST recovery 2:50 55 b/min 150/85 mmHg	Peak exercise 3:31 126 b/min	Test end recovery 14:30 61 b/min 180/90 mmHg
I	0.15 mm -0.47 mV/s	-1.20 -1.60	-1.00 0.09	-0.40 -0.48
II	0.55 -0.61	-2.35 -2.83	-1.65 2.00	-0.55 -0.46
III	0.40 -0.52	-1.15 -1.21	-0.60 1.72	-0.20 -0.61
aVR	-0.35 0.13	1.80 0.56	1.35 -1.43	0.45 0.06
aVL	-0.10 -0.23	0.00 -0.36	-0.20 -1.10	-0.10 -0.42
aVF	0.45 -0.50	-1.75 -2.03	-1.15 1.84	-0.35 -0.54

Lead	Baseline exercise 0:01 54 b/min	Max. ST recovery 2:50 55 b/min 150/85 mmHg	Peak exercise 3:31 126 b/min	Test end recovery 14:30 61 b/min 180/90 mmHg
V1	0.35 0.19	0.40 0.38	0.20 -0.14	0.65 0.25
V2	0.80 0.21	-0.80 -0.87	-0.70 0.03	0.55 0.31
V3	0.75 0.23	-2.00 -2.40	-1.45 0.17	0.00 0.17
V4	0.65 0.16	-2.80 -3.64	-2.00 -0.17	-0.40 -0.04
V5	0.45 0.08	-3.05 -3.81	-2.15 -0.14	-0.70 0.05
V6	0.35 0.10	-2.65 -3.54	-2.30 0.20	-0.60 -0.01

Fig.19.2 (a)

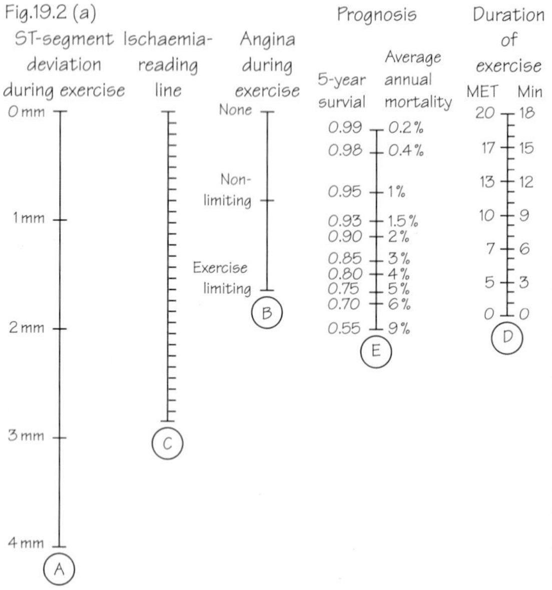

(b)

Duke Treadmill Score risk category		% dead at 1-year	0 VD	1 VD	2 VD	3 VD or LM
Men	Low	0.9	52.6	22.4	13.6	11.4
	Medium	2.9	17.8	15.6	27.9	38.7
	High	8.3	1.8	9.1	17.5	71.5
Women	Low	0.5	80.9	9.4	6.2	3.5
	Medium	1.1	65.1	14.2	8.3	12.4
	High	1.8	10.8	18.9	24.3	46

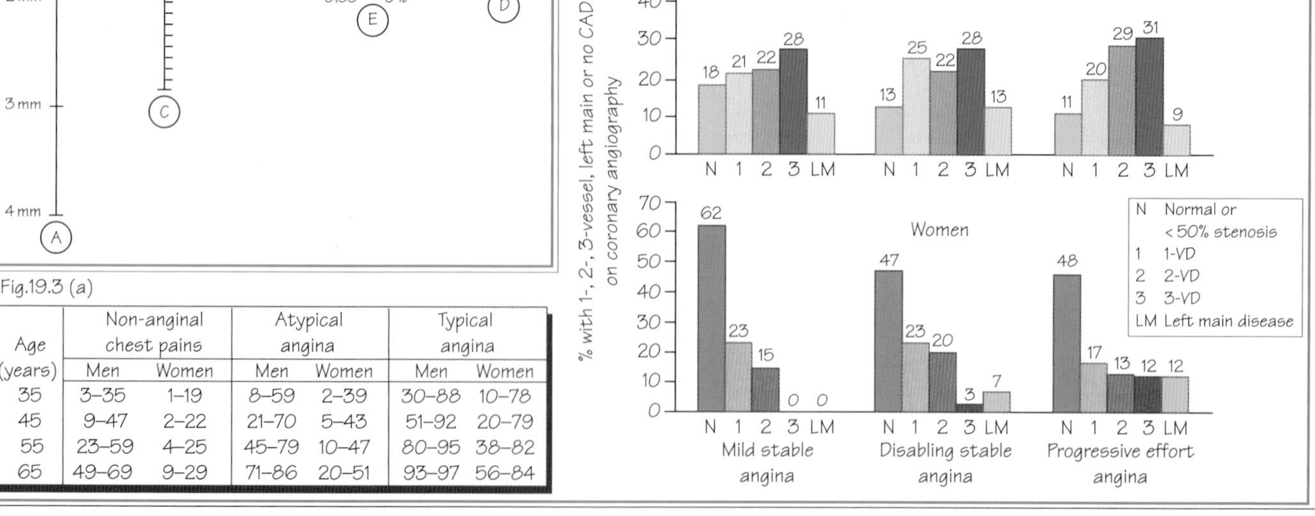

Fig.19.3 (a)

Age (years)	Non-anginal chest pains		Atypical angina		Typical angina	
	Men	Women	Men	Women	Men	Women
35	3–35	1–19	8–59	2–39	30–88	10–78
45	9–47	2–22	21–70	5–43	51–92	20–79
55	23–59	4–25	45–79	10–47	80–95	38–82
65	49–69	9–29	71–86	20–51	93–97	56–84

The distinction between acute and chronic chest pain is arbitrary: most clinicians understand acute chest pain to be new onset (≤ a few weeks) symptoms which may indicate an acute coronary syndrome, whereas chronic chest pain has been present for ≥ 4–6 weeks and, while the differential diagnosis is wide, the main concern is whether chronic stable angina is present. So, it is important to establish: (a) whether or not angina is present; (b) if it is, what is the prognosis; and (c) if angina is not present, what is the diagnosis?

Diagnosis of chronic stable angina

Features suggesting chronic stable angina include:

• *Demographics*. The more ischaemic heart disease (IHD) risk factors present, the more likely is angina: increasing age (the dominant risk factor), diabetes, smoking, hypertension, hyperlipidaemia, adverse family history (IHD in a first degree relative ≤ 65 years), high body mass index (BMI), central obesity, psychological stress.

• *Clinical features*. Typical angina increases the chance of angina and comprises: (i) a retrosternal ache ('pressure', 'heaviness', 'discomfort'); (ii) provoked by effort, possibly radiating to the neck, jaw, left arm (sometimes only there) sufficiently intense to lead to exercise lessening, or stopping; (iii) rapidly (≤ 1–2 min) relieved by rest. The amount of effort required to provoke symptoms is reproducible, reduced in the cold and after meals. The more symptoms differ from this the less likely are they to be angina. The more other symptoms (e.g. aches/pains elsewhere, tiredness, etc.) are present, the lower the chance of organic disease.

• *Physical examination*, for vascular disease (bruits/diminished arterial pulses), complications of IHD (heart failure, etc.) and other causes of angina (aortic stenosis, pulmonary hypertension) and effort dependent chest tightness (e.g. asthma), though rarely shows diagnostic abnormalities.

The ECG in stable angina

• The resting ECG is normal in stable angina, however severe the coronary disease, unless there has been previous infarction, when there may be T wave changes, loss of R wave height regionally, or pathological Q waves.

• The exercise ECG is the mainstay of diagnosis, and allows estimation of prognosis (Figs 19.1–19.3). For diagnosis, one requires typical symptoms and ECG changes (planar or downsloping ST depression) during effort and, after exercise, typical ischaemic repolarization changes. The more the exercise test differs from this, the less likely is IHD. The exercise test is a fallible guide, no more! A 'normal' test can be associated with critical coronary disease, and an abnormal test with normal epicardial coronary arteries (see Chapter 64)!

Prognosis in chronic stable angina depends on:

• Age, worse when older.

• Left ventricular (LV) function: a normal ECG likely indicates normal LV function. Anterior Q waves suggest LV dysfunction, as do extensive Q waves elsewhere. A non-specifically abnormal ECG can indicate poor or good LV function, a dilemma resolved by cardiac ultrasound.

• The more symptoms, the worse the prognosis.

• Exercise tolerance test (ETT) findings (Fig. 19.2).

• Control of risk factors.

• Presence of previous instability, especially if adverse features present including (but not limited to) a troponin rise (the greater the rise the worse the outlook).

Fig. 19.1 Exercise test in severe coronary disease. The exercise phase is indicated. Left ventricular function is likely to be good, given the good R waves. Exercise lasted 3 min 31 s (not long!) due to severe chest pain. Haemodynamic data (blood pressure [BP]/heart rate [HR]) is important (symptoms/ST changes occurring at a lower HR–BP indicate a higher probability of severe coronary disease). Peak ST depression occurred in recovery (after 2 min 50 s) with every lead, except aVR and V1 developing marked downward sloping ST depression (first number by the lead = millimetres of ST depression; second number = slope of the ST depression: negative number = downsloping; positive = upsloping). These changes are termed 'post-exercise repolarization changes' and are not typical here as there is much more ST depression than usual. When ECG recording finished at 14 min 30 s, the ECG was still abnormal with ongoing ST flattening infero-laterally. This test shows a very poor work capacity due to angina, with severe ECG changes, and severe prolonged post-exercise ST changes. The likelihood is very high that this patient has severe coronary disease. A severe left main stenosis with a blocked right coronary artery was found.

Fig. 19.2 (a) The Duke normogram. An exercise test using the Bruce protocol is undertaken. To obtain the risk of dying, a ruler is held between the mark for the amount of ST depression, and the presence or otherwise of angina during the test. A point is obtained on the ischaemia reading line; this point is then connected with a ruler to the duration of exercise column, allowing the 5-year survival rates to be obtained. The formula for the Duke normogram is Duke treadmill score = exercise time – (5 × max ST depression in millimetres) – (4 × angina index), where the angina index is: 0 = no angina; 1 = non-limiting angina; 2 = exercise limiting angina. Values between –25 (high risk) and 15 are obtained, and translated into 5-year mortality (b)VD, vessels significantly diseased with stenosis 75%; LM, left main stem disease.

Fig. 19.3 (a) Pre-test probability of significant coronary artery disease (percentage with significant coronary artery disease). The first number is the percentage of patients without diabetes, smoking or hyperlipidaemia, and the second is for the same patients with these three risk factors. This data assumes normal resting ECGs; the probability of coronary artery disease (CAD) with abnormal resting ECGs is higher than here. The probability of coronary disease increases with increasing age, increasing number of CAD risk factors, and increasing typicality of classic anginal symptoms. Women have lower risks for coronary disease at every stage. (b) Severity of CAD related to symptoms. There clearly is a relationship, but it is surprisingly weak. This data emphasizes the need for additional risk stratification (e.g. exercise stress testing) beyond evaluating symptoms in managing chronic stable angina.

20 Acute breathlessness

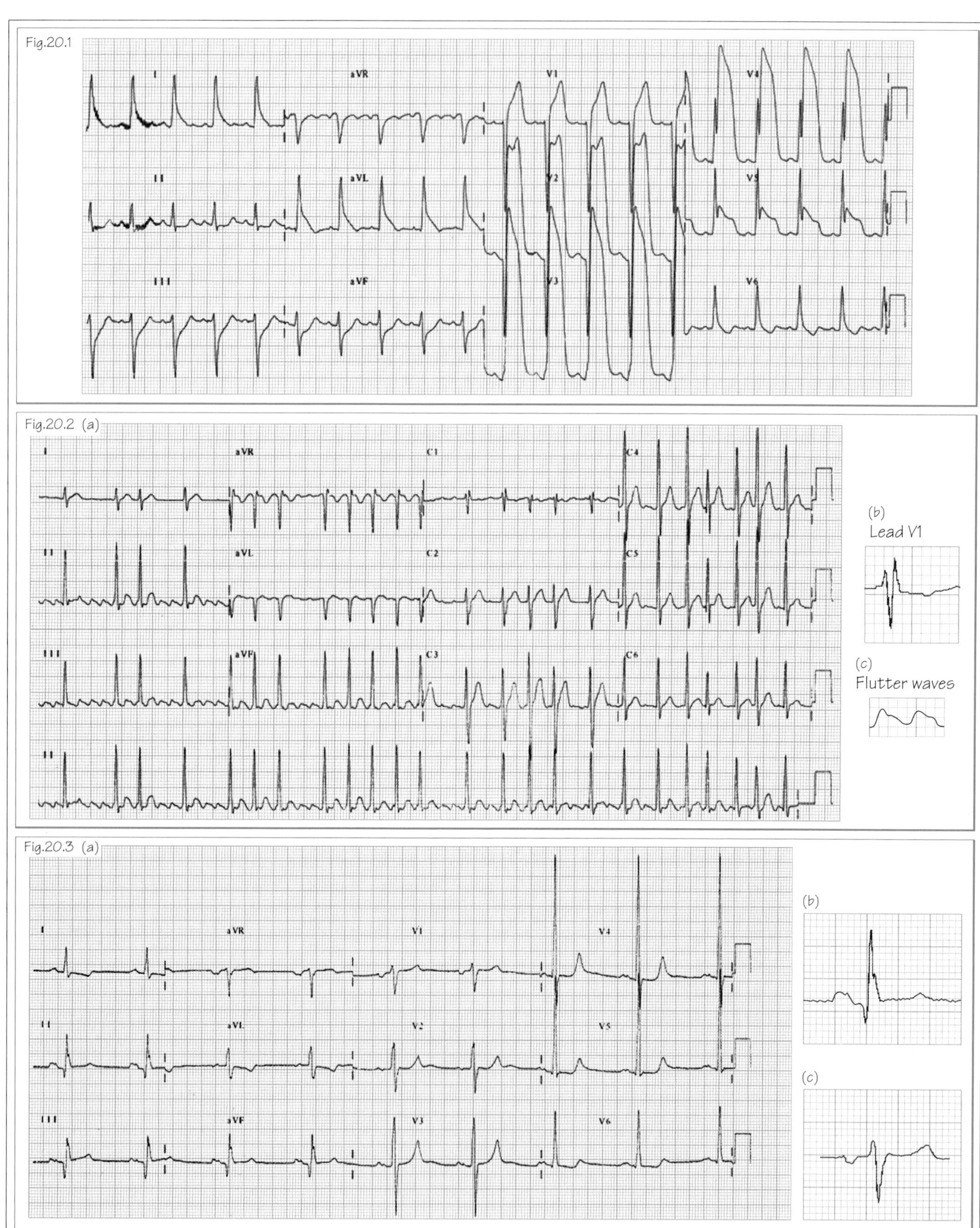

The cause of new onset severe breathlessness can usually be identified from the history, physical examination, and simple tests including the ECG, spirometry/peak flow, chest X-ray and blood gases. Brain natriuretic peptide (BNP) has an increasingly important role.

Acute left ventricular failure The patient is usually obviously breathless especially on lying flat, and is cold, sweaty, tachycardic (proportional to severity) and cyanosed, and in life-threatening pulmonary oedema, pink frothy sputum. The causes are:

• Acute myocardial infarction (AMI), common, suspected from typical cardiac quality pain (retrosternal chest discomfort, 'tightness', 'squeezing' or 'heavy' sensation, sometimes radiating to the neck, and/or left or both arms) with sweating and/or nausea. The ECG maybe 'classic', i.e. ST elevation (Fig. 20.1); however, equally and not infrequently, the ECG may show 'only' ST depression, left bundle branch block, or less specific signs despite a new myocardial infarction (MI) being present. *One should always have a high index of suspicion that a new MI underlies acute left ventricular failure (LVF).*

• Multivessel coronary disease without major infarction, not uncommon. The ECG usually shows widespread ST depression, which normalize with LVF treatment. Subsequent troponin release is often low, and left ventricle (LV) function, once LVF has resolved, is reasonable. Angiography confirms multivessel coronary artery disease and guides treatment.

• Decompensated chronic heart failure, often from a remote MI, with a more recent event, such as atrial fibrillation, fluid retention from a non-steroidal anti-inflammatory agent (NSAIA), or anaemia, etc. The ECG shows evidence of old damage, e.g. anterior lead Q waves, left bundle branch block, etc.

• Aortic stenosis, often first suspected from finding left ventricular hypertrophy (LVH) on the ECG (as the murmur is very quiet during acute LVF); the differential diagnosis of pulmonary oedema with an ECG showing LVH includes hypertensive heart disease, and ischaemically mediated heart failure.

Pulmonary embolus There are four distinct presentations of a pulmonary embolus with different ECG findings (Table 20.1).

Arrhythmias It is unusual for tachyarrhythmias to cause heart failure, unless they are very fast, there is damage to LV function, or severe valvar heart disease is present. The commonest arrhythmias causing heart failure are atrial fibrillation in a patient with pre-existing LV dysfunction. Occasionally atrial fibrillation results in very fast ventricular heart rates, and breathlessness; the commonest cause of this is the Wolff–Parkinson–White syndrome.

Pneumonia Is a common cause of breathlessness. Patients experience malaise, fever, and cough, breathlessness and occasionally chest pain or haemoptysis. The ECG is either normal, or shows the results of sepsis – sinus tachycardia, sometimes with non-specific ST changes. Pneumonia increases the risk of MI in subsequent weeks threefold.

Airways disease **Asthma** patients have acute attacks of wheezing with breathlessness. The ECG shows sinus tachycardia during the episodes, proportional to severity. **Chronic obstructive pulmonary disease**, usually (not always) smoking related, results in a gradual decline in effort tolerance over years. The clinical course can be punctuated by acute exacerbations. The ECG may show the consequences of pulmonary arterial hypertension (right atrial enlargement, right axis deviation, dominant R wave in lead V1, due to right ventricular hypertrophy or to right bundle branch block) though is often unremarkable.

Pneumothorax This results in sinus tachycardia.

Dysfunctional breathing Is a common cause of breathlessness. Sinus tachycardia may (infrequently) occur; low levels of carbon dioxide (CO_2) in the blood increase the pH, altering the physiology of repolarization. Widespread ST changes can occur, ST flattening, and ST depression being the most common. Clearly these changes also occur with coronary disease, or left ventricular dysfunction from many causes, e.g. cardiomyopathy, so these diseases may need to be ruled out before concluding the ECG changes are due to hyperventilation alone.

How to analyse the ECG in an acutely breathless patient

There are many different ways to analyse the ECG in the setting of acute breathlessness, and everyone needs to find the approach that suits them best. One approach to this situation (the same as in most illnesses) is as follows:

1. Check the name, date and time on the ECG. Many ECGs float around hospitals, and not infrequently find there way into the wrong

Fig. 20.1 Anterior wall myocardial infarction. The patient presented with severe chest pain, followed by severe breathlessness. They were found to be in life-threatening pulmonary oedema, with this ECG. Sinus tachycardia, heart rate 113 b/min. Normal P wave, PR interval. QRS complexes unremarkable in the standard leads (I to III, aVR to aVF), not clearly visible in the chest leads. ST elevation in leads I, aVL and V1–5, gross in the chest leads (> 5 cm in lead V3), ST depression inferiorly (III and aVF) and laterally (V6). This is a very large anterior wall ST segment elevation myocardial infarction (STEMI), complicated by acute left ventricular failure. Very aggressive reperfusion is required.

Fig. 20.2 Heart failure. The patient had mild effort breathlessness and then suddenly became much more breathless. (a) The ECG shows a well organized atrial arrhythmia (look at the rhythm strip and Fig. 20.2c), probably atrial flutter, and a fast QRS rate, overall around 140–150 b/min. The QRS axis is rightward shifted (equidominant R wave lead I, i.e. R = S wave, and dominant R wave lead II and III), according to the computer, +89°. (b) The QRS complex is unremarkable aside from a RSR′ pattern in lead V1, indicating partial right bundle branch block (RBBB). Normal T waves. Heart failure is often provoked by the onset of atrial flutter/fibrillation. A secundum atrial septal defect (with pulmonary to systemic blood flow of 4 : 1) underlay the heart failure, the clues here being right axis deviation, and partial RBBB.

Fig. 20.3 (a) Left atrial enlargement ((b) bifid P wave in lead II, (c) late negative deflection in lead V1) marked left ventricular hypertrophy (LVH) with repolarization changes. The standard leads show unremarkable voltages, the chest leads greatly increased (S V3 = 18 mm, R V4 = 43 mm, together 61 mm, markedly raised). Laterally (I, aVL, V5 and V6) 'reverse-tick' ST depression ('LVH-associated repolarization changes', in old terminology 'LVH with strain'). The patient had critical aortic stenosis, though from the ECG could equally have hypertensive heart disease.

Table 20.1 Different presentations of a pulmonary embolus with different ECG findings.

Syndrome	Incidence	Symptoms/signs	Signs	ECG findings
Small PE	++++	Pleuritic chest pain	None	Normal
Moderate PE	++	Sudden onset breathlessness ± pleuritic chest pain	↑Heart rate Clinically obvious cyanosis	Sinus tachycardia
Large PE	+	Sudden SOB	Cold, obvious cyanosis ↑Heart rate ↓BP, ↑JVP	↑Heart rate ± QRS complex right axis deviation → S1Q3T3 ± Right bundle branch block
Chronic PE	+	Gradual onset SOB over months	Normal heart rate ↑JVP, RV hypertrophy	RA and RV hypertrophy Right bundle branch block

BP, blood pressure; JVP, jugular venous pressure; PE, pulmonary embolus; RA, right atrium; RV, right ventricle; SOB, shortness of breath.

set of notes. Be aware of this, and *always* check these details on *every* ECG you examine.

2. Define the illness from the history and clinical examination. This is crucially important, as it guides your eye in examining the ECG. By definition, obvious findings will leap out at you, and you will not need any real understanding of the patients illness to find these. However, such obvious findings may have quite different interpretations depending on the clinical situation. For example, right bundle branch block (RBBB) in many ECGs is not of great significance, but in the setting of acute breathlessness it may indicate a pulmonary embolus. Subtle clues must be looked for, and you will only find these clues if you know what you are looking for. An example is a dominant T wave in lead V1, often not of great significance, but in a patient suspected of having an acute coronary syndrome it may well indicate an acute lesion in the circumflex coronary artery. Relatively small posterior wall myocardial infarcts, associated with similar subtle ECG changes, are occasionally complicated by papillary muscle rupture, and acute severe mitral regurgitation. You may need to be quite alert to pick up these clues.

3. Determine the heart rhythm (see Chapters 40 and 41). Clearly this will usually be sinus. If it is atrial fibrillation (AF), it's relevance to breathlessness depends on the heart rate, and whether or not there is underlying heart disease (if there is no history of chest pain, there are no murmurs, and the rest of the ECG is normal, then there is unlikely to be any heart disease). In the absence of any heart disease, and with a heart rate <120 b/min it is unlikely to be the sole explanation.

4. Determine heart rate. This is crucially important. Many (but not all) patients with a immediately life threatening cause for their acute breathlessness have a tachycardia, itself proportional to the severity of the illness. This is particularly true for acute heart failure (though beware in interpreting this, if they are on a beta-blocker), pulmonary embolus, pneumonia and asthma. Severe breathlessness with a normal heart rate raises the possibility that the breathlessness is not organic in nature.

5. Determine the shape of the P wave (see Chapter 7) and in particular, whether there is any evidence for left atrial enlargement (the most sensitive sign for which is a dominant negative P wave in lead V1, see Chapter 33). The finding of ECG evidence for a large left atrium increases the chance that breathlessness relates to left heart failure (though does not at all make this inevitable). If the ECG is otherwise normal, consider mitral stenosis/regurgitation. If the QRST complexes are abnormal, consider other diagnoses (see below).

6. Determine the QRS axis (see Chapter 10). Normal or leftward axis is usually not of great diagnostic help, but a rightward axis shift may indicate the right heart is operating under strain. The common causes for this include chronic obstructive pulmonary disease (COPD) and a pulmonary embolus.

7. Determine whether there is any evidence of conducting tissue disease (see Chapter 11). Left bundle branch block (LBBB) is often not of great help diagnostically, though as it is associated with left ventricular disease, it is a pointer that the diagnosis may be heart failure. In the setting of chest pain having the characteristics of myocardial ischaemia, it increases the probability the symptoms actually being due to myocardial ischaemia. Right bundle branch block likewise is often not of great diagnostic utility, though in a few acutely breathless patients does indicate acute right heart strain due to a pulmonary embolus (PE). Partial RBBB can be caused by an atrial septal defect (ASD), and this may be the only ECG clue (though be aware that most patients with partial RBBB have normal hearts).

8. Determine whether there are any Q waves, or regional loss of R wave height (see Chapter 9) such as may indicate a remote MI. These findings are clearly clues that the diagnosis may be heart failure.

9. Examine the ST segments (see Chapters 13 and 14). ST elevation may indicate an AMI; ST depression may indicate myocardial ischaemia. Either of these findings is likely to indicate a need for urgent angiography and revascularization.

10. Examine the T waves (see Chapters 15 and 16). Diffuse flattening may indicate a cardiomyopathic process, whereas flattening in the distribution of a coronary artery may indicate coronary disease. Deep T wave inversion often indicates a critical coronary lesion, though sometimes a form of hypertrophic cardiomyopathy. 'Reverse-tick' T wave inversion (see Chapter 16) occurring laterally (Fig. 24.2(b)) often indicates left ventricular hypertrophy (which in turn may relate to aortic stenosis – listen for a murmur, or hypertension, usually revealed by the history).

Try to summarize the clinical situation and ECG findings in 1–2 sentences: for example, 'A 35-year-old man, with a family history of DVT, presents acutely breathless following a plane flight. Examination shows anxiety and tachycardia, his ECG shows right axis deviation, and inverted T waves V1–3, I suspect the diagnosis is a large pulmonary embolus.'

21 Chronic breathlessness

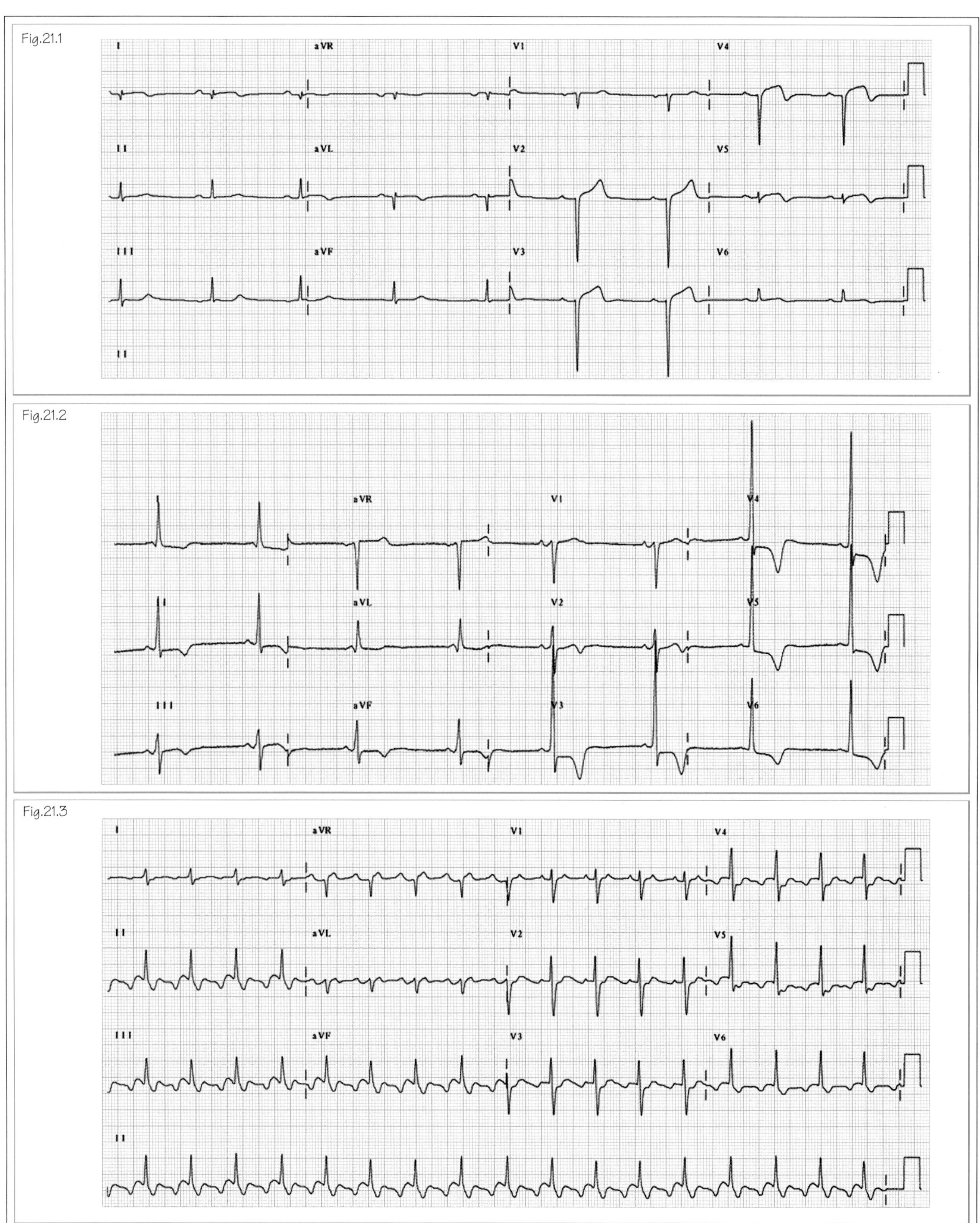

The cause of long-standing breathlessness can be identified from the history, physical examination, and simple tests including the ECG, spirometry, chest X-ray and brain natriuretic peptide (BNP). Occasionally more sophisticated tests are necessary, including cardiac magnetic resonance (MR), cardiac catheterization and specialized lung tests.

Heart failure is diagnosed from: (i) identifying a predisposing cause (e.g. rheumatic fever, hypertension, valvar heart disease, previous myocardial infarction [MI] [Fig. 21.1]); (ii) resulting in effort breathlessness without wheeze, orthopnoea, ankle oedema; (iii) physical examination – large heart, third heart sound, bibasal inspiratory lung crepitations, raised venous pressure, ankle oedema; and (iv) investigations – cardiac ultrasound, ECG and BNP. Most patients have ECG abnormalities, depending on aetiology (Table 21.1): (i) *ischaemic heart disease*, heart failure relates to a previous MI and the ECG shows pathological Q waves or regional loss of R wave height; (ii) *aortic stenosis*, the ECG shows left ventricular hypertrophy (LVH); (iii) *cardiomyopathy*, often idiopathic dilated cardiomyopathy (DCM), the ECG often shows atrial fibrillation (AF), small QRS complexes and diffuse ST changes, and, rarely, hypertrophic cardiomyopathy (HCM) (Fig. 21.2). The severity/extent of the ECG changes in heart failure often relate to the severity of cardiac damage, though there are many exceptions. Heart failure with a normal ECG is possible, but unlikely. If the ECG is normal, then causes other than heart failure should be considered first.

Chronic obstructive airways disease (COPD) causes slowly progressive effort breathlessness with wheeze, no orthopnoea, with exacerbations, and, when the right heart fails ('cor pulmonale'), peripheral oedema. The ECG may show the consequences of the destruction of the pulmonary arterial circulation, and the difficulty the right ventricle has in pushing blood into the lungs – right ventricular hypertrophy, with deviation of the QRS axis to the right and/or a dominant R wave in lead V1. Surprisingly the ECG often shows neither of these changes, despite dramatic increases in pulmonary artery pressure. The commonest findings in COPD are: (i) low voltage QRS complexes, due to the increased lung volume decreasing the transmission of electricity to the chest wall; and (ii) non-specific ST flattening, often throughout the ECG leads.

Obesity is usually obvious. The ECG shows small PQRST complexes, but no T wave abnormalities. Anterior wall myocardial infarction also often shows small QRS waves, though often with flat or inverted T waves. Thus changes in the T wave are useful to tell 'straightforward' obesity apart from myocardial damage.

Physical deconditioning has no pathognomonic ECG changes, but the history is suggestive. Resting heart rate and QT interval increase with unfitness though, in those without cardiac disease, are still often within the normal range. An exercise test shows a low work capacity, due to breathlessness, with a very brisk increase in heart rate, but no ECG changes.

Anaemia suspected from the physical examination, and confirmed by a blood count. The ECG is unremarkable.

Arrhythmias usually do not cause breathlessness, unless there is pre-existing left ventricular dysfunction, or the arrhythmias have resulted in left ventricular impairment, or the arrhythmias are very fast or very (≤ 30 b/min) slow. The ECG is diagnostic (Fig. 21.3).

Fig. 21.1 Old anterior wall myocardial infarction (MI) – pathological Q waves in leads I, aVL, V1–4. Upright anterior chest T waves suggests that the anterior wall MI is likely to be ≥ 1 week old, and probably much older. Anterior MI is strongly but not invariably associated with substantial impairment to left ventricular function.

Fig. 21.2 Left ventricular hypertrophy (LVH). Substantial increase in the voltage of the leads looking at the left ventricle – the R wave in V5 = 33 mm (exceeding that for the diagnosis of LVH in many scoring systems – see Chapter 24). In addition, there are gross ST–T changes, with ST depression/T wave inversion in most of the chest leads (V3–6). There is also T wave inversion in the inferior leads (II, III, aVF). This ECG shows severe LVH with generalized repolarization changes, too extensive to be just due to acquired LVH. The diagnosis is therefore hypertrophic cardiomyopathy (HCM), or in addition to acquired hypertrophy (from hypertension or aortic stenosis) there is another process such as ischaemia from critical coronary disease. In fact, the patient had HCM.

Fig. 21.3 Atrial tachycardia. The rhythm is not immediately apparent. From lead V1 it is easy to miss the second P wave buried in the T wave. However, inspection of lead II shows two abnormally shaped P waves for every QRS complex. The differential diagnosis includes atrial flutter. However, as an iso-electric line is clearly seen between the P waves in lead II, not found in classic atrial flutter, it is more likely that this is an automatic atrial arrhythmia, such as atrial tachycardia.

Table 21.1 ECG findings in different causes of breathlessness.

	Normal	Mild 'non-specific' ST changes	ST elevation	Q waves	Prominent left-sided voltages	Dominant R wave V1	Small QRS complexes	Left bundle
Interpretation	LV dysfunction unlikely	Non-diagnostic ECG	Myocardial infarct	Myocyte necrosis unless very small Q's, when 'physiological'	Left ventricular hypertrophy	Right ventricular hypertrophy or old posterior wall myocardial infarct	Either very few functioning myocytes, or increased electrical insulation of heart	Damage to left bundle
Most likely diagnosis	Respiratory disease, e.g. asthma, or 'psychogenic' breathlessness	Any!	Pulmonary oedema	Heart failure due to previous MI	Heart failure due to aortic stenosis or end-stage hypertension	Pulmonary hypertension, due to COPD or heart failure (latter less likely)	Obesity (normal ST/T) Extensive myocardial damage (abnormal ST/T)	Many causes, but raises the possibility of heart disease
Cardiac disease	Unlikely 'Anginal equivalent' breathlessness	Certainly possible IHD DCM Valvar heart disease	Acute MI Pericardial disease	Previous MI DCM	As above Aortic regurgitation Mitral regurgitation	Mitral stenosis Old posterior wall MI Cardiomyopathy, e.g. due to Duchenne muscular dystrophy	Poor LV function Pericardial effusion	Poor LV Aortic stenosis IHD Hypertension
Respiratory disease	Asthma Dysfunctional breathing	Certainly possible Asthma COPD Interstitial lung disease	Unlikely	Unlikely, unless co-morbid disease present	Unlikely	Chronic fibrotic lung disease Chronic PE's	COPD (occasionally)	COPD
Other	Physical deconditioning	Interstitial lung disease			Thin patient, consider weight loss and physical deconditioning	Obesity	Hypothyroidism	Any systemic disease, e.g. vasculitis

COPD, chronic obstructive pulmonary disease; DCM, dilated cardiomyopathy; IHD, ischaemic heart disease; MI, myocardial infarctions; PE, pulmonary embolus; ST/T, ST/T wave changes; LV, left ventricular.

22 Palpitations

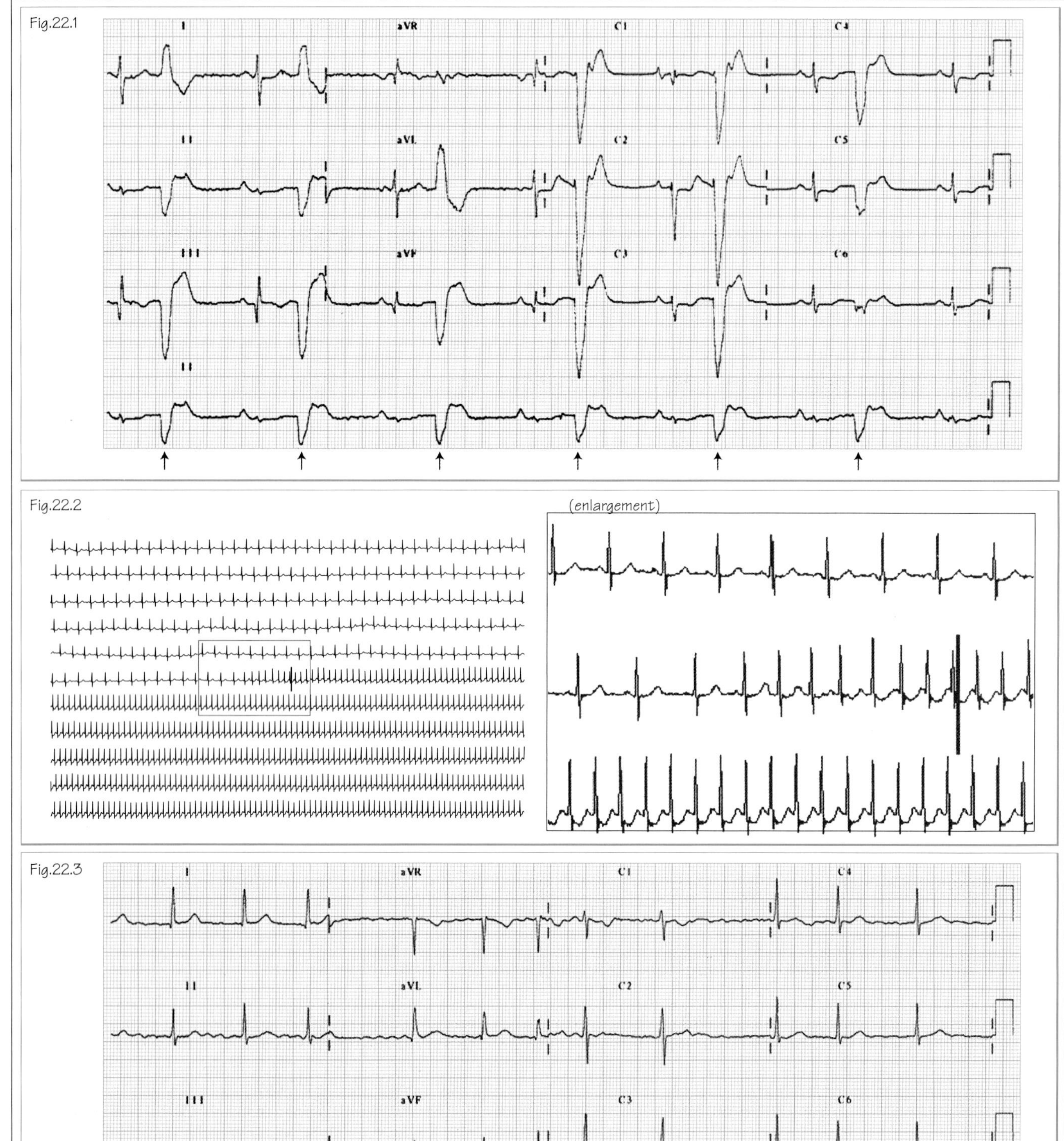

Palpitations are an abnormal appreciation of the heartbeat. The key to diagnosis is to obtain an ECG during an attack; which method is best depends on the frequency and duration of the symptoms (Table 22.1). The history provides a reasonable diagnostic guide:

• **Appreciation of the normal heartbeat** (e.g. almost always relating to emotional stress, rarely relating to thyrotoxicosis, and very rarely to phaeochromocytoma). Palpitations in this situation have a slow onset/offset over many minutes, ill-defined duration, usually last many hours, and have no response to vagotonic manoeuvres (Valsalva, neck pressure, cold drinks). They usually occur in the context of emotional stress.

• **Arrhythmia**. Palpitations due to arryhythmias usually are of sudden (instantaneous) onset, sudden/slow offset, duration well-defined and remembered by the patient, and they may have identified a response to vagotonic manoeuvres. Patients may have noticed post-event polyuria, although this is a relatively rare phenomenon. Bradyarrhythmias do not cause palpitations, tachycardias can:

  • Ventricular extrasystoles (VEs) cause brief symptoms (lasting only a few seconds') from the:

    (a) Extra beat itself ('extra' beats, 'heart all over the place' 'fluttering').

    (b) Increased gap between the VE and the following sinus beat ('as if the heart has stopped'). This is often the symptom that patients find the most worrying, as they are concerned that their heart may actually stop.

    (c) Increased strength of the beat following the extrasystole ('heart restarts with a great thud').

  Symptoms are commoner at slow heart rates, e.g. at night time. This is because some extrasystoles are more likely to occur when the cardiac action potential is prolonged. This occurs with low heart rates, and when vagal tone is high, conditions both found at night (Chapter 17). Atrial extrasystoles cause fewer symptoms than VEs (Fig. 22.1).

  • Re-entrant supraventricular tachycardia (SVT) (atrioventricular re-entrant tachycardia [AVRT] and atrioventricular nodal re-entrant tachycardia [AVNRT]) give rise to sudden onset fast (patients taps out a heart rate of 150–200 b/min) regular palpitations, of well-defined duration, usually (not always) with symptoms stopping as suddenly as the arrhythmia does. Symptoms other than palpitations are rare, unless there is associated heart disease (e.g. coronary disease, left ventricular dysfunction, etc.). Associated heart disease is relatively rare, as the common age of presentation for many SVTs is 20–50, whereas most structural heart disease occurs in an older age group.

  • Atrial fibrillation (AF) results in sudden onset fast palpitations, differentiated from re-entrant SVTs by their irregularity ('all over the place') and from VEs by the heart rate (fast in AF, normal in VES). Atrial fibrillation is associated with structural heart disease, so breathlessness and (rarely) angina may occur. Atrial fibrillation terminates abruptly, so symptoms usually stop suddenly. Many re-entrant tachyarrhythmias (e.g. AVNRT or AVRT) last only a number of minutes, only relatively rarely lasting many hours, whereas AF, while it certainly can last only a number of minutes, not infrequently lasts many hours or even days. Occasionally sinus disease underlies AF. If so, when AF terminates the sinus node takes 3–5 s to restart, when sinus arrest occurs and cardiac output ceases, some patients may feel faint or actually blackout.

  • Ventricular tachycardia (VT) gives rise to three distinct syndromes: (i) sudden onset fast regular palpitations, ± near blackouts; (ii) blackouts, which maybe preceded by fast regular palpitations; (iii) sudden cardiac death, when VT degenerates to ventricular fibrillation. The clue to VT being the diagnosis is knowing or finding structural heart disease, or finding an abnormal inter-attack ECG. Though most such ECGs show obvious abnormalities, be aware that there are a few conditions where the ECG signs can be quite subtle, and these include right ventricular cardiomyopathy (where subtle repolarization changes in leads V1 to 3 may occur, though this is not a universal finding at all), and Brugada syndrome (whose ECG appearance can come and go).

Alarm signals

Though most palpitations are due to benign conditions, a few are the harbinger of sudden cardiac death from a serious arrhythmia. Much of the data alerting one to the possibility that there may be a risk of death comes from the clinical history and the inter-attack ECG. The warning signals are:

1 Adverse family history of sudden cardiac death at an early age. The younger the relatives are affected, the more worrying are palpitations in any close relative. These mandate full investigation to elucidate their mechanism. Many conditions (though not quite all) are associated with an abnormal ECG in *affected* family members. The common conditions to consider include hypertrophic cardiomyopathy (see Chapter 34), and inherited channelopathies, of which the commonest are hereditary long QT syndrome (see Chapter 39) and Brugada syndrome (see Chapter 39). The chance of finding an inherited predisposition to sudden death in someone with a completely normal 12-lead ECG is there, but is very low.

2 High risk for coronary disease, a common cause of sudden cardiac death. Coronary disease, even when very severe, can be associated with

Fig. 22.1 Ventricular extrasystoles (VEs) (arrowed) alternating with sinus beats, best seen in the rhythm strip as broad beats (as they arise from the ventricle and are conducted slowly). Left bundle branch shape, so right ventricular origin, and directed towards lead I, away from leads II/III, so arising inferiorly. The underlying ECG shows biatrial enlargement (prominent up and down P wave in lead V1), borderline right axis deviation, deep Q wave in lead III (not lead II or aVF, so possible rather than certain old inferior myocardial infarction). The anterior chest leads show non-specific ST changes, with downsloping ST depression. There are many causes for this ECG, including ishaemic heart disease (IHD) and cardiomyopathy. The patient had severe inoperable coronary disease, and severely impaired left ventricular function.

Fig. 22.2 Twenty-four hour ECG, in a patient with brief bursts of regular palpitations. Initially sinus rhythm, then a fast regular narrow complex tachycardia, with ST segment depression, becoming more pronounced over the next 30–40 beats. A few beats into the arrhythmia there is a bold line, the patient activated marker, confirming when symptoms occur. This ECG looks like atrioventricular nodal re-entrant tachycardia (AVNRT).

Fig. 22.3 This patient had infrequent prolonged irregular palpitations. ECG recorded during an attack. Atrial fibrillation (AF) – no discernible P wave, irregular baseline, especially in lead II, fine fibrillatory f waves, and an irregular QRS response. Well-controlled QRS rate of 75 b/min; unusual, as most patients have a high heart rate at AF onset, around 120–150 b/min. A lower heart rate suggests: (i) atrial fibrillation has been present longer than realised; (ii) underlying atrioventricular (AV) conduction disease; (iii) the patient is taking drugs to slow AV conduction; or (iv) high vagal tone, e.g. physical fitness. The underling QRST complexes are normal.

Table 22.1 How to obtain an ECG during an attack of palpitations.

Duration of attack	Frequency	Best method	Description
> 30 min	Any	12-lead ECG	Attend A&E department when palpitations start (and obtain a photocopy of the ECGs). Always ask whether palpitations were present when the ECG was taken
< 30 min	Daily	24-h ECG	See Chapter 63. Recording duration = 24 h
> few min	Weekly	24-h ECG or external event recorder (EER)	EER = solid-state device applied to chest wall during symptoms, so recording a 10–20 s single channel ECG, transmitted telephonically to the cardiology department
< few min	Weekly	24-h ECG Prolonged external recording (continuous or loop)	Prolonged continuous external recording = 3–5 chest leads, to solid-state device, worn on a cord around the neck (R test evolution™ device, Novacor), 8 days of continuous ECG recording External loop recorders obtain ECG recordings from 3–5 chest leads, and 'capture' the last 40–50 min of ECG activity; 'frozen' by pushing a button on the device, analysed later
> few min	Monthly	External event recorder	As above
< few min	Monthly	Internal event recorder	Solid-state device implanted subcutaneously in the left pectoral region; battery life ± 18 months. Continuously records ± 40 min ECG activity, frozen by patient application of electronic 'wand'. Programmed to store events with heart rates ≥ or ≤ than specified levels. Useful for evaluating dangerous syncope.

A&E, accident and emergency.

a completely normal resting ECG; this is perhaps the one important exception to the basic rule that most patients with palpitations and a normal 12-lead inter-attack ECG are at low risk of sudden cardiac death. Accordingly, if the patient is at increased risk for coronary disease, it may be appropriate to consider performing an exercise stress test (see Chapter 64) or other investigations to clarify whether or not coronary disease actually is present.

3 Regardless of the family history, ECG evidence of such genetic/acquired pro-arrhythmic conditions and Wolf-Parkinson-White syndrome with an obvious delta wave (see Chapter 12).

4 Underlying heart disease. This may well come out of the history and physical examination (angina, murmurs, signs of heart failure, etc.). The ECG signs to look for include:

- Those relating to a previous MI. The ECG signs indicating a remote MI for include Q waves (see Chapter 9), especially anteriorly (as anterior infarcts are associated with the greatest damage to left ventricular function, and the degree of damage relates to the propensity to ventricular arrhythmias). Other ECG signs include regional loss of R wave height (see Chapter 9). It is held that sustained regular palpitations occurring after but not before an acute MI should be assumed to be due to VT until proved otherwise. Vigorous investigation in this situation is required to ascertain whether or not VT is the cause of palpitations, as such VT can be the harbinger of sudden cardiac death.
- Those indicating left ventricular hypertrophy LVH (see Chapters 8 and 24). The ECG signs of LV hypertrophy include: increased left-sided voltages, left axis deviation of the QRS complex, and lateral lead repolarization changes (T wave flattening, or frank 'reverse-tick' ST depression, see Chapter 00). LVH is important, as it is in itself an pro-arrhythmic condition (promoting the development of VT), and also a pointer to aortic stenosis, and, much more rarely, hypertrophic cardiomyopathy.
- Diffuse ST/T wave changes, which may indicate a cardiomyopathic process, such as T wave flattening, or frank ST depression. However, be very cautious in interpreting the ST/T wave in patients with palpitations. Many such patients do not have an arrhythmia underlying their symptoms, rather having an anxiety condition. Anxiety itself, and the associated hyperventilation, not infrequently causes ST/T wave changes. Thus, while realizing that ST/T wave changes in this setting may be a pointer to a myopathic process, and so a more serious cause to the symptoms, be aware that in most patients they mean no more than that they are anxious. Once patients are labelled as having heart disease, it may be a very difficult to remove this diagnosis.

5 Syncope with palpitations.

23 Syncope

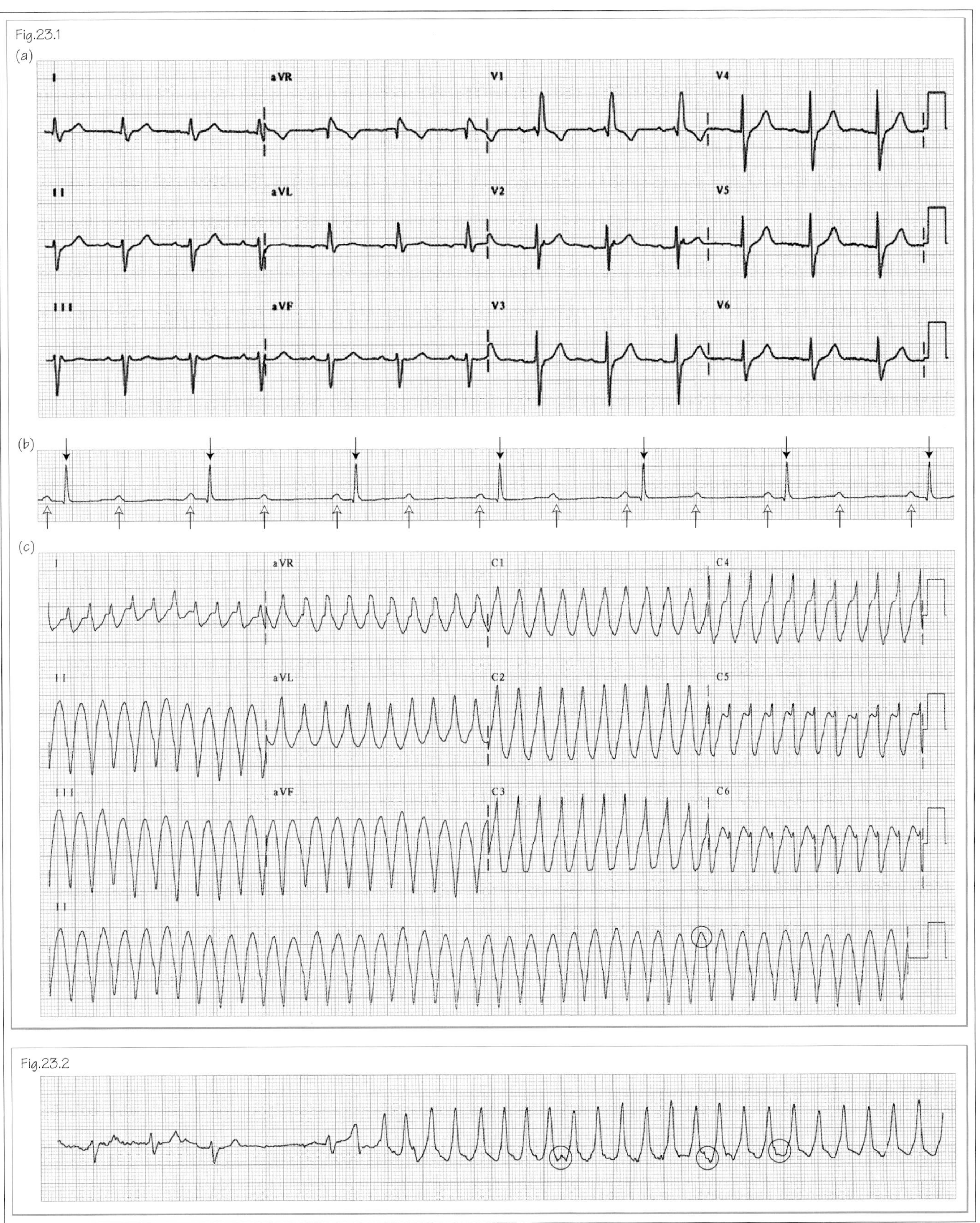

Fig.23.1
(a)
I
aVR
V1
V4
II
aVL
V2
V5
III
aVF
V3
V6
(b)
(c)
I
aVR
C1
C4
II
aVL
C2
C5
III
aVF
C3
C6
II
Fig.23.2

Syncope is 'loss of consciousness with loss of postural reflexes'. The key to diagnosis is to record an ECG (and preferably blood pressure) before and during a spontaneous attack. This is often quite a difficult thing too, although sometimes ambient monitoring allows this. Equally, on occasions, it is sometimes possible to induce an attack to obtain this data. Good clues to the diagnosis can be obtained from the history, physical exam and ECG alone (Table 23.1):

'Vasomotor' syncope relates to altered circulatory control lowering blood pressure (Table 23.2). The clues to this diagnosis are: (i) warning before an attack; (ii) gradual collapse (i.e. some protective reflexes remain intact); (iii) brief loss of consciousness; (iv) injury is very rare; (v) syncope may be situation specific, e.g. only occur in church, etc.

Bradyarrhythmias usually pauses of ≥ 4 s are required to cause syncope, e.g. sinus node disease, heart block. The clues to the diagnosis include: (i) older age patient, often > 70 years; (ii) no warning; (iii) injury as a consequence of the event is comon.

Tachyarrhythmias need to be fast to cause syncope ≥ 250–300 b/min; e.g. atrial fibrillation (AF) with Wolff–Parkinson–White (WPW) syndrome, associated with structural heart disease (e.g. ventricular tachycardia [VT] with moderate left ventricular [LV] dysfunction, AF with severe LV dysfunction), or ventricular and completely disorganized (torsade-de-pointes). The clues to the diagnosis include: (i) palpitations often (not always) felt before the syncope; (ii) injury common; (iii) most patients (not all) either are known to have structural heart disease (e.g. previous myocardial infarction), or have an abnormal inter-attack ECG.

Left ventricular outflow tract obstruction effort-induced syncope occurs in severe aortic stenosis, diagnosed from the physical exam and ECG (LV hypertrophy). Hypertrophic obstructive cardiomyopathy causes similar symptoms, with a bizarre ECG. Cardiac ultrasound defines either condition. The clues to the diagnosis are that symptoms of near or actual syncope occur on effort (see below).

Pulmonary hypertension needs to be severe (≥ 80–100 mmHg) to cause effort-induced syncope. The ECG may show right ventricular hypertrophy.

Epilepsy is usually so obvious that there is no doubt as to the diagnosis. Occasionally undiagnosed arrhythmias underlie seizures e.g. hereditary long QT syndrome.

Situations mimicking syncope include hyperventilation and psychogenic causes.

Table 23.1 Inter-attack ECG in syncope.

	Interpretation	Further management
Normal	Arrhythmia unlikely, not excluded	If vasomotor syncope likely – tilt-table test; if unlikely, and injury present – Reveal® device
RBBB	Non-specific	Exclude Brugada syndrome (consider ajmaline flecainide challenge)
Long PR interval	Heart block possible; other causes should still be considered	If history of Stokes–Adams attack, permanent pacemaker; if CAD, consider EP study to: (i) measure AH, HV intervals; (ii) to exclude inducible VT; otherwise Reveal® device
Trifasicular block*	Heart block likely	Pacemaker
Q waves	VT related to the scar of the old MI	Ventricular stimulation study or Reveal® device
LVH	Aortic stenosis, hypertrophic cardiomyopathy. If hypertensive, VT may underlie syncope	Cardiac ultrasound AVR for aortic stenosis; specialist management for HCM; otherwise Reveal device®
Long QT interval	Polymorphic VT	(i) Exclude relevant drugs; (ii) beta-blockers; (iii) ICD; (iv) family screening

*, Long PR interval + RBBB and L or R axis deviation.
AH, atrial – His conduction time; AVR, aortic valve replacement; CAD, coronary artery disease; EP, electrophysiology; HCM, hypertrophic cardiomyopathy; HV, His – ventricular conduction time; ICD, implantable cardioverter defibrillator; LVH, left ventricular hypertrophy; MI, myocardial infarction; RBBB, right bundle branch block; VT, ventricular tachycardia.

Fig. 23.1 (a) Bifascicular block (which can lead to higher-grade atrioventricular [AV] block). Sinus rhythm, 60 b/min, normal P waves, PR interval. Full right bundle branch block (RBBB) (late large positive deflection in lead V1) with left axis deviation (positive QRS in lead I, negative in leads II, III), indicating damaged anterior fascicle of the left bundle (see Chapter 10). (b) A 2 : 1 heart block. P waves = small arrows; QRS complexes = large arrows. Every second P wave does not conduct through to fire the ventricle. The underlying QRS complex is narrow and unremarkable. (c) Ventricular tachycardia (VT). No clear-cut P waves; very fast QRS rate (240 b/min); the QRS complex is broad (145 ms), i.e. broad complex tachycardia, which can be VT or supraventricular tachycardia (SVT) with aberrancy (i.e. R/LBBB). The features here strongly suggest VT: the general shape, i.e. it doesn't look like right or left bundle, confirmed by the extreme QRS axis (+260°). Possibly, independent P waves (look for small occasional irregularities that may be P waves, circled). This ECG came from a patient with a remote myocardial infarction (MI) and syncope.

Fig. 23.2 Rhythm strip from monitoring in recent syncope. The heart slows, then a run of ventricular tachycardia (VT) starts (fast broad complex tachycardia, showing independent P wave activity). Syncopal VT due to structural heart disease.

Table 23.2 Vasomotor syncope.

	Vasovagal syncope	Neurocardiogenic syncope	Carotid sinus hypersensitivity	Micturition syncope	Postural hypotension
Age	Usually young	Any age; commoner in middle age	Usually elderly	Usually elderly; only occurs in men	Common in the elderly, diabetic
Position when syncope occurs	Upright	Almost always upright; after standing still, e.g. when out shopping	Usually when standing, can occur when sitting	Passing urine, in the middle of the night ± alcohol	Standing – immediately
Preceding symptoms	Modest warning	Pre-syncope = 'near' syncope = 'as if about to blackout', for 10–30 s	Often none	Often none	Presyncope very common
Diagnostic test	Usually none required; if intrusive tilt-table test	Tilt-table test • Bradycardic: symptoms with ↓heart rate • Vasodepressor: symptoms with ↓SBP • Mixed	Bradycardia (≥ 3 seconds asystole) ±/or hypotension (≥ 50 mmHg fall) on carotid sinus massage, done while lying or standing	History of prostatism	Postural blood pressure

Table 23.3 Investigations in syncope.

	Comments	Diagnostic yield
12-lead ECG	See Table 23.2	Very low
24-h ECG	Rarely useful; best for: (i) sinus node disease; (ii) frequent complex VPCs or non-sustained VT, which may indicate sustained VT	2%
External loop recording	Useful for frequent syncope – attacks > every week	20%
Internal loop recording	Often very useful; expensive	83–94%
Tilt table test	Use in vasomotor syncope; low reproducibility, often fails to guide therapy	11–87%
Exercise stress test	Useful for exercise related symptoms	Low
Carotid sinus massage	Useful in the elderly	Low
Electrophysiological study – no structural heart disease	Rarely useful	6%
Electrophysiological study – structural heart disease	Most useful in IHD	41%
Genetic analysis	Useful in suspected Brugada syndrome, hereditary long QT syndromes	High in pre-selected groups

VPC, ventricular premature contraction; VT, ventricular tachycardia.

Alarm signals

Most syncope is vasomotor and benign. Some, however, is due to malignant arrhythmias and leads to sudden cardiac death. Clearly, it is vitally important to distinguish the dangerous causes, which by definition need early treatment, from the much more common benign causes that rarely require any treatment. The clues to a dangerous diagnosis are:

• Older age increases the probability of a dangerous cause.

• Adverse family history, i.e. family history of sudden death at an early age, the younger the relatives affected, the more worrying.

• Syncope on effort is a high-level alert signal, as this either means an obstruction to cardiac output (e.g. aortic stenosis, hypertrophic cardiomyopathy, pulmonary hypertension) or an malignant arrhythmia induced by effort. Conversely, syncope occurring after effort is rarely due to a dangerous cause, and often relates to 'vagal switch on'. Syncope occurring in response to sudden noises (e.g. an alarm clock) may indicate hereditary long QT syndrome (a dangerous genetic illness, see Chapter 39).

• Structural heart disease, especially impaired LV function, cardiomyopathy

• Older age plus Stokes-Adams type symptoms, i.e. sudden syncope without warning, with injury, appearance during the episode 'as if dead', afterwards full prompt restoration of all faculties.

• Certain abnormalities on the inter-attack ECG: Q waves, long QT interval, Brugada pattern, extensive conducting tissue disease (e.g. long PR plus bundle branch block, full left bundle, etc.). Mild abnormalities of the inter-attack ECG, especially in older patients, is often of little diagnostic significance.

Investigations in syncope

See Table 23.3.

24 Hypertension

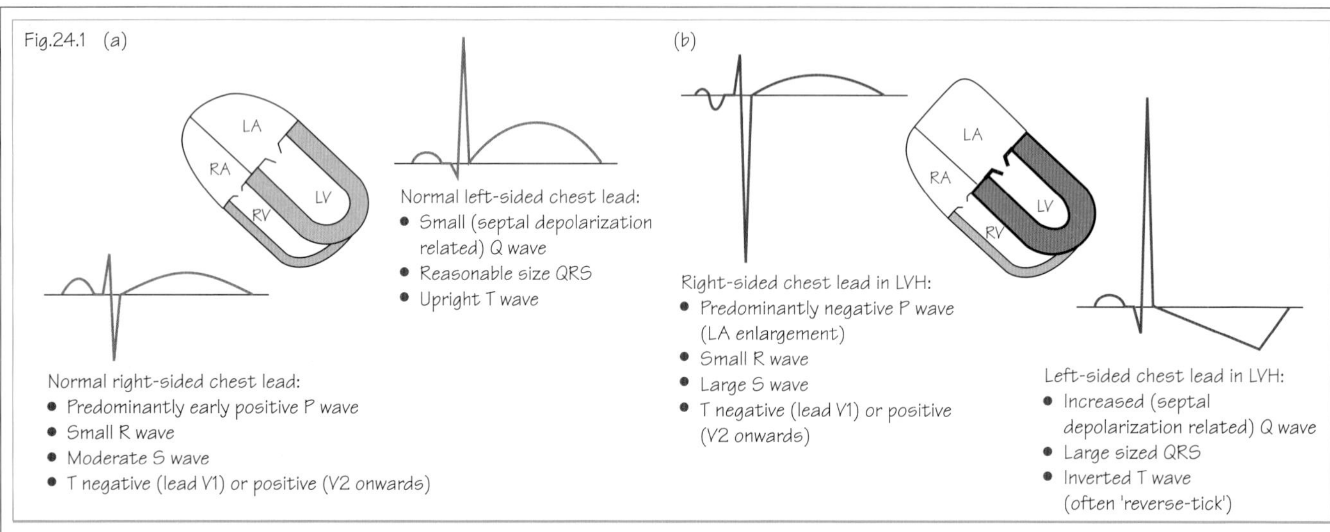

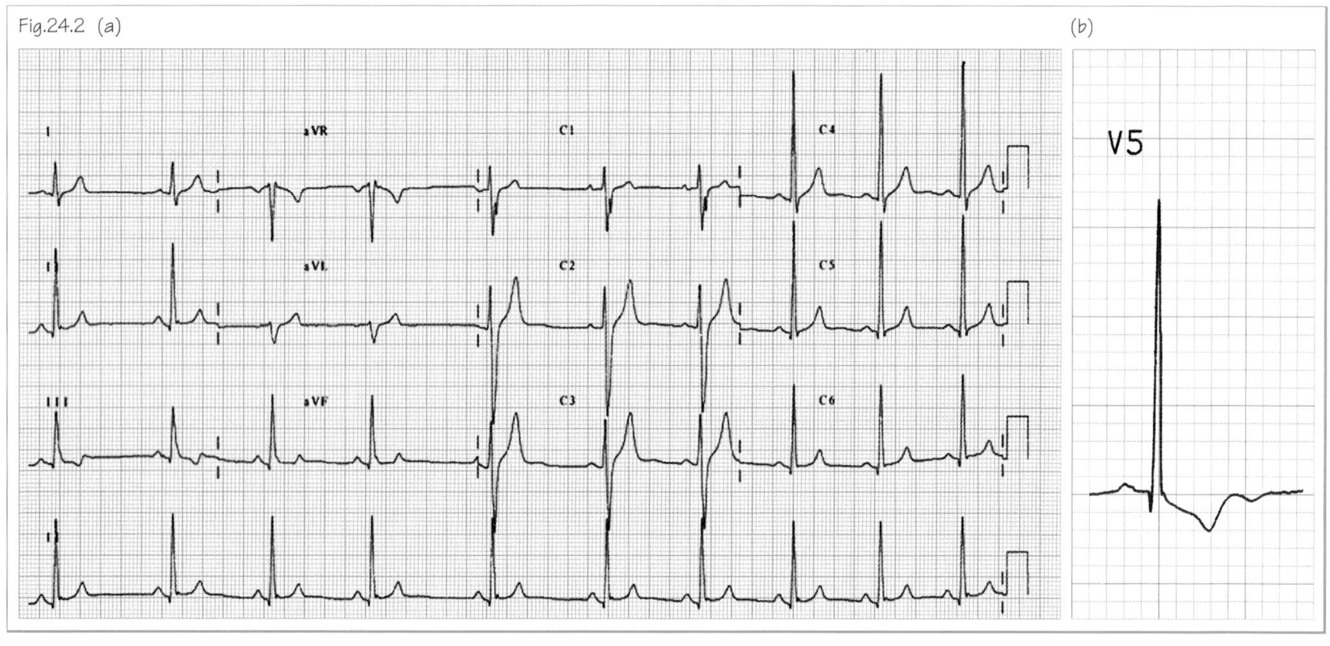

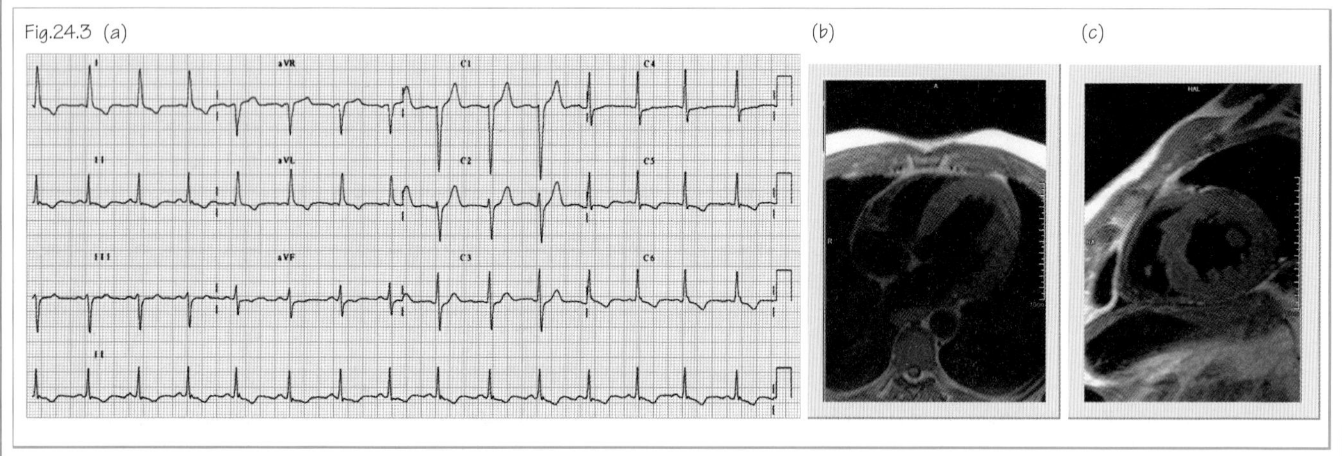

Fig.24.1 (a)

Normal right-sided chest lead:
- Predominantly early positive P wave
- Small R wave
- Moderate S wave
- T negative (lead V1) or positive (V2 onwards)

Normal left-sided chest lead:
- Small (septal depolarization related) Q wave
- Reasonable size QRS
- Upright T wave

(b)

Right-sided chest lead in LVH:
- Predominantly negative P wave (LA enlargement)
- Small R wave
- Large S wave
- T negative (lead V1) or positive (V2 onwards)

Left-sided chest lead in LVH:
- Increased (septal depolarization related) Q wave
- Large sized QRS
- Inverted T wave (often 'reverse-tick')

Fig.24.2 (a)

(b)

V5

Fig.24.3 (a)

(b)

(c)

Hypertension, though difficult to define, diagnose and treat, underlies many strokes, myocardial infarcts and much heart failure. The ECG is useful in measuring:

- The severity of hypertension induced vascular damage (ECG left ventricular hypertrophy [LVH]).
- The response to treatment, by measuring the decrease in ECG LVH, and normalization of repolarization abnormalities.
- Arrhythmic complications.

Hypertension-induced vascular damage assessment

The extent of vascular damage is determined by age, sex, cholesterol, blood pressure, diabetic status, smoking, etc., which interact together in a complex manner. In part, the extent of damage (and the likelihood of an adverse event) is determined by how long and how far the blood pressure has been elevated, i.e. the integral of blood pressure × time duration. The heart, like any muscle, hypertrophies if it works harder in proportion to the amount of work done. So, the amount of LVH is a marker of the blood pressure–time integral (and so of prognosis). It can be measured:

- From the ECG; increased tissue mass in LVH increases current flow during depolarization, increasing R wave height in left ventricular (LV) leads, used to diagnose LVH (Table 24.1) though the relationship between LV mass and ECG voltage is not close, due to: (i) variable chest wall insulation altering the current that reaches the observing electrode – in part overcome by examining the standard leads, which are unaffected by the chest wall; (ii) the fact that similar mass ventricles generate different current levels – due to known factors (e.g. age – younger hearts generate more voltage for any given mass than do older hearts) and unknown ones. This causes problems with the ECG diagnosis of LVH; there are no ideal cut-off values for LVH. Low values increase sensitivity (i.e. reduce false negatives) at the expense of specificity (i.e. increase false positives); high cut-off values increase specificity (few false negatives) at the expense of sensitivity (i.e. many patients with LVH are missed).
- By the presence of 'repolarization abnormalities'. Hypertrophy preferentially prolongs action potential duration in epicardial cells, so reversing the normal direction of LV repolarization (which now proceeds from the endocardium to the epicardium), so inverting the T wave in the LV leads. Repolarization abnormalities occur only in severe hypertrophy, and are associated with a worse outlook. Their resolution with treatment is associated with an improved outlook.
- Cardiac ultrasound is better than the ECG in diagnosing LVH, but is not as cheap and so is less readily available.
- Cardiac magnetic resonance imaging (MRI) is the most sensitive way to measure LVH – highly reproducible and expensive.

Table 24.1 Left ventricular hypertrophy.

Voltage criteria
Limb leads
• R wave in lead I + S wave in lead III > 25 mm
• R wave in lead aVL > 11 mm
• R wave in lead aVF > 20 mm
• S wave in lead aVR > 14 mm
Praecordial leads
• R wave leads V4, V5 and V6 > 26 mm
• R wave leads V5 or V6 + S wave in praecordial leads > 45 mm
Non-voltage criteria
• Delayed ventricular activation time ≥ 0.05 s in leads V5 or V6
• ST depression and T wave inversion in the left praecordial leads

Arrhythmias in hypertension

Left ventricular hypertrophy is a powerful substrate for: (a) atrial fibrillation (AF); (b) ventricular arrhythmias. The presence of hypertension requiring treatment in AF greatly increases the risk of thromboemboli, particularly stroke. Those patients with hypertension and LVH definitely require hypotensive treatment, so finding ECG LVH in those with AF equates with a need for warfarin. In LVH and normal LV systolic function, non-sustained ventricular arrhythmias are common, e.g. ventricular extrasystoles, non-sustained ventricular tachycardia. Progression of the hypertrophic process leads to a reduction in LV function, which greatly increases the chance of more sustained ventricular arrhythmias, both monomorphic and especially polymorphic ventricular tachycardia (e.g. in conjunction with pro-arrhythmic drugs, hypokalaemia). During a myocardial infarction, the presence of LVH greatly increases the risk of ventricular fibrillation.

Fig. 24.1 The ECG in left ventricular hypertrophy (LVH): (a) normal; (b) LVH. In health, neither the right nor the left atrium dominates the P wave; in LVH, left atrial enlargement is common, seen as a prominent late negative deflection in lead V1 P wave. LV causes the right-sided leads to deepen their S waves (as the bulk of the left ventricle depolarizes away from these leads – this geometry is not well illustrated here). The left lateral leads often develop some deepening of the physiological Q waves associated with septal depolarization. The QRS complexes increase in height, sometimes massively. The T waves become inverted with severe hypertrophy. Occasionally these repolarization changes are the only signs of LVH, and increased left-sided lead voltages do not develop. LA, left atrium; LV, left ventricle; RA, right atrium; RV, right ventricle.

Fig. 24.2 (a) Left ventricular hypertrophy (LVH), not associated with repolarization changes. Sinus rhythm, normal P wave, PR interval, QRS axis (+80°). Lead II = 20 mm, S in V2 + R in V5 = 47 mm (normal ≤ 45 mm). No ST/T changes. ECG from a man with severe hypertension. (b) Left ventricular hypertrophy with repolarization changes. Lead V5 from a patient with hypertensive heart disease. This complex shows a slightly broad P wave, normal PR interval. Prominent Q wave, due to septal depolarization, great increase in R wave size (40 mm), and 'reverse-tick' T wave inversion. These three findings are pathognomonic for LVH.

Fig. 24.3 (a) Left ventricular hypertrophy (LVH), repolarization criteria, no voltage criteria. Sinus rhythm, normal P wave, PR interval. QRS complex normal size throughout. Lateral lead 'reverse-tick' T wave inversion (lead I, II, aVL, ±V4, V5/6). This ECG could have come from a patient with an acute coronary syndrome, but coronary angiography was normal. Cardiac magnetic resonance imaging (MRI) (b,c) shows gross increase in left ventricular mass to twice normal size.

25 Shock

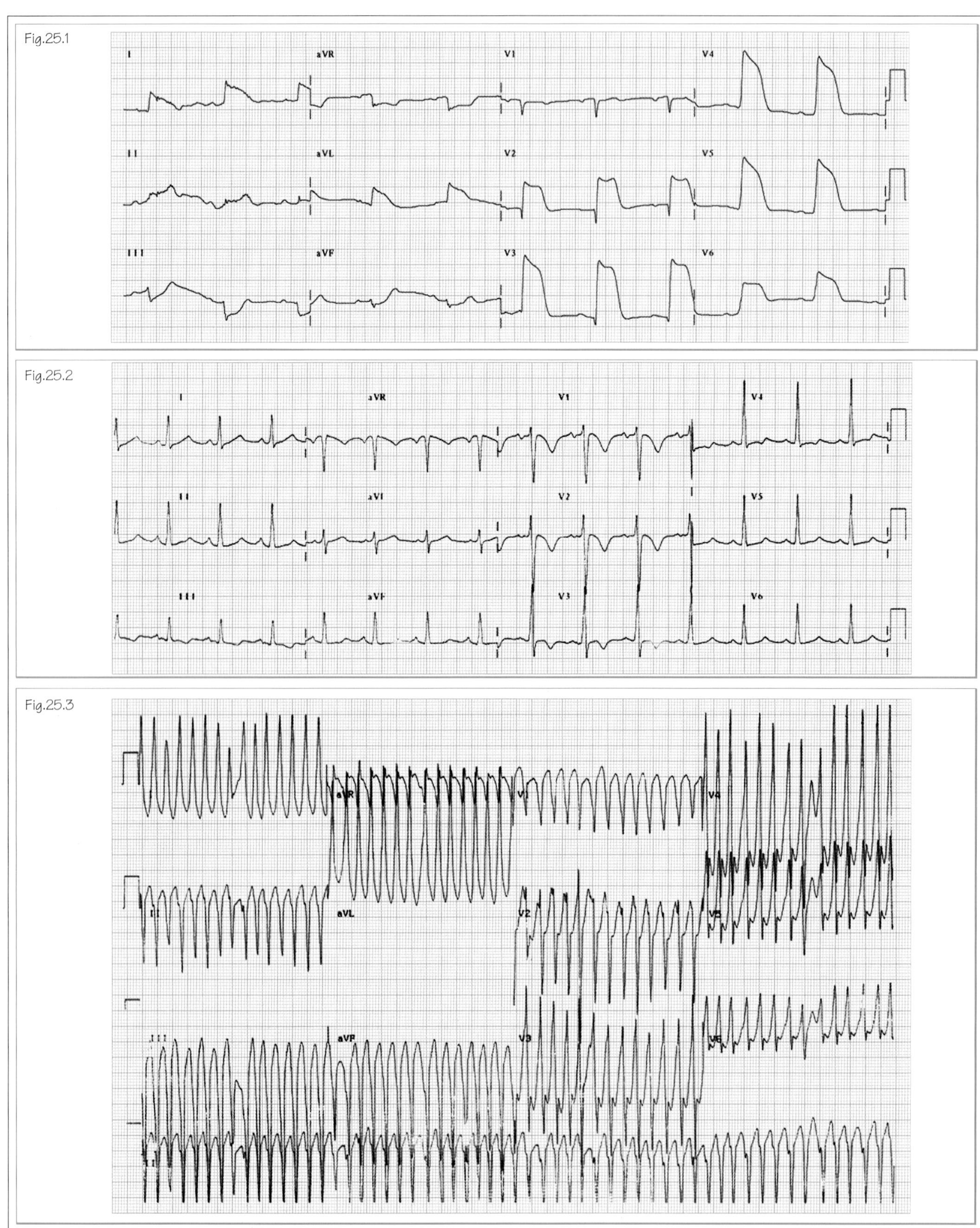

Fig.25.1
I
aVR
V1
V4
II
aVL
V2
V5
III
aVF
V3
V6
Fig.25.2
I
aVR
V1
V4
II
aVL
V2
V5
III
aVF
V3
V6
Fig.25.3
aVR
V1
V4
II
aVL
V2
V5
III
aVF
V3
V6

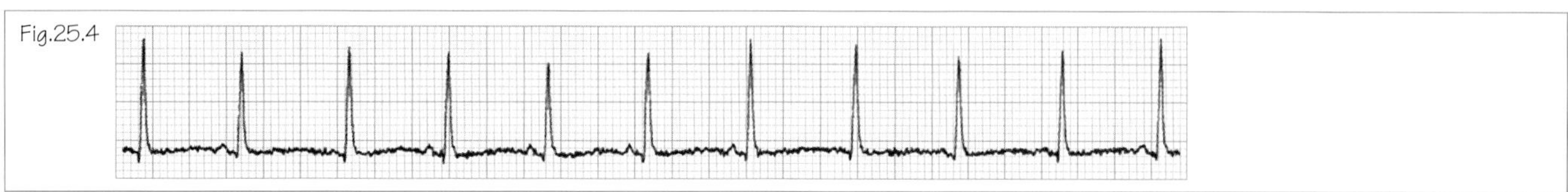

Shock is 'low blood pressure with evidence of organ malperfusion'; recognized by cold skin, confusion and low urine output. It is common and has a high mortality. The causes include:

- Primary cardiac causes, with a low cardiac output. The patient is cool, with high left atrial pressures (pulmonary oedema and breathlessness) and right-sided pressures (increased jugular venous pressure; peripheral oedema). Causes include valve disease (acute, e.g. rupture of aortic or mitral valve due to endocarditis, or chronic, e.g. decompensated aortic stenosis, myocardial infarction [MI], pericardial effusion with tamponade, and pulmonary emboli).
- Sepsis, especially gram-negative septicaemia.
- Hypovolaemia, especially from gastrointestinal bleeding.
- Miscellaneous causes including Addisonian crisis and spinal trauma.

Management

The key principle is to rapidly establish the cause and institute treatment. For diagnosis, in addition to the history and physical examination, investigations help particularly the ECG, cardiac ultrasound and blood tests.

The ECG in shock

- Normal: a cardiac cause is unlikely.
- Sinus tachycardia, a common non-specific finding. Patients with septic shak often feel warm, whereas in cardiogenic shock they often have cool skin. Occasionally shock relates to myocarditis (Fig. 25.2), where the diagnostic clue is a tachycardia out of proportion to the haemodynamic disturbance. The ECG usually shows other changes, including ST flattening/depression, T wave inversion, conducting tissue disease or, much more rarely, ST elevation.
- Arrhythmias commonly complicate but infrequently cause shock (unless other factors are present):
  (a) Very fast heart rate in some cases of atrial fibrillation (AF) with Wolff–Parkinson–White (WPW) syndrome (Fig. 25.3).
  (b) Ventricular tachycardia (VT) with structural heart disease (e.g. post-MI monomorphic VT) or if very disorganized (e.g. polymorphic VT).
  (c) Modest arrhythmias may cause shock if there is pre-existing cardiac dysfunction e.g. AF with severe left ventricular (LV) dysfunction.
  (d) Profound bradycardia, e.g. heart block. Drugs (beta-blockers, etc.) can cause shock with bradycardia if myocardial depression is also present (e.g. drug overdose, severe intrinsic myocardial disease). Hypothermia causes shock with bradycardia and a prominent late notch on the QRS complex, the 'Osborne wave'.
- Acute myocardial infarction is a common cause, easily recognized if ST elevation or widespread Q waves are present (Fig. 25.1), less easily diagnosed if the infarction is posterior (ECG changes can be subtle) or in the 70% of infarcts not associated with ST elevation (non-ST segment elevation myocardial infarctions [NSTEMIs]), which have a lower but still significant chance of progressing to shock than a ST segment elevation myocardial infarction (STEMI), especially in the elderly or diabetics (see Chapters 30 and 31). It is important to determine the mechanism of shock, as some forms are treatable: (i) balloon angioplasty with stent insertion, supported with an intra-aortic balloon pump, or coronary artery bypass graft (CABG) for myocardial ischaemia; (ii) mitral valve surgery for acute mitral regurgitation; (iii) surgical/percutaneous closure for a ventricular septal defect.
- Left ventricular hypertrophy may indicate aortic stenosis (in shock the typical murmur may be very quiet or absent, and the real clue to the diagnosis is from the ECG), hypertensive herat disease or cardiomyopathy. A cardiac ultrasound usually clarifies the diagnosis, and should be undertaken immediately, as aortic valve replacement in decompensated aortic stenosis is life saving.
- Small QRS complexes, with a sinus tachycardia (more rarely, atrial fibrillation) may indicate a pericardial effusion and cardiac tamponade (Fig. 25.4). A rare sign of pericardial tamponade is QRS alternans, i.e. beat-to-beat variation in the size of the QRS complex, due to the beat-to-beat swinging of the heart in the fluid-filled pericardial space.
- Left bundle branch block is a common finding, and does not give any aetiologic clues. It may indicate underlying heart muscle disease (dilated cardiomyopathy, advanced ischaemic heart failure or indeed LV dysfunction of any aetiology), acute MI, or just coincidental conducting tissue disease.
- Right bundle branch block often has no particular meaning, but may indicate a pulmonary embolism (look for sinus tachycardia, right axis deviation), or, more rarely, an atrial septal defect.

Fig. 25.1 Gross anterior wall myocardial infarction, major ST elevation in leads I, aVL, leads V2–6. ST depression in leads III and aVF ('reciprocal' changes). The patient had cardiogenic shock due to a proximal occlusion of the left anterior descending (LAD) coronary artery and underwent a successful primary percutaneous coronary intervention (PCI).

Fig. 25.2 Myocarditis. Sinus tachycardia, heart rate 91 b/min, non-specifically abnormal P wave, normal PR interval, good voltage QRS complexes throughout. T wave inversion, deep, in leads V1–3; ST depression V4–6. This ECG could have many causes, including ischaemic heart disease, pulmonary emboli (sinus tachycardia, and right heart strain appearance in leads V1–3). However, this patient had a severe myocarditis.

Fig. 25.3 Not an easy ECG. Gross tachycardia, heart rate ±180 b/min, irregular, suggesting atrial fibrillation. Broad QRS of 200 ms. Slurred upstroke in leads V5/6, left axis deviation, apparent Q waves in the inferior leads. This is Wolff–Parkinson–White syndrome, with 'pre-excited' atrial fibrillation. The heart rhythm and low blood pressure responded to DC cardioversion.

Fig. 25.4 Rhythm strip showing varying height of the R wave, termed QRS alternans, due to a large pericardial effusion with cardiac tamponade.

26 Stroke

Fig.26.1

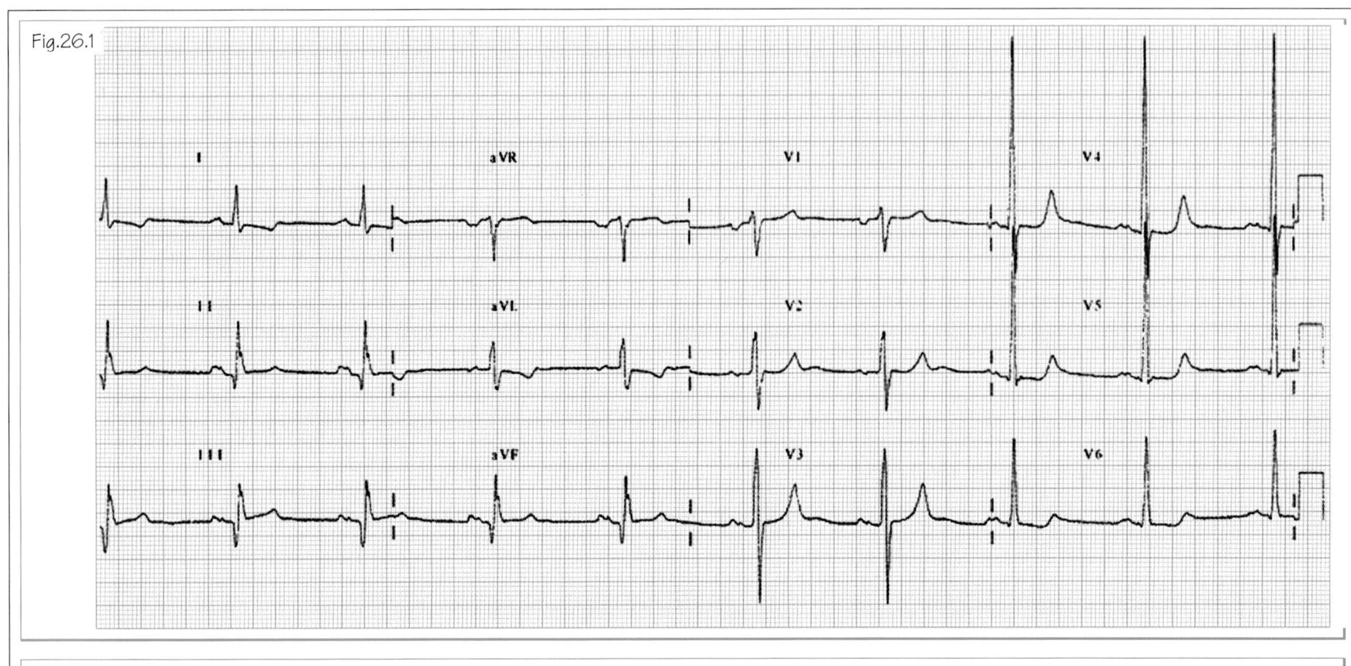

Fig.26.2

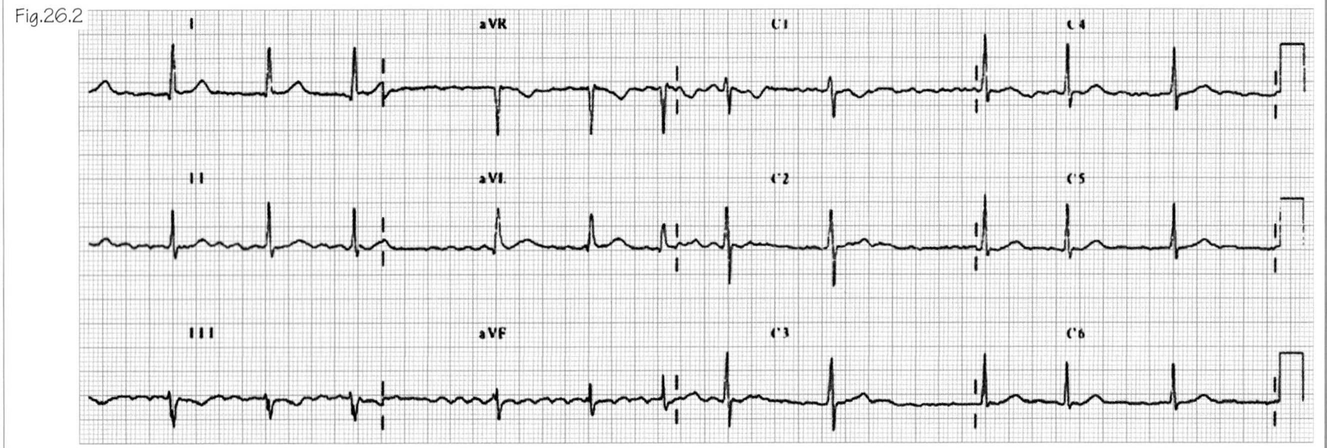

Fig.26.3

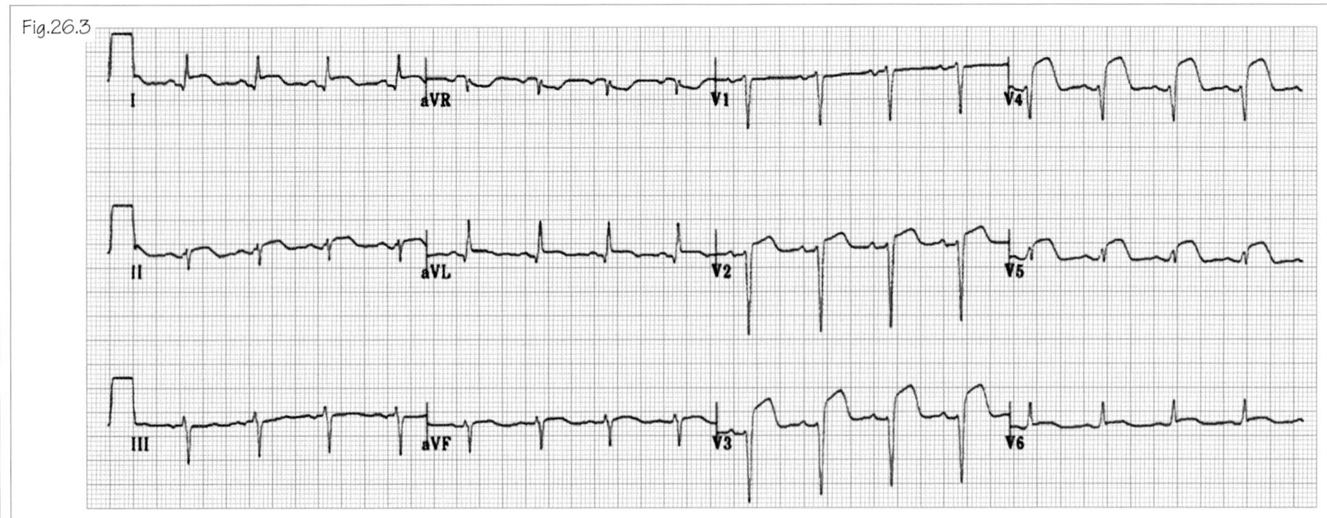

Stroke is a common disabling condition. The ECG can help determine aetiology; sometimes it changes as the consequence of stroke.

Aetiological clues to stroke from the ECG

• Left ventricular hypertrophy (LVH) (Fig. 26.1) is an important risk factor for stroke, partly as it is very strongly associated with prolonged hypertension (itself associated with stroke), and partly for other little understood reasons (meta-analyses suggest that LVH is an risk factor for stroke, independent of other confounders such as hypertension).

• Atrial fibrillation (Fig. 26.2) is a powerful risk factor for stroke, particularly in the elderly, those with hypertension, and those with structural heart disease. It usually needs to be present for ≥ 24 h to cause stroke. It is often present at the time of hospitalization for the acute stroke though some data suggests that it may be intermittent, and should be screened for in all those who present with stroke with an initial ECG showing sinus rhythm.

• Myocardial infarction (MI), especially transmural infarction in the early stages, is a potent risk factor for stroke (Fig. 26.3). Usually the MI is obvious, and causes typical symptoms, and either ST elevation or Q waves are seen on the ECG. Sometimes it is silent, and the ECG changes may be subtle; loss of R wave height, or ST/T wave changes only.

• Left ventricular (LV) dysfunction, especially if associated with heart failure, is another important risk factor for stroke. The ECG clues to LV dysfunction are:

(a) The ECG is not normal or nearly normal! Most cases of systolic LV dysfunction have major ECG abnormalities, the absence of which makes LV dysfunction unlikely.

(b) Q waves are present.

(c) Conducting tissue is present – this is particularly so in the dilated cardiomyopathies. This can be right or more typically left bundle branch block.

• Patent foramen ovale (PFO) is a risk factor for stroke, especially in the younger patient, if associated with an atrial septal aneurysm with right to left shunting (demonstrated on transthoracic cardiac ultrasound bubble study imaging). Though most patients with PFOs have a normal ECG, a small number have a curious M-shaped bifid notch on the ascending branch, or on the zenith, of the R wave in inferior ECG leads (II, III, aVF), called 'crochetage'.

ECG consequences of stroke

A stroke can induce ECG changes. This is reputed to be commonest with sub-arachnoid hemorrhage (SAH), where widespread pan-anterior deep T wave inversion (mimicking a so-called proximal left anterior descending [LAD] -pattern ECG) may occur, reputedly due to the rapid increase in cardiac catecholamines induced by the SAH.

ECG accompaniments to a stroke

Stroke usually occurs in patients with a heavy burden of pre-existing vascular disease. Thus patients who are shown on exercise testing to have asymptomatic ST depression on community screening have a higher risk of strokes than those without such silent myocardial ischaemia. Furthermore, if patients, once they have recovered from the cerebrovascular accident (CVA), undergo exercise stress testing, a high proportion are found to have silent myocardial ischaemia. This emphasizes the need for general cardiovascular risk factor control.

Fig. 26.1 Left ventricular hypertrophy (LVH). Sinus rhythm, broad P wave in lead II, with bifid appearance (P mitrale), and late prominent negative deflection in lead V1, indicating left atrial enlargement. Normal PR interval, normal QRS axis 60°. Increased left ventricular voltages, with R in V4 = 40 mm, in V5 = 34 mm, S in V3 = 18 mm (so R V5 + S V3 = 52 mm); the voltage criteria for LVH in the praecordial leads are substantially exceeded (see Chapters 8 and 24) though interestingly not in the standard leads. Repolarization abnormalities with 'reverse-tick' ST depression in leads I, II, and early changes in leads V5/6. Prominent inferior lead (II, III, aVF) Q wave, which here are part of the hypertrophic process and do not indicate an old myocardial infarction. Long-standing severe hypertension.

Fig. 26.2 Atrial fibrillation (AF). Marked irregularity to the baseline, with no discernable P waves, and an irregular QRS response indicate that the rhythm is atrial fibrillation. Heart rate, 75 b/min. Unremarkable QRS complexes. Conclusion is AF with no other ECG evidence of heart disease.

Fig. 26.3 Myocardial infarction (MI). Sinus rhythm, unremarkable P waves, normal PR interval. QRS complex show left axis deviation (–38°; positive in lead I, negative in lead II and III). Very deep S wave in leads V1–4, with just a tiny preceding R wave – in practical terms, these are the same as pathological Q waves. ST elevation in lead I, II (just), aVL, V2–5, indicating an evolving antero-lateral MI. Conclusion: recent (≤ 1 or 2 days) anterior wall MI. Some 1% of untreated MIs are complicated by a stroke, a risk reduced by streptokinase.

27 Emotion and the ECG

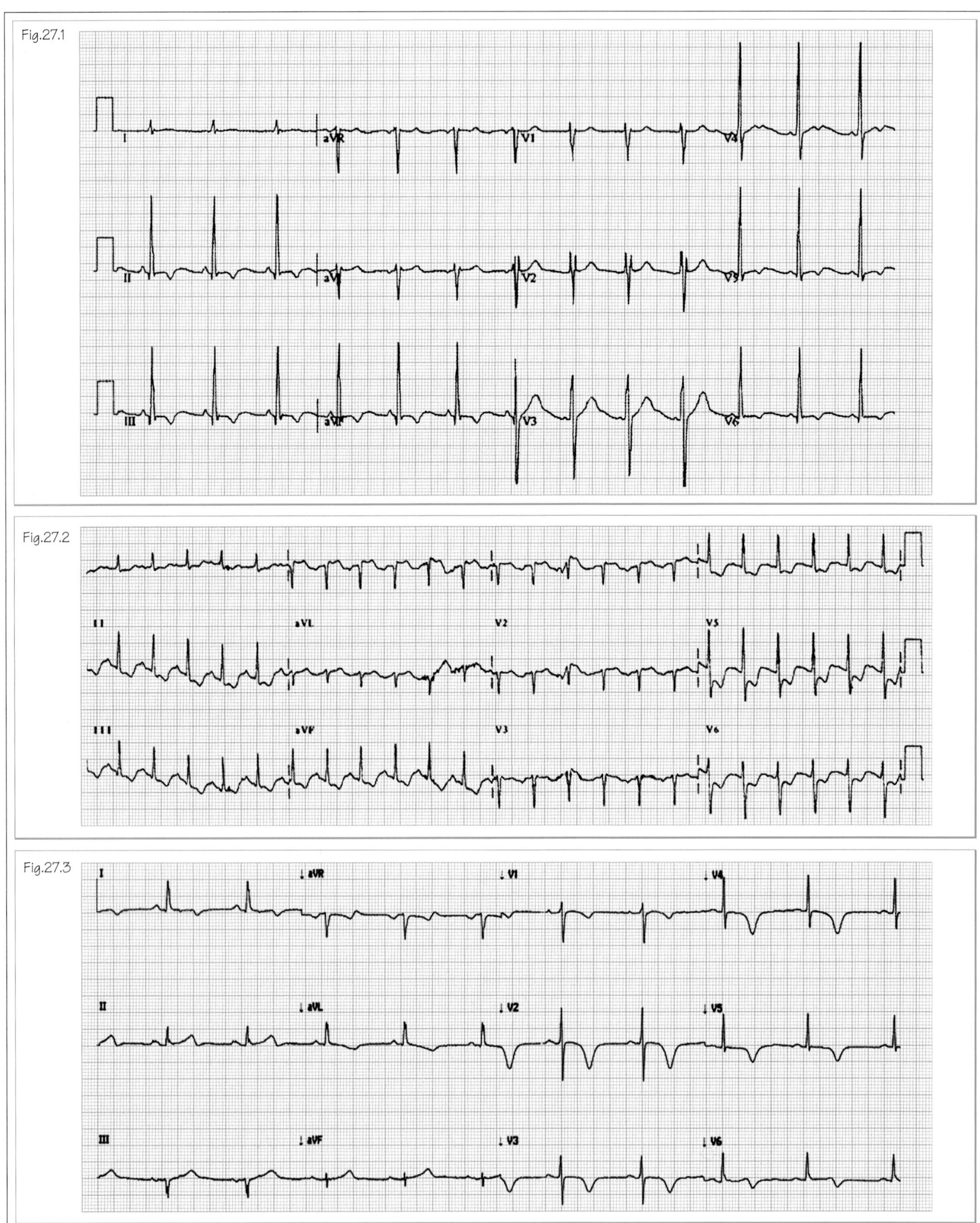

Emotion can affect the ECG

Emotion can affect the ECG two ways:

- Firstly, by causing asymptomatic ECG changes, leading to an erroneous diagnosis of heart disease. These changes are limited to ST/T wave changes (i.e. not involving the development of a Q wave, or changes to the QRS complex).
- Secondly, much more rarely, by causing 'organic' cardiac disease, such as 'standard' myocardial infarction, arrhythmias or the syndrome of transient left ventricular dysfunction.

Diagnostic difficulties

An extraordinary common difficult problem in clinical practice is to decide whether an abnormal ECG reflects cardiac pathology or not, with the ECG changes being explained by anxiety or hyperventilation.

Anxiety-related ECG changes

Anxiety can profoundly alter the ECG, probably via changes in autonomic nervous system function, as evidenced by the ECG normalizing with manoeuvres that normalize autonomic function (reassurance, rest, and anxiolytics and beta-blockers), with catecholamine infusion producing similar ECG changes. The ECG changes in anxiety are:

- ST flattening, the commonest finding.
- Frank ST depression; not rare, especially in hyperventilation.
- T wave inversion

How does one differentiate anxiety-induced changes from those reflecting cardiac disease? Fully assessing demographics (age, sex, etc.) and symptomatology are the keys to a correct diagnosis. Though one can often be fairly confident that some patterns are due to anxiety, one cannot always be 100% certain, so it is not uncommon to undertake further limited investigations to exclude heart disease, always explaining beforehand that the result is likely to negative, and the test is required only for reassurance.

ST elevation and emotion

1 Emotion can provoke ST segment elevation myocardial infarctions (STEMIs) in pre-existing coronary artery disease.

2 Tako-tsubo syndrome: rare, in elderly women, where stress induces reversible left ventricular dysfunction of a specific pattern extending beyond the territory supplied by one coronary artery (affecting parts of the anterior wall and apical region) giving the appearance of a Japanese octopus pot, the Tako-tsubo. The syndrome is not due to atheromatous/thrombotic coronary disease. It is provoked by emotional or physical stress and results in chest pain, hospital admission, sometimes cardiogenic shock. The admission ECG shows ST segment elevation in leads V3–6, evolving in 3 days to deep T wave inversion, T wave flattening, and then further deepening at 2–3 weeks (Fig 27.3). Cardiac specific enzyme rise is low and left ventricular dysfunction improves ≤ 2 weeks.

Hyperventilation-related ECG changes

The ECG can change markedly with hyperventilation:

- Ten per cent of normal subjects who forcibly hyperventilate develop some form of T wave inversion, characteristically biphasic T waves, symmetrically inverted T's, and downsloping ST segment depression.
- In coronary artery disease hyperventilation leads some to develop ST depression.
- In severe coronary disease with spontaneous chest pain and ST elevation, deliberate marked hyperventilation provokes painful episodes with ST elevation in 50%. Ten per cent of similar patients develop coronary spasm and ST elevation with physical stress, e.g. hard handgrip exercises or placing their forearm in ice water.
- In patients with spontaneous chest pain with ST segment elevation, and angiographically normal coronary arteries (Prinzmetal angina), hyperventilation can induce angina, chest pain and, at angiography, diffuse coronary spasm.

Hyperventilation syndrome

Patients with the acute hyperventilation syndrome (AHS) present obviously breathless, agitated, with weakness, parasthesias and possibly syncope. Chest pain (atypical for angina) may occur. Examination may show distress, visible hyperventilation and carpopedal spasm. The ECG can show prolonged QT interval, ST elevation or depression, or T wave inversion. Arterial blood gases are diagnostic.

In chronic hyperventilation syndrome (CHS) the overbreathing is not overt; patients present with breathlessness and chest pain ('neurocirculatory asthenia'), with multiple other symptoms and negative investigation. Arterial blood gas is abnormal in two thirds, with low $P\text{CO}_2$ and normal pH due to renal compensation. The ECG changes are as for AHS.

Arrhythmias and emotion

- Long QT interval dependent arrhythmias can be provoked by emotion/stress (e.g. auditory). Sudden noise (e.g. an alarm clock), on top of sleep-induced bradycardia prolonging an already long QT interval in hereditary long QT syndrome, results in an alerting response, a catecholamine surge and torsade-de-pointes type ventricular tachycardia, resulting in syncope or death.
- Extreme anxiety can cause sudden cardiac death from malignant ventricular arrhythmia), both in subjects with normal hearts (though occult pro-arrhythmic genetic diseases may be present) and in pro-arrhythmic conditions, especially left ventricular dysfunction.

Fig. 27.1 Anxiety-induced ST changes/QT interval prolongation. Non-cardiac chest pain and anxiety. Sinus rhythm, normal P wave, prominent QRS voltages (young/thin patient), abnormal ST segments with inferior lead (II, II and aVF) T wave inversion, extending laterally (V5/6), and bizarre bifid T wave in lead V4, with a long QT interval (520 ms, corrected to 620 ms). Interpretations to this ECG that should be actively excluded: left ventricular hypertrophy, infero-lateral ischaemia (? right coronary artery), long QT syndrome (possibly genetic). After further investigation, it was concluded that the T wave/QT changes were induced by hyperventilation.

Fig. 27.2 Anxiety-induced ST depression. Sinus tachycardia heart rate 150 b/min, with a P wave preceding each R wave. Normal P wave, PR interval, QRS complexes. Dramatic downward sloping ST depression laterally (V4–6), and inferiorly (II, III, aVF). There are many explanations of such an ECG. The patient was prone to anxiety, recovering from orthopaedic surgery when this ECG was taken; pulmonary emboli is a real possibility, as is myocardial ischaemia, and these must both be excluded. The diagnosis turned out to be anxiety induced ECG changes, with the immediate post-episode ECG being normal.

Fig. 27.3 Tako-tsubo syndrome. Woman with chest pain, small troponin rise. Pan-anterior (I, aVL, V1–6) deep symmetrical T wave inversion. High-grade left anterior descending (LAD) lesion *must* be angiographically excluded; the ventriculogram confirmed the typical contractile abnormality.

28 Sudden cardiac death

Fig.28.1

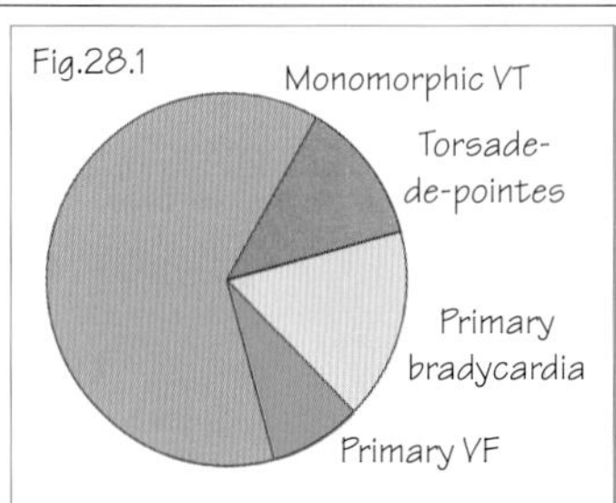

Fig.28.2

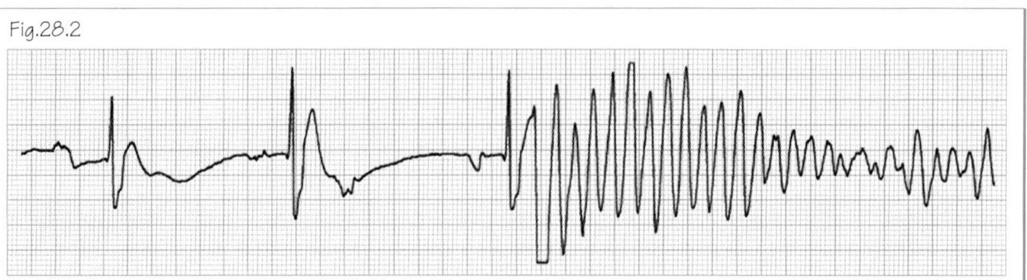

Fig.28.3

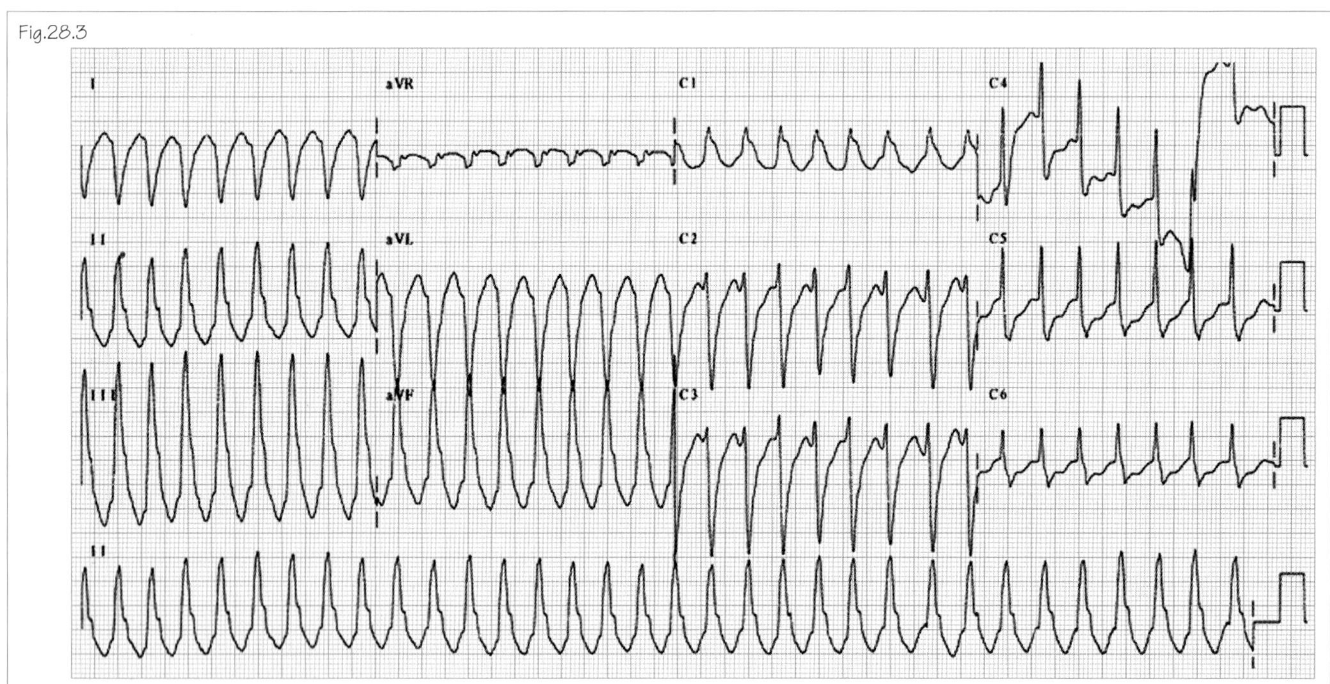

Fig.28.4

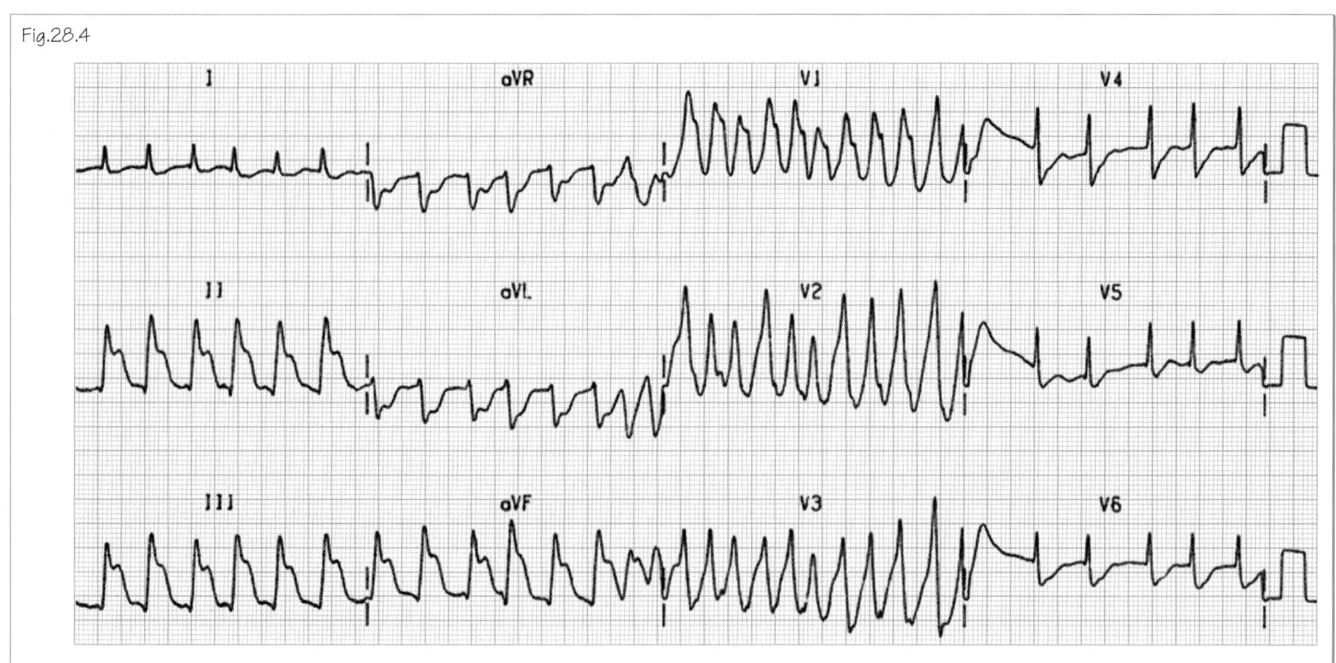

Sudden cardiac death (SCD) arises from a sudden loss of heart function, resulting in death within 1h. It accounts for 50% of cardiac deaths.

Mechanisms and management of SCD

Most SCD relates to ventricular arrhythmias. A few cases relate to primary bradyarrhythmias (Fig. 28.1). Most ventricular tachycardia/ ventricular fibrillation (VT/VF) relates to coronary disease, 25% to heart failure/cardiomyopathy and 5% to aortic stenosis. Other rarer non-arrhythmic causes of SCD include pump failure from large myocardial infarctions (MIs), pulmonary embolisms and exsanguination or pericardial tamponade from aortic dissection. Some non-cardiac conditions cause sudden death, but by definition not sudden *cardiac* death, e.g. large strokes, brisk gastrointestinal bleeds, etc.

All arrhythmias associated with a loss of cardiac output clearly require immediate treatment. A few can be resuscitated: those due to bradyarrhythmias require pacing, those with tachyarrhythmias require determination of the underlying cardiac disease and requirement for specific treatment, and often also anti-tachycardic device therapy.

Cardiac conditions underlying SCD

- Ischaemic heart disease (IHD) without previous infarction underlies SCD either when new infarction/ischaemia provokes VT/VF (more likely in those with left ventricular hypertropy [LVH]) or causes the loss of so much myocardium that cardiac output cannot be sustained.
- Ishaemic heart disease with remote MI:
  - The MI-related scar provides a substrate for a re-entry circuit allowing sustained monomorphic VT, which degenerates into VF. Such a scar delays normal depolarization and marginally prolongs the QRS complex. This can be seen as a late positive deflection on a highly amplified averaged QRS complex (a '*late potential*' from a signal averaged ECG [SAECG], where 100–1000 beats are averaged to improve the signal to noise ratio). Most patients with monomorphic VT have late potentials; most patients with late potentials do not have VT. Factors in addition to late potentials are needed for VT, including new ischaemia, hypokalaemia (possibly through QT interval lengthening), and abnormal autonomic function, amongst others.
  - The chance of VT/VF relates inversely to LV function.
- Left ventricular dysfunction from any non-IHD cause is a powerful substrate for VT/VF, though the risk is less than for those with post-MI LV dysfunction.
- Aortic stenosis.
- Cardiomyopathy (hypertrophic, right ventricular and other rare ones).
- Primary electrical abnormalities, including long QT syndromes, Brugada syndrome and Wolff–Parkinson–White syndrome.
- Pro-arrhythmic drugs are a common and under-recognized cause of ventricular arrhythmias, especially in acquired long QT syndrome.

ECG risk-markers for SCD

The greatest individual risk is in those with impaired LV function and:

- Prolonged QRS duration, the broader the higher the risk.
- Prolonged QT interval, if marked, is associated with an arrhythmic tendency.
- Frequent ventricular arrhythmias; VPC rate correlate weakly with SCD post-MI; non-sustained VT correlates more strongly.
- 'Late-potentials', a necessary but not sufficient condition in post-MI related SCD.
- Autonomic imbalance, as measured by low 24-h heart rate variability (see Chapter 63), identifies an 'at-risk' population.
- Electrophysiology studies: in those with impaired LV function, ambient non-sustained VT and inducible VT not suppressible with drugs, the subsequent risk of SCD is high.

Long QT syndromes

Long QT syndromes underlie SCD due to torsade-de-pointes (TDP) ventricular tachycardia. The QT interval reflects action potential duration (APD), and when APD is prolonged, QT interval lengthens. Pathological APD prolongation promotes afterdepolarizations (see Chapter 38) that provoke or underlie sustained ventricular arrhythmias (especially TDP). Afterdepolarizations are commonest when the QT interval is longest, i.e. low heart rate or at night and are promoted by adrenergic switch-on. There are two forms of long QT syndrome:

1 *Hereditary long QT syndrome*, rare, affects 1 in 10 000; crucially, you must think of this condition not to miss this dangerous diagnosis (see Chapter 39).

2 *Acquired long QT syndrome*, common. Often due to a process/demographics (e.g. LV dysfunction, critical coronary disease, hypokalaemia, renal failure/old age, female sex, etc) when a QT interval-lengthening drug is added. Torsade-de-pointes in long QT syndromes is unrelated to arrhythmic scars, and so occurs in those without late potentials. A common 'initiating' sequence for TDP in long QT syndromes is 'short, long, short'; i.e. 'short' due to an ectopic, long from the post-extrasystolic compensatory period (which lengthens an already long QT interval), short from the first TDP beat. Treatment is cardioversion for TDP, removal of any underlying cause in acquired long QT syndrome. TDP can sometimes be prevented by a pacemaker, by preventing long RR intervals. Perhaps paradoxically, beta-blockers are used, especially in hereditary long QT syndrome, emphasizing the importance of adrenergic stimuli in provoking arrhythmias.

Fig. 28.1 The majority of the arrhythmias underlying sudden cardiac death are ventricular tachyarrhythmias, largely sustained monomorphic ventricular tachycardia (VT), though with a significant contribution from torsade-de-pointes VT and primary ventricular fibrillation (VF) (primary = arrhythmia that occurred first, secondary = arrhythmia following on from the primary arrhythmia). A small number are due to high-grade heart block.
Fig. 28.2 Coronary care unit (CCU) monitoring showing bradycardia, rhythm uncertain (possibly sinus with a long PR interval, possibly heart block), then a very fast and disorganized ventricular arrhythmia, losing amplitude quickly and degenerating into ventricular fibrillation.
Fig. 28.3 Broad complex tachycardia. P waves cannot be seen. The ventricular complexes are of one shape (monomorphic), broad with right axis deviation. The V1 complex is positive (i.e. shows a positive not negative deflection), with the initial deflection being the most positive (quite unlike right bundle branch block, where there is a late large positive deflection). These appearances are virtually pathognomonic of ventricular tachycardia
Fig. 28.4 Initial rhythm uncertain, possibly atrial fibrillation (fast slightly irregular RR intervals). Massive ST elevation inferiorly (leads II, III, aVF) indicative of inferior ST segment elevation myocardial infarction (STEMI). When the ECG recording of leads V1–3 was made, a fast, moderately organized arrhythmia occurred – this is a burst of ischaemically mediated ventricular tachycardia.

29 Acute coronary syndromes

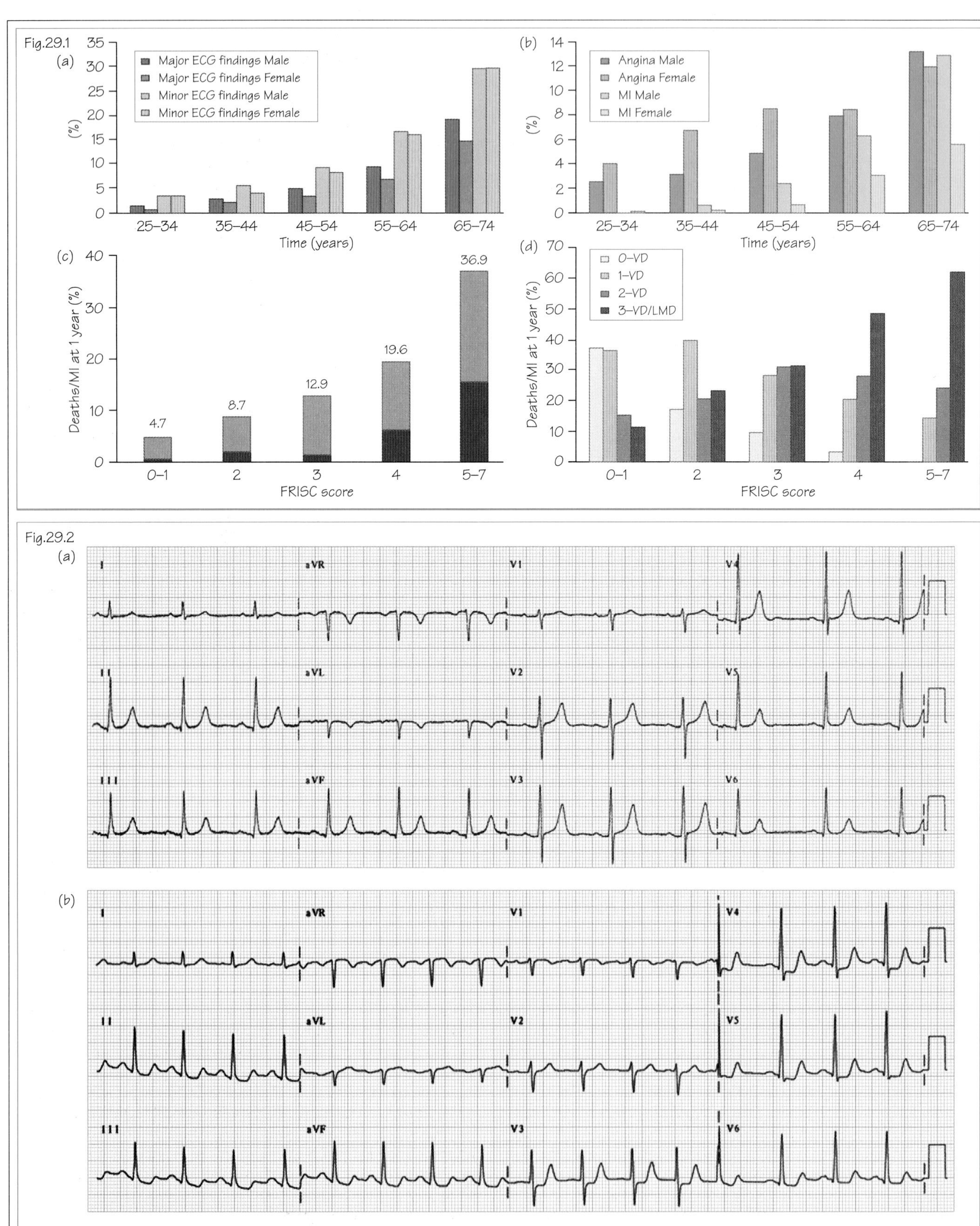
Fig.29.1
(a)
Major ECG findings Male
Major ECG findings Female
Minor ECG findings Male
Minor ECG findings Female
(%)
0
5
10
15
20
25
30
35
25–34
35–44
45–54
55–64
65–74
Time (years)
(b)
Angina Male
Angina Female
MI Male
MI Female
(%)
0
2
4
6
8
10
12
14
25–34
35–44
45–54
55–64
65–74
Time (years)
(c)
Deaths/MI at 1 year (%)
0
10
20
30
40
4.7
8.7
12.9
19.6
36.9
0–1
2
3
4
5–7
FRISC score
(d)
0-VD
1-VD
2-VD
3-VD/LMD
Deaths/MI at 1 year (%)
0
10
20
30
40
50
60
70
0–1
2
3
4
5–7
FRISC score
Fig.29.2
(a)
I
aVR
V1
V4
II
aVL
V2
V5
III
aVF
V3
V6
(b)
I
aVR
V1
V4
II
aVL
V2
V5
III
aVF
V3
V6

Acute coronary syndromes (ACSs) are due to thrombus within a coronary artery that: (i) transiently or permanently occludes the vessel; and (ii) can break up, so embolizing fragments to the distal myocardium. Vessel occlusion and distal embolization account for the cardinal clinical feature, ischaemic chest pain *at rest*. Though the thrombus can resolve spontaneously without harm, the clot has the potential to abruptly close the vessel, leading to infarction and death. Some ACSs have a high mortality, others only a small increase; the ECG is one factor that can be used: (i) to diagnose the presence of an ACS; and (ii) to differentiate risk. A basic scheme of ACS, depending on the presentation ECG and troponin levels, is as follows:

- Troponin negative ACS, associated with any ECG finding except ST segment elevation.
- Non-ST segment elevation myocardial infarction (NSTEMI), by definition troponin is raised. Any ECG change can occur, including transient *self-resolving* ST segment elevation.
- ST segment elevation myocardial infarction (STEMI) where, by definition, ST elevation due to myocardial ischaemia occurs. Without treatment, usually, a full thickness Q wave myocardial infarction (MI) occurs. If resolution occurs without Q waves or loss of R wave height, and no/minor troponin release (a rare occurrence) then the syndrome is a 'threatened STEMI' (no treatment given) or 'aborted STEMI' (treatment given). If the ST elevation gives way to significant loss of R wave height without Q waves, it is a 'partial thickness MI', whereas if the STEMI proceeds to Q waves, it is a 'full thickness' MI.

The ECG in ACS

The ECG in suspected ACS is used to confirm or refute the diagnosis, to guide therapy, and to estimate prognosis.

Diagnostic role of the ECG

Though it can be exceptionally easy to diagnose an ACS, it can be very difficult. The clinical features increasing the probability of ACS are:

- Major risk factors for vascular disease, or cocaine use.
- Pain typical for myocardial ischaemia, i.e. retrosternal tightness/heaviness, possibly radiating to the neck, arm(s), the back. Sweating with pain increases the chance of an MI.
- If symptoms are similar to previous unequivocal MI, or clear cut effort dependent angina then the diagnosis is easy.
- Pain occurs in episodes lasting < 20 min; longer than this, and either a myocardial infarction is occurring (the ECG is abnormal), or the pain is non-cardiac (the ECG is often normal).
- Abnormal ECGs raise the probability of an ACS, but rarely 'clinch' the diagnosis (the exception is in STEMI). ECG abnormalities are more diagnostically helpful in younger patients, as older people often have non-relevant ECG abnormalities (Figs 29.1a–d & 29.2a,b).
- An exercise test reproducing symptoms with ECG changes (e.g. planar or downsloping ST depression). On occasions it can be difficult to know if symptoms arise from the heart; this may need further evaluation by coronary angiography.

Therapeutic role of the ECG

Acute coronary syndromes with ST segment elevation benefit from thrombolysis; all other ACSs do not, rather requiring intense anti-platelet therapy. If the risk of an adverse outcome is high (see Fig. 29.1c) then early angiography with a view to revascularization is appropriate.

Prognostic role of the ECG

It is crucial to estimate prognosis in ACSs, using risk-scoring systems. Factors associated with an adverse outcome are:

- Increasing age, male sex, diabetes.
- Resting ECG changes (see Fig. 29.1a–d): ST depression and elevation have surprisingly similar and adverse outcomes. In those with normal ECGs, further risk stratification is obtained from the exercise ECG.
- Troponin rise.

Fig. 29.1 (a) ECG findings in the general population. Major ECG changes (ST depression, T wave inversion, second or third atrioventricular (AV) block, complete left or right bundle branch block, frequent premature beats, atrial fibrillation or flutter) and minor changes (borderline Q wave, left or right axis deviation, QRS high voltage, borderline ST segment depression, T wave flattening, QRS low voltage) increase with age. (b) Incidence of angina and myocardial infarction (MI); both increase with age. Note high rates of angina in young women, with low MI rates; much anginal-type chest pain in women does not relate to ischaemic heart disease (IHD). Ischaemic heart disease incidence is lower than major/minor ECG changes, i.e. ECG abnormalities are not exclusively related to IHD, so minor changes cannot be relied on to confirm a diagnosis of IHD. (c) Outcome in acute coronary syndromes (ACS) from the FRISC (fragmin during instability in coronary disease) study. One point for each of: age > 70 years, male sex, diabetes, previous MI, ST segment depression on admission ECG, increased concentrations of markers of myocardial damage or inflammation. Outcome plotted against risk score (death in dark purple shade, MI in light purple shade); the higher the score, the worse the outcome. (d) Patients with higher scores have more severe coronary disease at angiography. Troponin (like the ECG) is just one amongst many risk factors, i.e. troponin negative patients can still be at high risk, as can patients with a normal resting ECG. Some patients at low risk have severe coronary disease, and indeed an adverse outcome. VD, vessels significantly diseased; LMD, left main stem disease.

Fig. 29.2 ECG in acute coronary syndromes (ACSs). A patient admitted with acute chest pain, initially pain free (a); later in pain (b). Admission ECG virtually normal; there is a dominant (i.e. upright) T wave in lead V1 (sometimes this indicates an acute circumflex lesion). The ECG during chest pain shows widespread ST depression, downsloping in the inferior leads, planar in the antero-lateral leads. In ACS, ST depression of 1 or 2 mm increases 1-year mortality respectively by six and 10-fold. The ST depression here is 1 mm, is extensive and involves the anterior chest leads (another independent predictor of poor outcome). With such ECG changes, regardless of other risk factors, early angiography with a view to revascularization is appropriate.

30 Non-ST segment elevation myocardial infarction

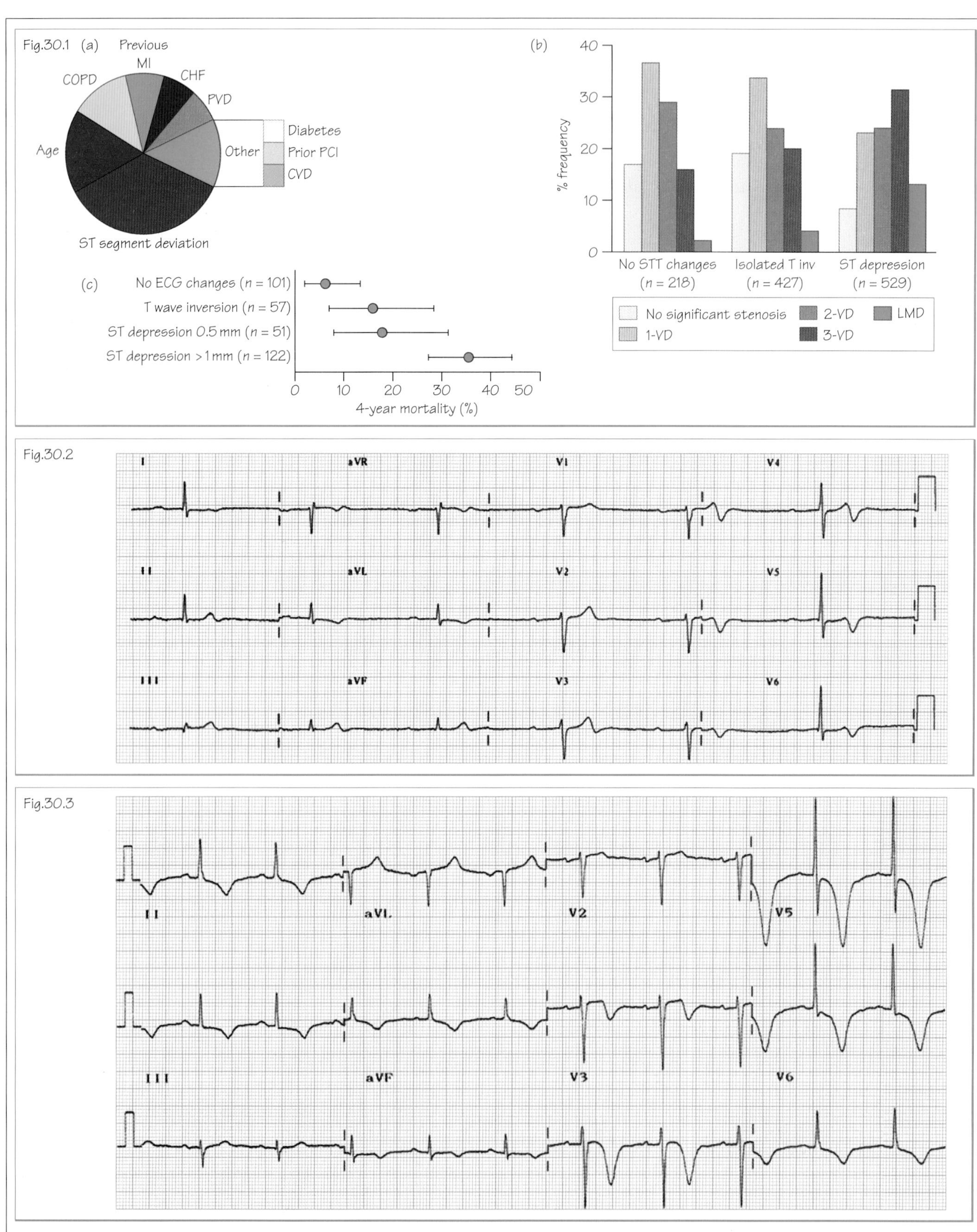

Non-ST segment elevation myocardial infactions (NSTEMIs) are diagnosed when a patient presents with ischaemic chest pain, occurring at rest, associated with a raised troponin. The ECG can show any pattern, except ST elevation (the diagnosis is then ST segment elevation MI [STEMI] – see Chapter 31). It is important to repeat the ECG frequently in NSTEMIs, as:

- This can help confirm the diagnosis – patients with fluctuating ECG changes are more likely to have an acute coronary syndrome (ACS) than those with an unchanging ECG (regardless of whether the ECG is 'fixed' in a normal pattern, or 'fixed' in an abnormal pattern). However, be aware that some fluctuating ECG changes relate to anxiety, and the metabolic disarray induced by hyperventilation.
- Patients can develop an ST elevation syndrome despite initially presenting with a non-ST elevation syndrome. ST elevation merits immediate aggressive reperfusion therapy (thrombolysis or percutaneous intervention).

ECG patterns in NSTEMIs

- Normal ECG is possible (and increasingly recognized due to the widespread availability of highly sensitive markers of myocardial necrosis). A normal ECG maybe due to the involvement of a small branch of the coronary circulation or to posterior wall ischaemia. Do not assume however that a normal ECG with a raised troponin is due to minor or single vessel coronary artery disease (CAD), always investigate for more major coronary disease. However be aware that a persistently normal ECG with frequent episodes of chest pain raises the possibility that the pains are not due to myocardial ischaemia. If the troponin is not raised, then there is a wide differential diagnosis, with gastro-oesophageal pain being high up on the list. If the troponin is raised, consider pulmonary emboli (the ECG clue are a sinus tachycardia, or more rarely, atrial fibrillation), renal failure and sepsis syndromes.
- T wave flattening, which usually occurs in the distribution of a coronary artery (see Chapter 15).
- T wave inversion, which also occurs in the distribution of a coronary artery. It can be of any severity, though the most typical is deep symmetrical T wave inversion. If it affects leads 1, aVL, V(1)2 to lead V5(6), it is often due to a high-grade stenosis in the proximal part of the left anterior descending (LAD) coronary artery, and is known as a 'LAD syndrome' ECG (Figs 30.2 and 30.3).
- ST depression on the presenting ECG is an ominous sign. It is associated with a high mortality. It can occur in any leads, though usually the distribution reflects the distribution of the coronary arteries. It often fluctuates; as myocardial ischaemia is lessened (nitrates, beta-blockers) the ST segment depression likewise resolves.
- Left bundle branch block is a much more difficult ECG to interpret as this renders the rest of the ECG uninterpretable.

Risk stratification in NSTEMI

There are numerous risk scores available, including the thrombolysis in myocardial infarction (TIMI) NSTEMI score, the global registry of acute coronary events (GRACE) score, the platelet glycoprotein IIb/IIIa in unstable agina; receptor suppression using integrilin therapy trial (PURSUIT) score, the fragimin during instability in coronary disease trial (FRISC) score and the TIMI risk index. All have analysed large databases (trial or registry based) and reached essentially the same conclusion (Fig 30.1); that NSTEMI ACS risk depends on: (i) ECG changes – ST depression is a high-risk situation, the greater the cumulative amount, the higher the risk. (ii) Older age, (iii) lower blood pressure, and (iv) higher heart rate are adverse prognostic features. (v) Troponin relates to outcome, and interacts with age and ECG changes. (vi) Extensive extra-cardiac vascular disease worsens outcome, as do (vii) other co-morbidities (renal failure, chronic obstructive pulmonary disease [COPD]).

Fig. 30.1 (a) This pie chart shows the relative importance of factors influencing long-term mortality and re-infarction in post-myocardial infarction patients (data from the pre-troponin era). Thirty-five per cent of the variation in risk relates to changes in the ECG; simply deduced clinical variables explain much of the remaining risk. CHF, congestive heart failure; COPD, chronic obstructive pulmonary disease; CVD, cardiovascular disease; MI, myocardial infarction; PCI, percutaneous coronary intervention; PVD, peripheral vascular disease. (b) Relationship between ECG changes and angiographic finding in acute coronary syndrome (ACS). ST depression is most likely to be associated with severe coronary disease. VD, vessels significantly diseased; LMD, left main disease. (c) Mortality risk in ACS and ECG findings. ST depression has the highest mortality risk and those with the greatest depression have the highest mortality.

Fig. 30.2 ECG in non-ST segment elevation myocardial infarction (NSTEMI). Sinus bradycardia, heart rate 40 b/min. The P wave shows a late predominantly negative deflection in lead V1 (left atrial enlargement). PR interval markedly lengthened at 320 ms. QRS complexes unremarkable (perhaps generally a bit small). The T wave is flat in lead I, inverted (just) in lead aVL, and biphasic in leads V4–6, i.e. T wave changes laterally. The T wave in lead V1 is upright (as opposed to the normal inversion). This patient has T wave changes only, the distribution of which suggests an acute lesion in a major branch of the circumflex coronary artery, or less likely, a branch of the left anterior descending. The sinus bradycardia suggests good-going beta-blocker therapy (though the heart rate is too slow for beta-blocker therapy to be the only explanation), or sinus node disease (which often relates to disease of the sinus node branch of the right coronary artery). The long PR interval partly relates to the sinus bradycardia, but also suggests intrinsic conducting tissue disease, which could be due to fibrosis, or perhaps right coronary artery disease affecting the conducting tissue.

Fig. 30.3 Pan-anterior T wave inversion – the 'LAD syndrome' ECG. Sinus rhythm, heart rate 63 b/min, normal P wave. Normal QRS axis. Normal R wave height, no pathological Q waves. The T wave in leads I, II, aVL, and leads V2–6 are very abnormal, showing deep symmetrical T wave inversion. This ECG pattern is so suggestive as to be pathognomonic for a lesion in the left anterior descending coronary artery, often in the proximal portion, and is termed the 'LAD syndrome' ECG. It is also found in the very rare condition of Tako-tsubo syndrome (see Chapter 27).

31 ST segment elevation myocardial infarction

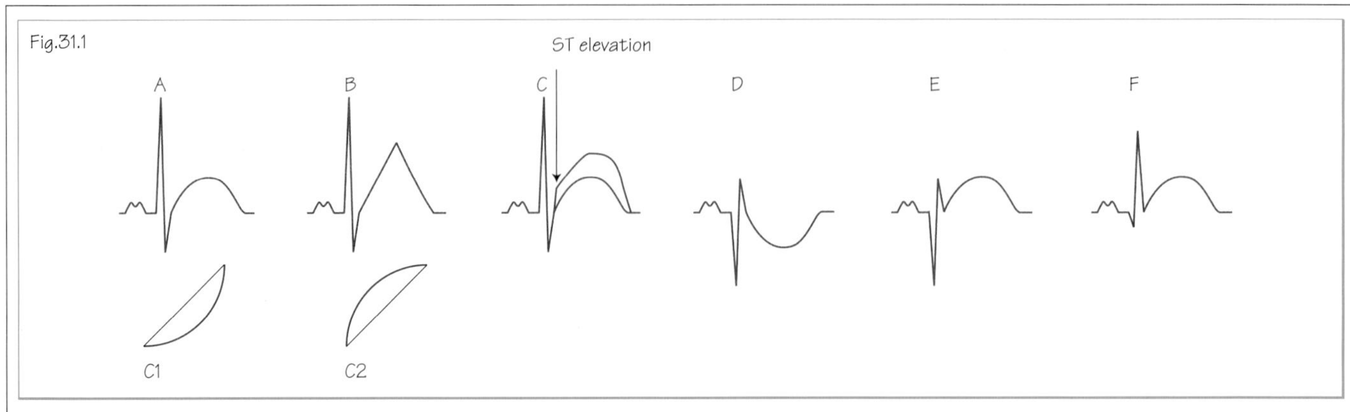

Fig.31.1
ST elevation
A
B
C
D
E
F
C1
C2

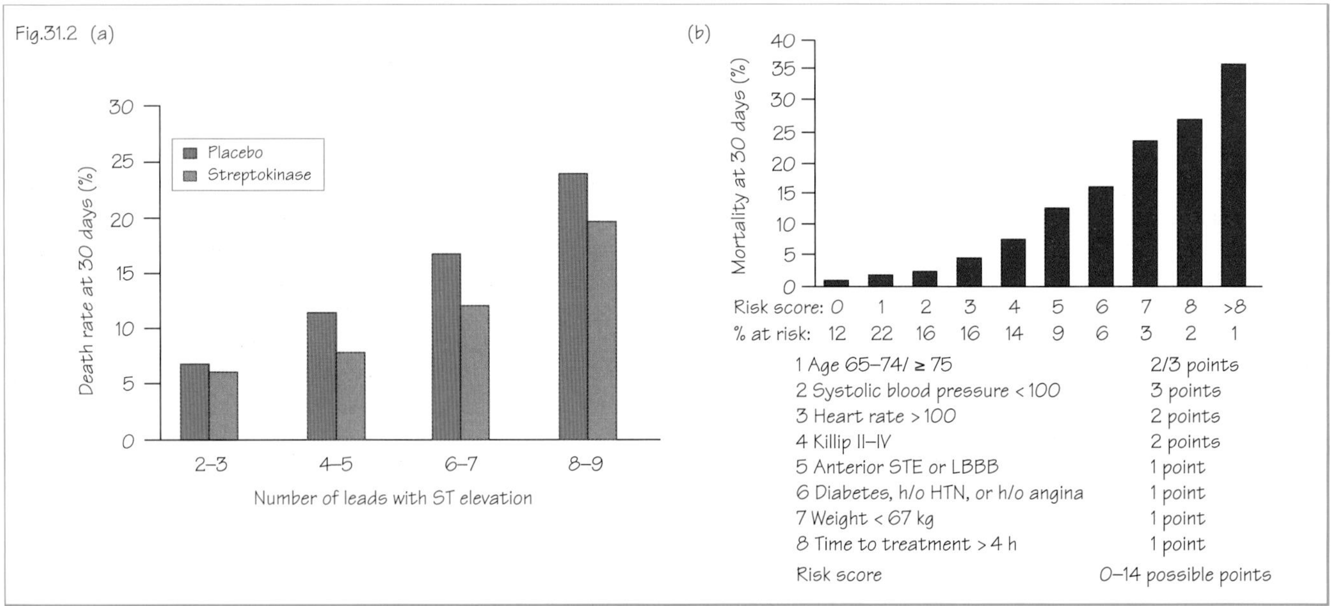

Fig.31.2 (a)
Placebo
Streptokinase
Death rate at 30 days (%)
Number of leads with ST elevation
2–3
4–5
6–7
8–9
(b)
Mortality at 30 days (%)
Risk score: 0 1 2 3 4 5 6 7 8 >8
% at risk: 12 22 16 16 14 9 6 3 2 1
1 Age 65–74/ ≥ 75 2/3 points
2 Systolic blood pressure < 100 3 points
3 Heart rate > 100 2 points
4 Killip II–IV 2 points
5 Anterior STE or LBBB 1 point
6 Diabetes, h/o HTN, or h/o angina 1 point
7 Weight < 67 kg 1 point
8 Time to treatment > 4 h 1 point
Risk score 0–14 possible points

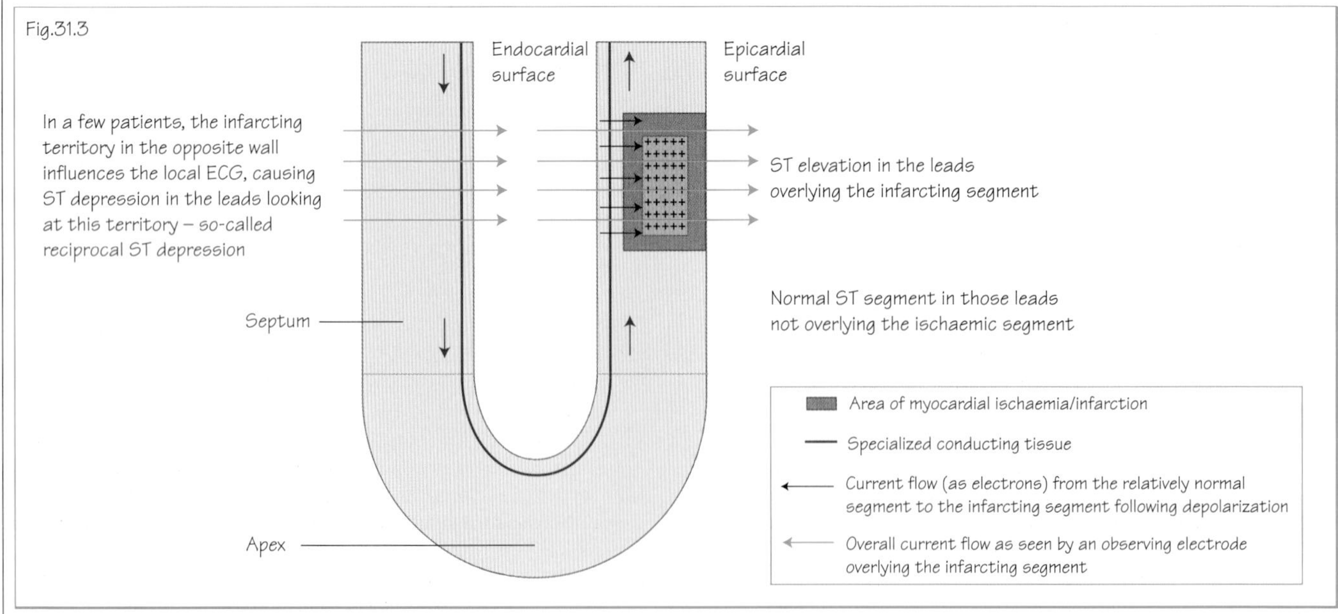

Fig.31.3
Endocardial surface
Epicardial surface
In a few patients, the infarcting territory in the opposite wall influences the local ECG, causing ST depression in the leads looking at this territory – so-called reciprocal ST depression
ST elevation in the leads overlying the infarcting segment
Normal ST segment in those leads not overlying the ischaemic segment
Septum
Apex
Area of myocardial ischaemia/infarction
Specialized conducting tissue
Current flow (as electrons) from the relatively normal segment to the infarcting segment following depolarization
Overall current flow as seen by an observing electrode overlying the infarcting segment

ST segment elevation myocardial infarctions (STEMIs) are dangerous and require early diagnosis and aggressive reperfusion therapy. They are recognized by characteristic ST elevation in the appropriate clinical setting, usually prolonged ischaemic chest pain, occasionally unheralded acute heart failure and, more rarely, arrhythmias (ventricular tachycardia [VT], ventricular fibrillation [VF], also atrial fibrillation [AF]). ST segment elevation myocardial infarctions are sometimes known as Q wave myocardial infarctions (MIs), or 'full-thickness' MIs, as they can progress to Q wave formation, though this is not inevitable.

The stages of a STEMI (Fig. 31.1)

Phase 0 (a non-classic phase): Not often talked about, is the onset of MI, when there maybe no ECG changes. This phase can be demonstrated during percutaneous coronary intervention (PCI) when prolonged balloon inflations sometimes (though not commonly) results in no ECG changes.

Phase 1: Hyperacute T waves (not ST elevation) are the earliest signs of a full thickness MI. They are recognized by finding tall peaked T waves. Their mechanism is unclear. This phase lasts perhaps just a few minutes, explaining why it is a rare finding in the emergency room.

Phase 2: ST elevation is the result of the sub-epicardium being more ischaemic than the sub-endocardium (Fig. 31.3) during occlusion of a major epicardial coronary artery. This leads to current flow from the endocardial to the epicardial region (then on to an observing electrode):
• ST elevation in STEMI is found in several leads next to one another (contiguous leads), not just one lead. These follow the known patterns of the coronary arteries (Table 31.1).
• ST elevation is frequently 'convex upwards' (Fig. 31.1, c2), in distinction to the 'concave upwards' pattern found in pericarditis (Fig. 31.1, c1). This can be a useful rule in distinguishing an MI from pericarditis – however this is only a guide, and exceptions can and do occur. If there is doubt from the ECG, this can be clarified by cardiac ultrasound (STEMI leads to a great decrease in the contraction of the affected segments, whereas in pericarditis the heart contraction is normal).
• Posterior infarction leads to ST depression in leads V1–3 (see Chapter 13). Additional clues that posterior infarction is the diagnosis are: (a) if an inferior MI is also present; (b) clinical features of infarction; and (c) cardiac ultrasound.

Phase 3: Is simultaneous resolution of the ST segment elevation (going on to T wave inversion) and the development of Q waves, indicating an electrical window due to myocyte death in that part of the heart (see Chapter 9). This phase occurs hours to days following the MI.

Phase 4: Is re-inversion of the inverted T waves, to the upright position, occurring several days to a week after the onset.

Phase 5: Another non-classic phase, occurring in very few patients, is late disappearance of the Q waves, occurring years or even decades later. The mechanism (cell migration, division or differentiation) is unclear.

The size of the myocardial infarct relates to prognosis and bears a relationship to ECG changes:
• The amount of ST elevation corresponds to the amount of tissue at risk. Furthermore, the more leads that show ST elevation, the worse the prognosis (Fig. 31.2).
• The speed with which ST elevation resolves with thrombolysis relates to how effective the treatment has been in opening up the artery, and hence to outcome. Though there are many methods, traditionally the amount of ST resolution in the lead with greatest ST elevation is examined 90 min after reperfusion therapy – resolution of ≥ 50% is strongly correlated with the infarct related artery being open.
• The absence of Q waves, or the loss of very little or no R wave height in the affected territory is associated with a smaller MI.
• Distribution; an anterior MI is usually larger than an inferior one, which is larger than a posterior one. There are exceptions to this 'rule'.

Prognosis in STEMIs relates to many factors (Fig. 31.1b); recent data suggests that the risk index (= systolic blood pressure × [age/100]/heart rate) is a good score.

Table 31.1 ST segment elevation myocardial infarctions (STEMIs).

Leads showing ST elevation	Infarct description	Artery occluded
I, II, aVL, V1–5/6	Antero-lateral	Proximal LAD
II, V1–3/4	Antero-septal	LAD
II, III & aVF	Inferior	Right coronary artery if ST elevation II > III, circumflex if III > II
I, II & V5/6	Lateral	Diagonal branch of LAD, OM branch of circumflex
V1–3 (ST depression)	Posterior	Circumflex

LAD, left anterior descending; OM, obtuse marginal.

Fig. 31.1 Sequence of ECG changes during an acute myocardial infarction. (A) ECG initially normal (< first few minutes). (B) Hyperacute T wave changes, very tall peaked T waves. (C) ST elevation, arising either from the downstroke of the QRS complex (i.e. as the R wave becomes an S wave), or from the continuation of the upstroke of the S wave) (minutes to hours). The ST elevation can be straight, concave up C1, or convex up C2. (D) Simultaneous resolution of ST elevation, formation of Q waves and T wave inversion (hours to days). (E) Late normalization of the T wave (days to weeks). (F) Rarely, restoration of the R wave (years to decades).

Fig. 31.2 (a) Data from GISSI 1, showing that more leads with ST elevation worsens outcome. This is true both for the index admission (data shown here), and also long term for those who survive the index event, i.e. for those who survive initially, the long-term outcome is best in those with fewest leads showing ST elevation at presentation. (b) Thrombolysis in myocardial infarction (TIMI) risk score for ST segment elevation myocardial infarction (STEMI). Age, haemodynamic data (heart rate, blood pressure) and haemodynamic status (Killip class) are amongst the most powerful adverse predictors of outcome.

Fig. 31.3 Mechanism of ST elevation in ST segment elevation myocardial infarction (STEMI) (see text).

32 Aortic valve disease and hypertrophic cardiomyopathy

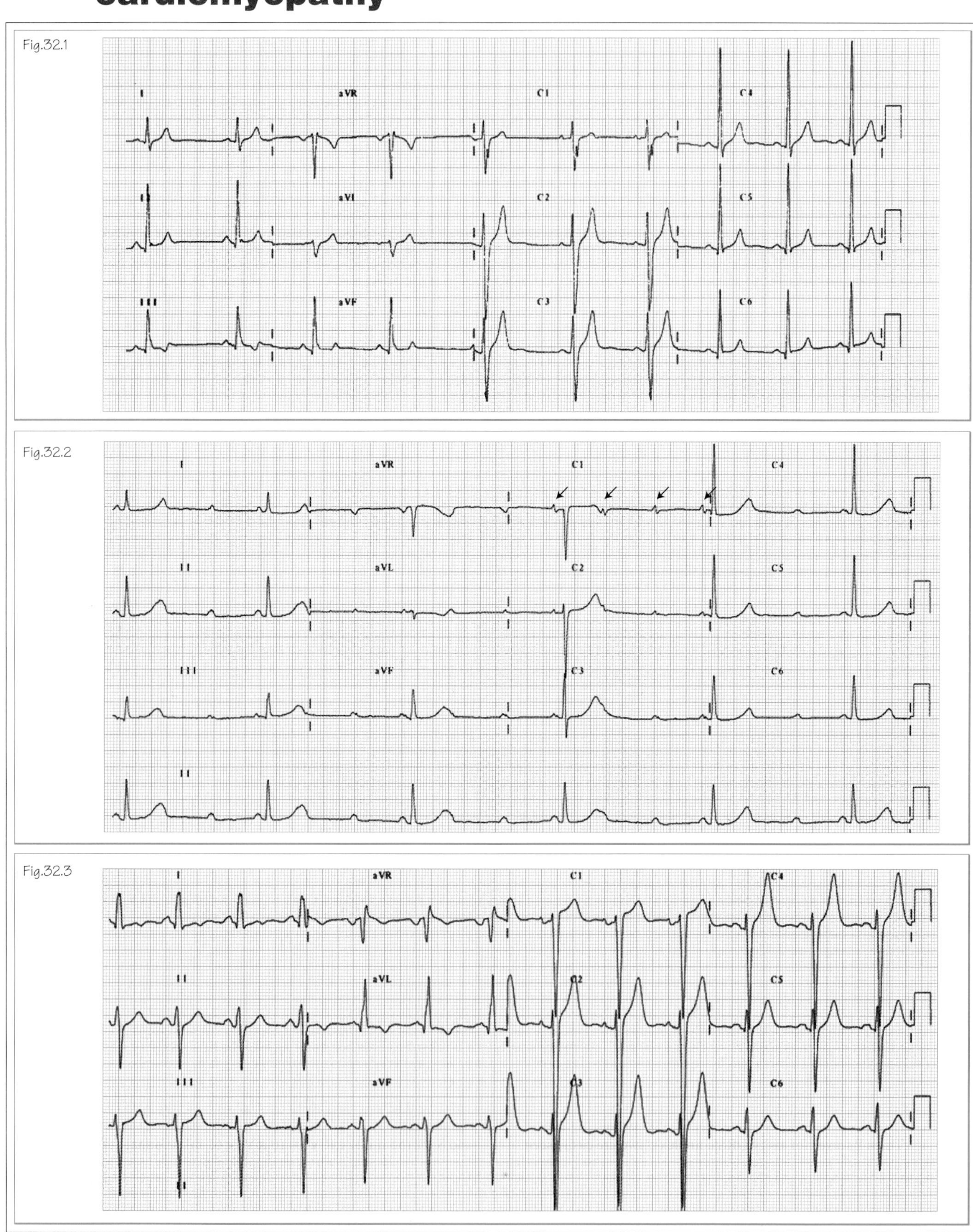

Aortic stenosis

Common and serious, aortic stenosis (AS) relates to:

- Rheumatic heart disease (very rare in developed countries), usually in young adults.
- Bicuspid aortic valve (1–2% of the population); the valve works well for years, then degenerates in middle age.
- Calcific degeneration in a previously normal valve, the commonest cause, relates to the same factors underlying coronary artery disease (age, cholesterol, vascular inflammation), very common in the elderly (≥ 65 years).

Prognosis and ECG findings

Aortic stenosis progresses slowly, with the peak pressure drop over the valve increasing by 4–6 mmHg/year. A gradient of ≥ 50 mmHg (valve area ≤ 1 cm^2) is required for symptoms (effort-dependent breathlessness, angina and syncope). Sudden cardiac death is very rare (1–2%) in asymptomatic severe AS, but common once symptoms develop. The prognosis *in the absence of surgery* with symptoms is poor; if angina is the presenting symptom (the case in 35%), half die by 5 years; if syncope (15%), half die by 3 years; and if dyspnoea (50%), half die within 2 years. Hence, once symptoms occur, surgery should be undertaken without delay. The ECG does not aid the timing of surgery as this is based on symptoms, possibly aided by the exercise stress test in highly selected *asymptomatic* patients.

The slow increase in the aortic valve narrowing allows increasingly substantial left ventricular hypertrophy (LVH) to develop. So, the ECG correlates of valvar AS are of increasingly obvious ECG LVH (Fig. 32.1). When symptoms occur, most (≥ 80%) patients have ECG LVH; many also show 'repolarization changes'; a few show only repolarization changes (usually the obese or elderly). A very few (especially the elderly) with symptomatic AS do not show ECG LVH and the ECG may be normal. This illustrates a general principle; stimuli to ECG changes are more likely to result in classic changes in the young than in the elderly. Calcific AS is associated with high-grade heart block (second/third degree) as the calcium burrows from the valve into the interventricular septum to disrupt the conducting tissue (Fig. 32.2), when it may lead to syncope. Asymptomatic complex ventricular ectopy is common.

Valvar AS needs to be differentiated from other causes of left ventricular outflow tract obstruction:

- Supra-valvar obstruction, exceptionally rare, presents in infancy.
- Infra-valvar obstruction:
  (a) Sub-aortic membrane, a very rare disease, found in infancy. The ECG shows very prominent LVH.
  (b) Hypertrophic cardiomyopathy (HCM), a condition affecting 0.2% of the population. A significant proportion have dynamic sub-aortic muscular obstruction. The ECG in HCM and AS both show LVH – the clue to HCM is the extent of repolarization abnormalities. In LVH from AS the repolarization abnormalities (flat/inverted Ts) are confined to the lateral leads (I, II, aVL, V5/6), whereas they are more extensive in HCM.

Aortic regurgitation

Aortic regurgitation (AR) has the same causes as valvar AS. Dilatation of the aortic root (hypertension, syphilis, Marfan and related syndromes) can lead to AR, as can damage to the valve from:

- Bacterial infection (infective endocarditis); the ECG may show a long PR interval from an aortic root abscess, which can proceed to complete heart block.
- Systemic lupus erythematosis, aortic valve damage is due to a sterile inflammation (Libmann–Sachs endocarditis). The ECG may be non-specifically abnormal (ST/T changes) from pericarditis.
- Rheumatic diseases (ankylozing spondylitis, Reiter's syndrome, anti-phospholipid syndrome).
- Marantic endocarditis ('*in situ*' thrombosis) rare, often due to the pro-thrombotic effects of malignancy. Aortic regurgitation and systemic emboli occur.

The ECG in long-standing AR shows LVH. The QRS complex is slightly broader than in AS, as the ventricle is larger (and so a greater distance for the depolarizing wave to travel). The T waves are more upright than in AS, i.e. early on, there are fewer 'repolarization' changes. However, in late severe chronic AR repolarization changes are common. One third of patients with chronic severe AR have incomplete left bundle branch block, ascribed to the regurgitant jet hitting and damaging the left bundle. In acute AR (e.g. *Staphylococcus aureus* infective endocarditis) the ECG may only show a sinus tachycardia.

Fig. 32.1 ECG in severe asymptomatic aortic stenosis (AS). Sinus rhythm, heart rate 62 b/min. P wave normal shape and duration. PR interval normal (145 ms). QRS duration normal (111 ms), axis +79°. QRS amplitude increased (lead II = 19, V2 S + V5 R = 47 mm); no LVH associated repolarization changes. This ECG could result from any process causing left ventricular hypertrophy (LVH) (hypertension, aortic valve disease etc.).

Fig. 32.2 Heart block in aortic stenosis (AS). Elderly female, breathless, severe AS. Three P waves for every QRS complex – two are easily seen, the third is at the end of the T wave, disguised in most leads, but well seen in lead V1. Each QRS has a preceding P wave with the same PR interval, i.e. the diagnosis is Mobitz type 2 heart block or '3 to 1 heart block'. QRS complex normal aside from borderline voltage criteria for left ventricular hypertrophy (LVH) – S V2 + R V5 = 42 mm (normal ≤ 35 mm). Cardiac ultrasound showed severe AS, moderate LVH.

Fig. 32.3 Hypertrophic obstructive cardiomyopathy, resting left ventricular outflow tract gradient 80 mmHg. Sinus rhythm, left atrial enlargement (prominent late negative deflection in lead V1), normal PR interval, left axis deviation (lead II and II negative, lead I positive; QRS axis –46°). QRS duration increased (123 ms), best shown in lead aVL. Gross left ventricular hypertrophy (LVH) (aVL = 15 mV, normal ≤ 11 mV; and S V2 (55 mm!) + R V5 = (6 mV) = 61 mV (normal ≤ 40 mV). Inverted T wave in lead aVL ('strain' pattern). Poor anterior R wave progression, partly due to left axis deviation. The LVH is extreme; this ECG could also be from a patient with aortic stenosis, or severe hypertension.

33 Mitral valve disease

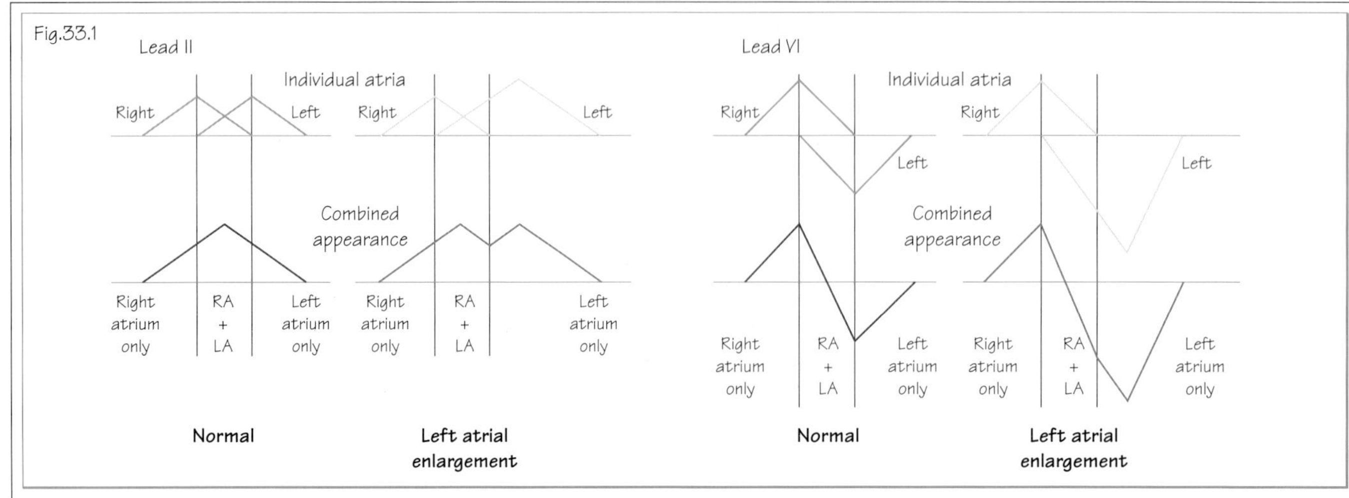

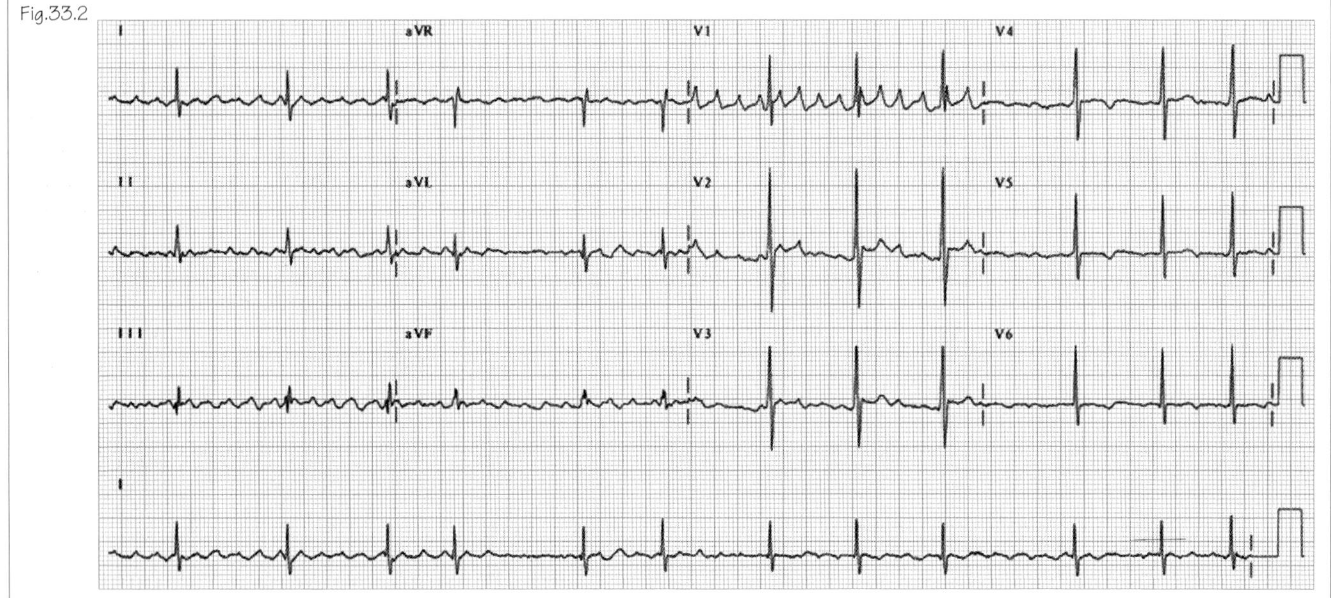

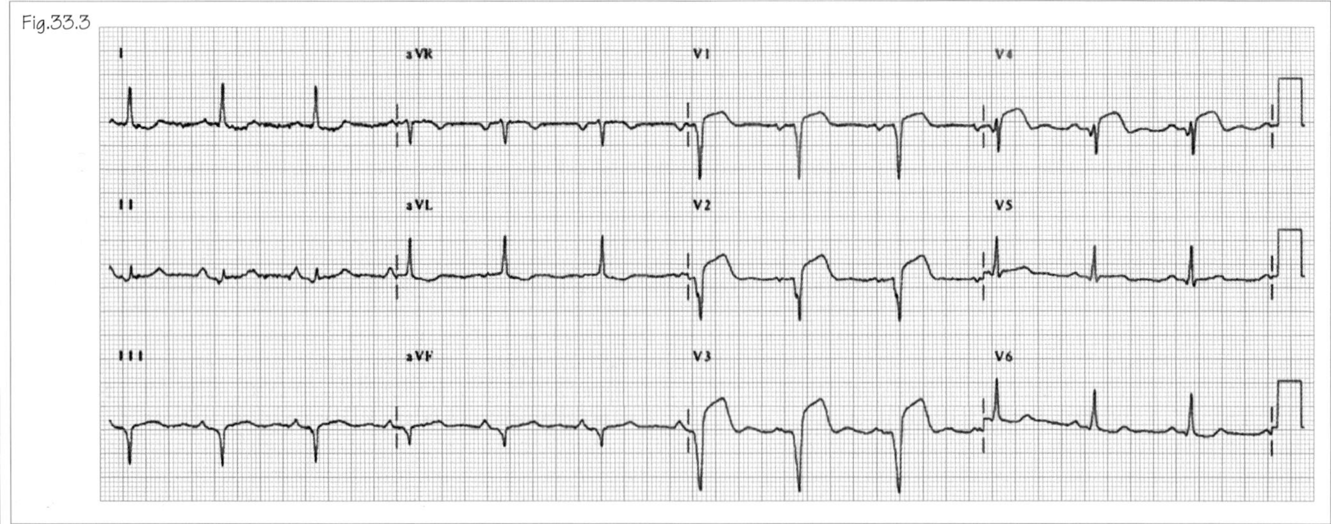

Mitral regurgitation

Mitral regurgitation (MR) is by far the commonest valve lesion. There are two causes:

• **Intrinsic disease of the mitral valve and its supporting apparatus** (termed 'organic' MR). The common causes are: rheumatic heart disease, mitral valve prolapse, papillary muscle dysfunction or rupture due to myocardial infarction (MI). Connective tissue diseases (Marfan, Ehlers–Danlos syndrome) cause a few cases, bacterial endocarditis is a rare cause, systemic lupus erythematosus (SLE) a very rare cause. The ECG signs of organic MR are:

(a) Left atrial enlargement (Fig. 33.1): the ECG signs are not as impressive as in mitral stenosis (MS).

(b) Atrial fibrillation is common.

(c) Left ventricular hypertrophy (LVH) occurs, but is much less common than in disease of the aortic valve (as the mitral regurgitant jet is expelled into the low pressure left atrium, the left ventricle does not work against pressure, and so there is less impetus to hypertrophy).

(d) Many – indeed most – patients with significant MR have unremarkable ECGs.

• **Dilatation of the left ventricle**, pulling on the mitral valve annulus (termed 'functional' MR). Any disease that damages and dilates the left ventricle leads to functional MR. The ECG changes are those of the underlying heart disease (e.g. Q waves in old myocardial infarction (Fig. 33.3), LVH in aortic stenosis, non-specific changes in dilated cardiomyopathy).

Mitral valve prolapse

The ECG findings in mitral valve prolapse relate to the severity of the MR: the more severe the regurgitation, the more likely there are to be signs of left atrial enlargement, atrial fibrillation and, occasionally, LVH (as above). ECG changes in mitral valve prolapse without significant MR are much debated, but both the symptoms (vague chest pains, tiredness, etc), and ECG changes (T wave flattening, QT interval changes) probably relate to co-incidental anxiety states, rather than to the mitral valve prolapse itself.

Mitral stenosis

Mitral stenosis is an increasingly rare lesion in the Western world, though still very common in less developed countries. It almost entirely relates to rheumatic heart disease. A very few cases relate to congenital MS, SLE, rheumatoid arthritis; an atrial myxoma can cause functional MS. The ECG findings are:

• Left atrial enlargement – MS can result in dramatically large left atrium, and very dramatic ECG evidence of left atrial enlargement.

• Atrial fibrillation is common (Fig. 33.2).

• Right ventricular hypertrophy (RVH) secondary to pulmonary hypertension occurs relatively late on in the natural history. Most patients with MS-induced pulmonary hypertension do not have convincing ECG signs of RVH (right axis deviation, increasing R wave size in lead V1 progressing to a dominant R wave, right bundle branch block).

The ECG in acute rheumatic fever

Rheumatic fever is caused by a humeral and cellular immunological reaction to a throat or skin infection with a group A *streptococcus*. Though inflammation occurs in the brain, joints, skin, it is the cardiac inflammation that gives rise to most concern. A 'pancarditis' occurs, i.e. endo-, myo-, and peri-carditis. The endocarditis most commonly involves the atrioventricular valve rings initially, then involves the valves directly (mitral most commonly, then the aortic, tricuspid and pulmonary valves), resulting in regurgitation acutely and sometimes heart failure. The ECG findings in rheumatic fever may be very non-specific; tachycardia is common, repolarization changes are not rare. PR interval prolongation (reflecting the myocarditis) is one of the criteria used in diagnosing rheumatic fever, but is not specific to rheumatic carditis (e.g. also occurring in diphtheria-related carditis).

Fig. 33.1 ECG findings in left atrial enlargement. This figure shows the classic ECG consequences of right and left atrial depolarization, individually (top line) and their combined appearance (bottom line), in normal hearts and in left atrial enlargement. The two principle consequences of left atrial enlargement are: (i) a broad bifid P wave in lead II; (ii) a prominent late negative deflection in lead V1. It is important to realise that an ECG diagnosis of left atrial enlargement does not always correlate with cardiac ultrasound findings – in other words, the ECG may suggest left atrial enlargement, whereas, left atrial enlargement is not present according to the ultrasound. Conversely, the ECG may be normal, whereas the cardiac ultrasound shows left atrial enlargement. LA, left atrium; RA, right atrium.

Fig. 33.2 ECG in a patient with mitral stenosis. Atrial fibrillation, with very coarse fibrillatory waves in lead V1 – these might be mistaken for an atrial tachycardia, but running one's eye along the rhythm strip at the bottom, one can see that the fibrillatory waves change continuously in appearance, which would not be the case with an atrial tachycardia. The QRS response is irregular, another hallmark of atrial fibrillation. Normal axis, but dominant R wave in lead V1 (due to pulmonary hypertension).

Fig. 33.3 Functional mitral regurgitation. Patient with old anterior wall myocardial infarction. Sinus rhythm, left atrial enlargement (prominent late negative deflection in lead V1 P wave). Q waves leads III, aVF and V1–4 (suggesting an left anterior descending [LAD] artery that 'goes round the corner', i.e. supplies some of the inferior wall). Persisting ST elevation in leads V1–4 suggest persisting occlusion of the infarct related artery, which increases the chance of finding a ventricular aneurysm.

34 Cardiomyopathy and myocarditis

Fig.34.1

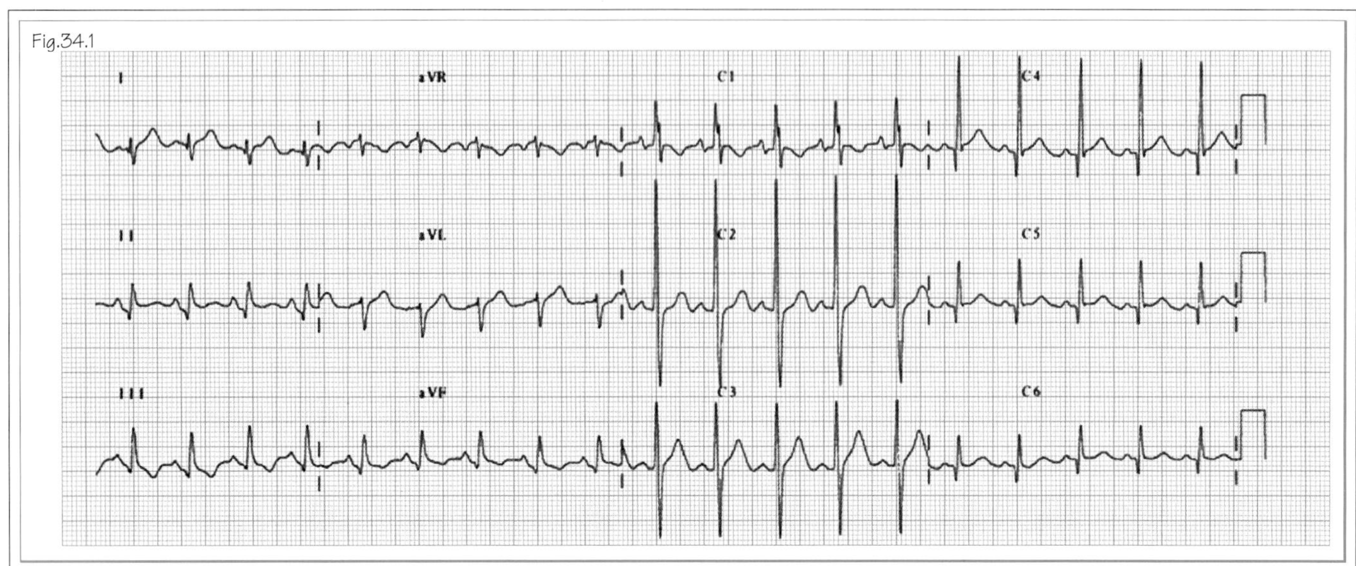

Fig.34.2

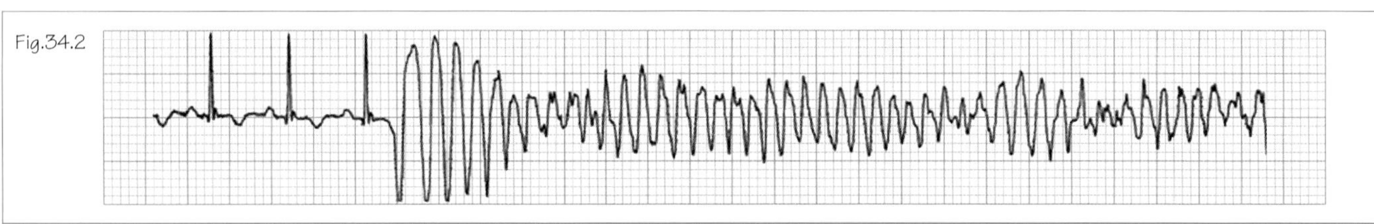

Fig.34.3

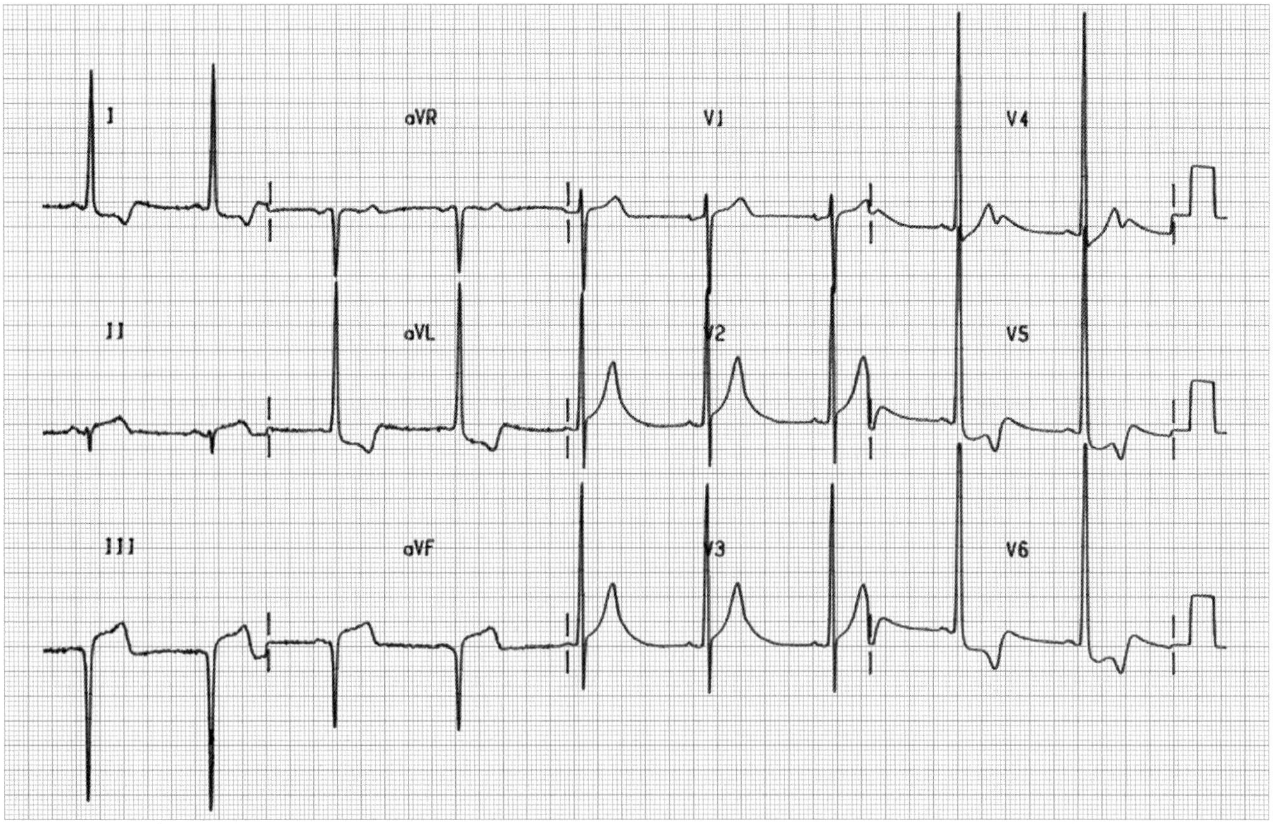

Cardiomyopathy is 'heart muscle disease', classified by ultrasound appearance and aetiology, though often first suspected from the ECG.

Hypertrophic cardiomyopathy

Hypertrophic cardiomyopathy (HCM), autosomal dominant, affects 0.2%, causes effort breathlessness, angina and sudden cardiac death (mainly from ventricular tachycardia [VT]/ventricular fibrillation [VF]). Left ventricular hypertrophy (LVH) occurs, characteristically of the septum; microscopically there is 'myocyte disarray' (the myocytes criss-cross each other randomly). In those with left ventricular outflow obstruction an ejection murmur occurs; in many there is no outflow gradient and no/few abnormalities on examination. Diagnosis is by cardiac ultrasound/magnetic resonance imaging (MRI)/genetic testing. The ECG is occasionally diagnostic, though in most the signs are non-specific:

- A normal ECG is rare (5–25%), usually in those diagnosed by genetic screening, they have mild LVH.
- ECG evidence of left atrial enlargement is common.
- Dramatic pathological Q waves are not infrequent, especially inferolaterally. Their origin is speculative.
- Left ventricle hypertrophy, sometimes massive, is common pathologically. Accordingly ECG signs of LVH, sometimes spectacular (*a clue to the diagnosis*) are common, but are by no means universal (Fig. 34.3).
- Diffuse ST/T wave abnormalities are common, including the classic distribution of repolarization changes associated with pressure/volume overload induced LVH, i.e. lateral T wave inversion (I, II, aVL, V5/6). ST/T wave changes can spread well beyond these leads, affecting any or all other leads and *the best clue to the presence of HCM* is finding LVH with widespread repolarization changes. Repolarization abnormalities (T wave inversion) restricted to the mid-chest leads are a feature of the 'Japanese' apical form of HCM.
- Arrhythmias are frequent; atrial fibrillation (AF), ventricular premature contractions (VPCs), and more sustained ventricular arrhythmias (Fig. 34.2).
- A small proportion has a short PR interval, from an accessory pathway (Wolff–Parkinson–White syndrome).
- ECG prognostic features: (i) survived cardiac arrest, known VT/VF confers extreme risk; (ii) non-sustained VT on a 24-h ECG; (iii) failure to increase blood pressure during an exercise test (reflecting abnormalities in the peripheral circulation).

Dilated cardiomyopathy

Dilated cardiomyopathy (DCM) is a common cause of heart failure. The cardiac ultrasound shows a dilated thinned left ventricle with poor systolic performance. There are numerous causes. The ECG is non-specifically abnormal:

- Arrhythmias: AF, VPCs and non-sustained VT are common as are sustained VT/VF in advanced heart failure.
- QRS broadening (including left bundle branch block) occurs frequently. The amount, and speed of increase, relate adversely to prognosis.
- QTc lengthening is common, as in all with left ventricular dysfunction.
- Small complex occur, especially late on. Conversely some patients demonstrate LVH, especially those with alcohol induced DCM or the more inflammatory forms, e.g. post-myocarditis.
- Occasionally Q waves are seen in non-ischaemic DCM, giving rise to confusion about aetiology.
- In the skeletal myopathies a dominant R wave in lead V1 (indicative of prominent posterior wall involvement, by the same mechanism as in posterior wall myocardial infarction) (Fig. 34.1).

Myocarditis

Acute myocardial infection results in: (a) no symptoms (mild cases); (b) ventricular arrhythmias, including sudden cardiac death (infrequently); (c) symptoms of pericarditis (rarely); (d) symptoms and signs of heart failure (occasionally). There are many causative organisms; the ECG usually shows non-specific findings, including sinus tachycardia (*tachycardia out of proportion to heart failure severity suggests myocarditis*) and ST/T wave changes. If the active process continues for ≥ few weeks then ECG evidence of LVH is common, though conversely in some loss of R wave height occurs. In very acute forms ST elevation develops (by the same mechanism as for ST segment elevation myocardial infarction [STEMI], i.e. epicardial involvement > endocardial involvement), which can progress to Q waves (again, by the same mechanism as in STEMI).

Restrictive cardiomyopathy

Restrictive cardiomyopathy is rare. The ECG shows low voltage complexes, possibly Q waves ('pseudo-infarction'), and commonly conducting tissue disease (right/left bundle branch block, long PR interval).

Fig. 34.1 Duchenne muscular dystrophy. Sinus tachycardia, 122 b/min, P wave shape reflects right atrial enlargement (prominent early deflection in lead V1). Normal PR interval, QRS duration. QRS axis deviated to the right (109°). Prominent Q waves lead II, V4–6 (too large to be physiological septal depolarization). Dominant R wave in lead V1, *the best clue to the actual diagnosis*. QRS complex is too narrow for this to be right bundle branch block (and the V1 morphology is wrong, showing too much positivity too early) or Wolff–Parkinson–White syndrome, and the shape is all wrong for Brugada syndrome, all causes of a dominant lead V1 QRS complex. The ECG could reflect pulmonary hypertension (lead V1 and the QRS right axis deviation are consistent with this); another less likely cause is an old true posterior wall myocardial infarction (MI). However, posterior wall MIs often have associated inferior wall MIs, not present here. The patient's age (21 years) and sex (male), even without physical examination makes the diagnosis of skeletal myopathy highly likely.

Fig. 34.2 Ventricular fibrillation. Sinus rhythm, giving way to a high frequency ventricular rhythm, whose amplitude falls quickly.

Fig. 34.3 Hypertrophic cardiomyopathy (HCM). Grossly abnormal ECG. Sinus rhythm, heart rate 58 b/min. Borderline abnormal P wave, broad in lead II, negative in lead V1, suggesting left atrial enlargement. QRS complex greatly increased in the left-sided leads (aVL = 29 mm, normal ≤ 11 mm; S wave in lead V2 = 8 mm, R wave in lead V5 = 41 mm, total 49 mm, normal = 35 mm), implying gross left ventricular hypertrophy (LVH). Left axis deviation (negative QRS in lead II, III, positive in lead I). Lateral leads show inverted T waves (I, aVL, V5/6), termed 'left ventricular (LV) strain'/'repolarization changes'. Gross inferior lead Q waves (leads III, aVF). This ECG could come from gross hypertensive heart disease or aortic valve disease, but *the LVH changes are so gross as to strongly suggest HCM*. The inferior lead Q waves might reflect an old inferior wall Q wave myocardial infarction (MI), but in the presence of such severe hypertrophy do not have to, and probably just reflect the LVH.

35 Pulmonary hypertension

Fig.35.1

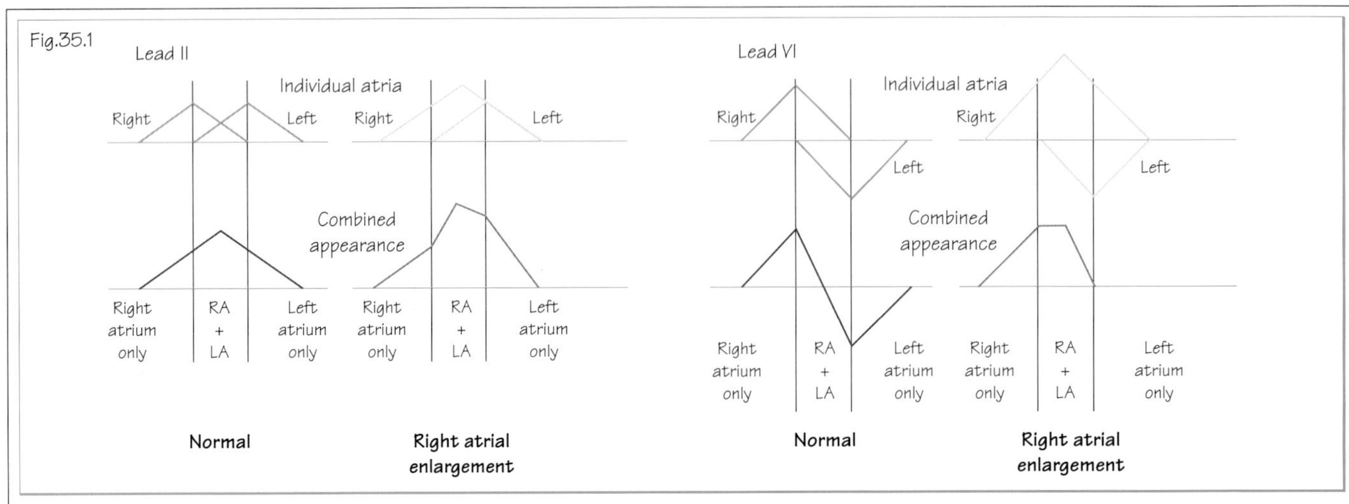

Fig.35.2

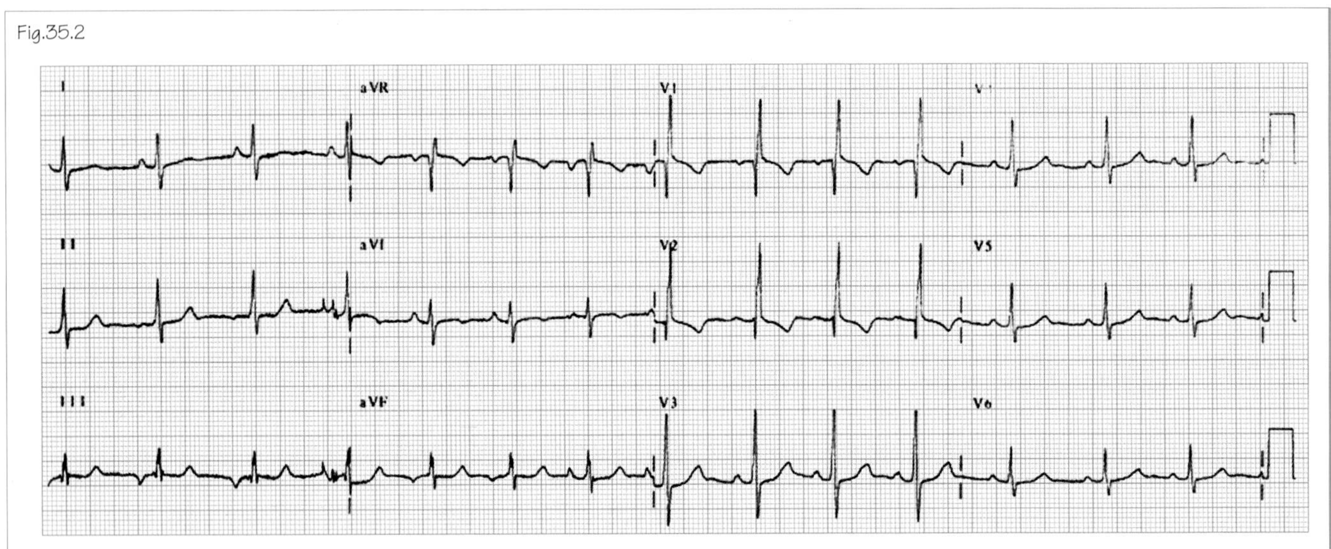

Fig.35.3

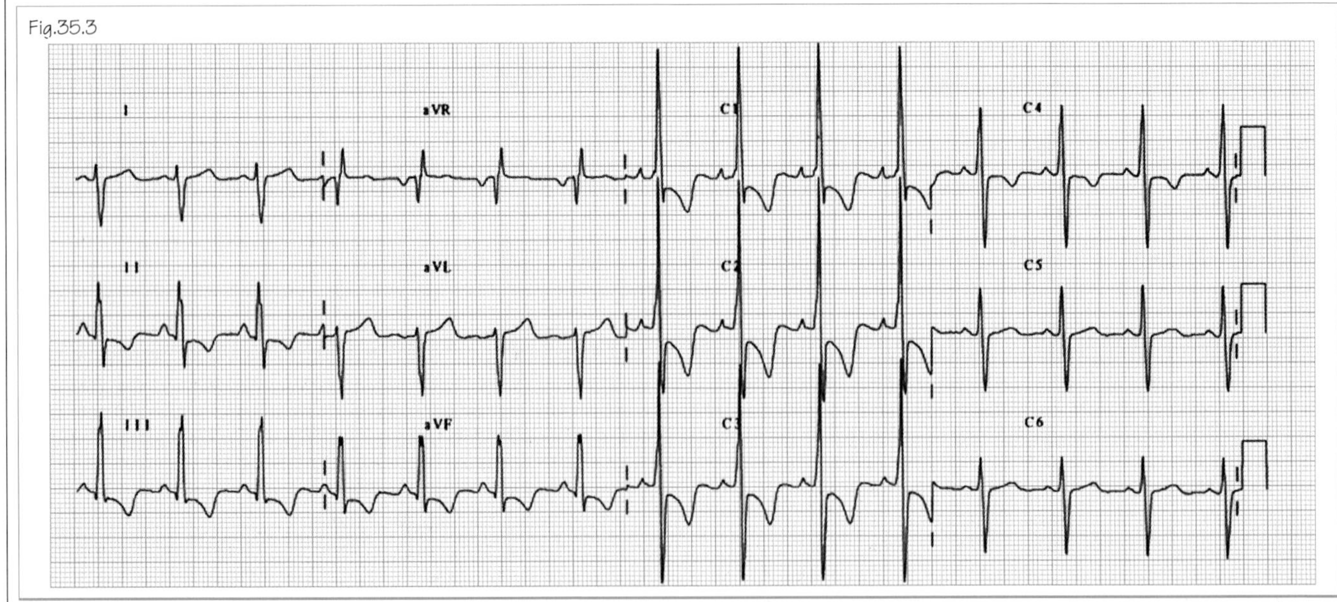

Pulmonary hypertension occurs when the pulmonary artery pressure rises above its normal value, of 30 mmHg systolic (Table 35.1). The causes are:

- Any left-sided cardiac disease sufficiently severe to cause heart failure, e.g. aortic/mitral valve disease, left ventricular dysfunction, hypertensive heart disease, etc. The ECG shows, in addition to any changes relating to pulmonary hypertension, left ventricular hypertrophy (LVH) (aortic valve/hypertensive heart disease), Q waves (ischaemic heart disease [IHD]), diffuse ST/T wave changes and loss of R wave height, or left bundle branch block (dilated cardiomyopathy).
- Lung diseases that destroys the pulmonary arterial circulation, e.g. chronic obstructive pulmonary disease (COPD), fibrotic lung disease (e.g. cryptogenic fibrosing alveolitis) or that result in hypoxic vasoconstriction (obesity related sleep apnoea syndromes).
- Thromboembolic lung disease
  (a) Acute pulmonary embolism (PE), which results in sinus tachycardia, and rarely right axis deviation, right bundle branch block. The features of chronic pulmonary hypertension (particularly a dominant R wave in lead V1) are not present.
  (b) Chronic PE, which often does not change the ECG, but may result in the classic findings of right ventricular hypertrophy (RVH) (see below). Sinus tachycardia is not a feature.
- Idiopathic (primary) pulmonary hypertension (PPH), a disease more common in women, with a genetic basis in some. Drug-related pulmonary hypertension should also be considered (e.g. from amphetamine-derived appetite suppressants). Patients with PPH usually present with an insidious decline in effort capacity, sometimes due to breathlessness, sometimes for non-specific reasons. There is clinical evidence of right heart hypertrophy; the venous pressure may be raised.
- Collagen vascular diseases; especially systemic lupus erythematosus (SLE) and scleroderma.

Table 35.1 Pulmonary artery systolic pressure.

Normal	≤ 30 mmHg
Mild	30–50 mmHg
Moderate	50–70 mmHg
Severe	≥ 70 mmHg

The ECG in many of the above conditions is dominated by the underlying pathology, or co-incidental pathology (for example, COPD occurs in smokers, many of whom have mildly abnormal ECG findings such as lateral T wave flattening due to clinically occult IHD). In 'pure' pulmonary hypertension the ECG may show evidence of RV hypertrophy and RA enlargement.

Right atrial enlargement

The ECG appearances of right atrial enlargement are of a tall, narrow, P wave in leads II and V1 (Fig. 35.1).

Right ventricular hypertrophy

The ECG appearances of RVH include:

- Right axis deviation, probably the commonest finding. This relates to the increased mass of the right ventricle pushing the QRS axis over to the right.
- A dominant R wave in lead V1 (Fig. 35.2). Lead V1 is normally dominated by the negative deflection induced by depolarization of the posterior wall of the left ventricle. However, in RVH, the rather small mass of the left ventricle posterior wall is overwhelmed by the now large mass of the right ventricle (Fig. 35.3).
- Right bundle branch block (RBBB). As the right ventricle hypertrophies, the hypertrophied myocytes interfere with the function of the right bundle, leading to right bundle branch block. Acute pulmonary hypertension, from acute massive pulmonary embolism, also causes right bundle branch block – the mechanism may be right ventricle stretch interfering with right bundle function or alternatively that acute PE-associated RBBB is due to infero-posterior wall ischaemia, caused by the stretched right ventricle compressing the right coronary artery, preventing adequate coronary perfusion.

Unfortunately many patients, even some with very dramatic elevations in right heart pressures, show none of the above signs. Thus the ECG cannot be used to rule in a diagnosis of pulmonary hypertension. If pulmonary hypertension is suspected, then either a cardiac ultrasound (to measure the velocity of the tricuspid regurgitant jet, from which an estimate of pulmonary artery [PA] pressure can be derived) or direct measurement of right heart pressures at cardiac catheterization is indicated.

Fig. 35.1 An idealized scheme explaining the morphology of the P wave in right atrial enlargement. Assumptions are that atrial depolarization passes equally towards lead II for both right and left atrial depolarization, and equally towards (for right atrial) and away (for left atrial) lead V1. The combined appearances are seen to be an amalgamation of the individual appearances. LA, left atrium; RA, right atrium.

Fig. 35.2 ECG of right ventricular hypertrophy (RVH). Unremarkable P waves. Normal PR interval. Borderline right axis deviation, QRS axis ≥ 90° (iso-electric R wave aVL, where R = S wave, and positive QRS leads III, aVF). Narrow complex QRS, generally normal aside from leads V1/2. In V1 there is a large Q wave, then a large R wave, which is termed dominant as the R wave ≥ Q/S wave. The T wave is inverted. Lead V2 shows similar abnormalities. There is a differential diagnosis of a dominant R wave in lead V1, which includes right bundle branch block (QRS too narrow here), Wolff–Parkinson–White syndrome (normal PR interval, QRS normal duration here), old posterior infarction (no inferior wall myocardial infarction here), skeletal dystrophy (which usually shows rather diffuse ST changes, not present here) and pulmonary hypertension (primary or secondary). This patient had congenital cyanotic heart disease.

Fig. 35.3 ECG of human immunodeficiency virus (HIV)-related pulmonary hypertension. P wave tall and peaked in lead II, V1 indicating right atrial enlargement. QRS axis swung to the right (123° by computer; negative in lead I, positive in leads II and III) and very dominant R wave in V1 (i.e. R wave much greater than S wave), both indicating right ventricular hypertrophy. Inverted T waves in leads V1–4 occur due to 'strain'. The ECG findings shown here are classical for severe pulmonary hypertension, though are rarely found: as a generalization, the younger the patient, the more likely are classic ECG findings, and vice versa, be it for pulmonary hypertension or any disease process. So, patients with congenital heart disease and pulmonary hypertension almost always show right axis deviation, and a dominant R wave in lead V1, whereas those with acquired pulmonary hypertension presenting in middle age or older rarely do. The ECG does not establish the cause of pulmonary hypertension.

36 Congenital heart disease

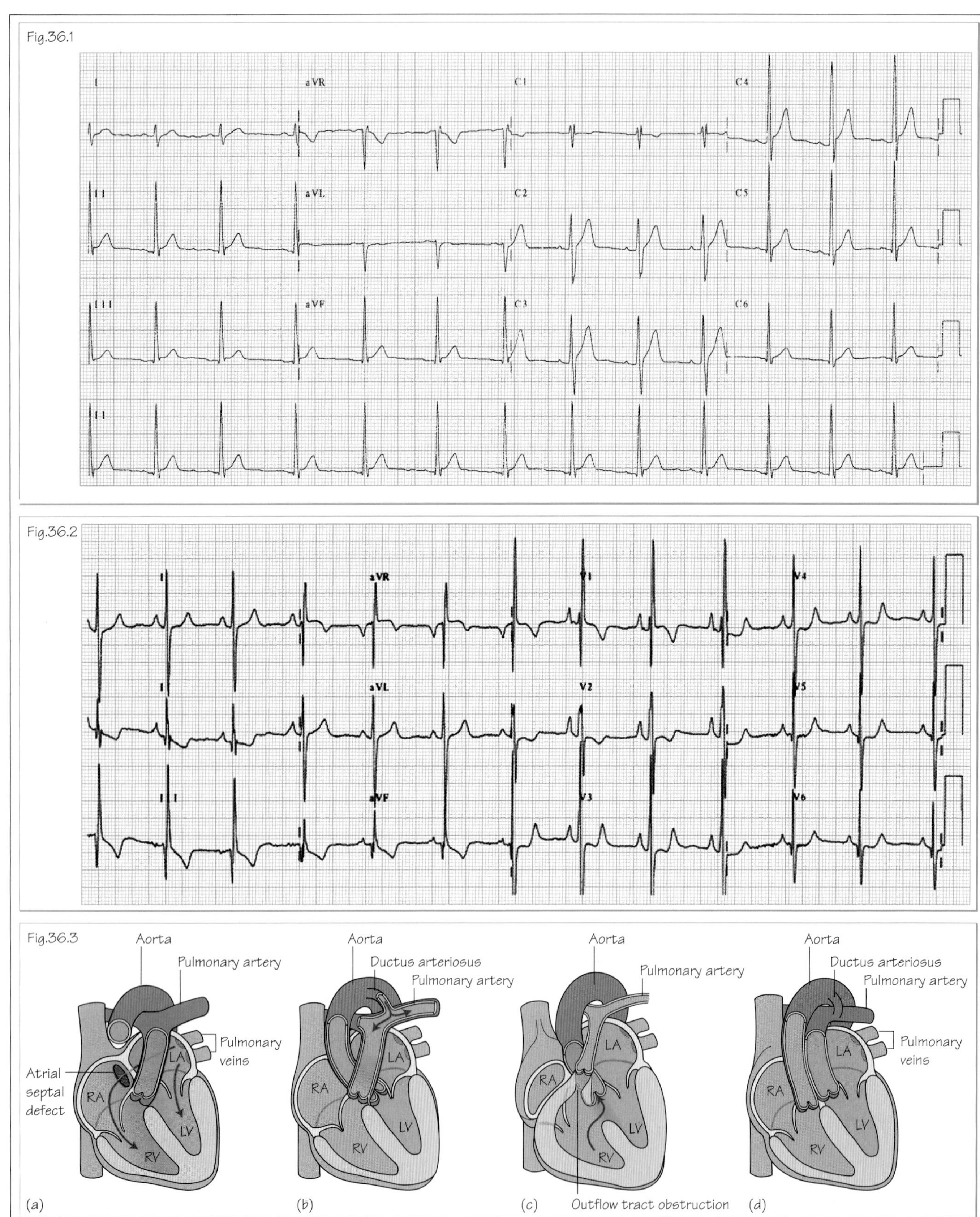

Congenital heart disease (CHD) is an increasing common condition in adults. The common forms are:

Bicuspid aortic valve

This has the same ECG pattern as calcific aortic stenosis (see Chapter 32).

Atrial septal defect

The ECG consequences of an atrial septal defect (ASD) relate to volume overload of the right heart (Fig. 36.1). The P wave (in 50%) shows right atrial enlargement; some patients have atrial arrhythmias (flutter, fibrillation), a consequence of right atrial stretch. The QRS axis is shifted to the right (right ventricular hypertrophy [RVH]), and there is usually a pattern of incomplete or complete right bundle branch block (RBBB) in lead V1. Diagnosis is confirmed by cardiac ultrasound/cardiac catheterization/magnetic resonance imaging (MRI). After closure, there remains a high atrial arrhythmia rate.

Ventricular septal defect

Ventricular septal defects (VSDs) account for 20% of CHD. The ECG signs depend of the size of the shunt and the pulmonary artery pressure:

- Small shunt; the ECG is normal.
- Moderate; left ventricular volume overload leads to ECG left ventricular hypertrophy (LVH). There may be RVH as well, manifest as an rsR′ in lead V1. As pulmonary hypertension develops the amplitude of the R′ wave increases.
- Large: there is ECG evidence of biventricular enlargement, with left atrial enlargement.
- Large VSD with little shunt due to pulmonary hypertension (Eisenmenger syndrome); the ECG shows evidence of RVH alone with no ECG evidence of LVH; QRS axis shift to the right, a deep Q wave and tall R′ wave in lead V1, and deep S wave in lead V6 (Fig. 36.2).

Tetralogy of Fallot

Comprises (functionally) a VSD with pulmonary stenosis. The ECG signs are dominated by right ventricular pressure overload; right axis deviation, and tall R waves in lead V1. Late on following corrective surgery arrhythmias are common; these include bradycardia due to atrioventricular (AV) block, atrial arrhythmias (flutter/fibrillation – in those with tricuspid regurgitation) and ventricular arrhythmias (in those with QRS duration in sinus rhythm of ≥ 180 ms, who usually have moderate–severe pulmonary regurgitation).

Patent ductus arteriosus

A patent ductus arteriosus (PDA) leads to LV volume overload, and the ECG signs comprise left axis QRS deviation, with deep Q waves and tall R waves in leads II, III, aVF, V5 and V6. If (flow-mediated) pulmonary hypertension occurs, RVH also develops.

Pulmonary stenosis

The ECG signs depend on the severity of the pulmonary narrowing; the more severe, the more likely is RVH, with right axis QRS deviation, incomplete right bundle branch block, and a dominant R wave in lead V1, There is often evidence of right atrial enlargement (tall spiked P wave in lead II).

Transposition of the great arteries

In D-transposition of the great arteries (TGA), the aorta arises from the right ventricle, and the pulmonary artery from the left ventricle. As the systemic veins drain into the right atrium, and on to the right ventricle (RV) (then into the systemic arterial circuit), and the pulmonary veins into the left atrium, then into left ventricle (LV) (and then into the lungs), there are two totally disconnected circuits which do not mix, unless there is a continuation of some form of the fetal circuit (found in two thirds), either the foramen ovale or ductus arteriosus. One third of patients have another defect allowing shunting and blood mixing (ASD, VSD, PDA, etc.). The ECG shows the consequences of the RV acting as the systemic ventricle, i.e. right axis deviation, RVH. If there is a co-existing large VSD or PDA or pulmonary stenosis also have LVH.

Eisenmenger syndrome

This comprises irreversible pulmonary hypertension due to (initially) a large left to right shunt (e.g. VSD) increasing pulmonary blood flow, so leading to changes in the pulmonary circulation that obliterate the pulmonary vasculature; the increased difficulty the RV has in pushing blood through the lungs leads to reversed flow (now right to left) through the shunt, cyanosis, ill-health and eventually death. The ECG is dominated by the increased work of the RV, showing right axis deviation and RVH.

Fig. 36.1 ECG from a patient with an atrial septal defect. Sinus rhythm, borderline right axis QRS deviation (at +90°), rSR′ pattern in lead V1. A fairly unremarkable ECG, though the patient had a large shunt (3 to 1).

Fig. 36.2 ECG from Eisenmenger syndrome due to a ventricular septal defect (VSD). Sinus rhythm, dramatic evidence of right atrial enlargement (best seen in lead V1 as a tall early peak to the P wave). Normal PR interval. QRS axis deviated to the right (look for the iso-electric standard lead – where the R wave = the S wave. aVR is the closest, so the axis is at right angles to this, either −60° or +120°. Inspection of lead III and aVF shows it must go towards lead III and away from lead aVL, i.e. +120°). The QRS complex in lead V1 shows a rsR′ pattern, i.e. a late and very large R wave i.e. a 'dominant' R wave (i.e. R wave > S wave). The right axis deviation with dominant R wave in lead V1 are fairly pathognomonic of right ventricular hypertrophy (RVH). There are inverted T's in V1–3, 'repolarization changes' or in old terminology 'RV strain'.

Fig. 36.3 Congenital heart disease. (a) Atrial septal defect; oxygenated blood returning from the lungs to the left atrium crosses over into the right atrium, increasing the work of the right ventricle, and pulmonary blood flow. (b) Patent ductus arteriosus. Oxygenated blood is passed from the aorta into the pulmonary circulation, increasing blood flow through the lungs and left ventricle. (c) Tetralogy of Fallot. Pulmonary stenosis prevents blood easily entering the lungs, and a ventricular septal defect allows blood to shunt right-to-left, causing cyanosis. (d) Transposition of the great arteries. The systemic and pulmonary circuits are separate, unless there is persistence of the foramen ovale, ductus arteriosus, or a more complex shunting lesion.

37 Endocrine disease and electrolyte disruption

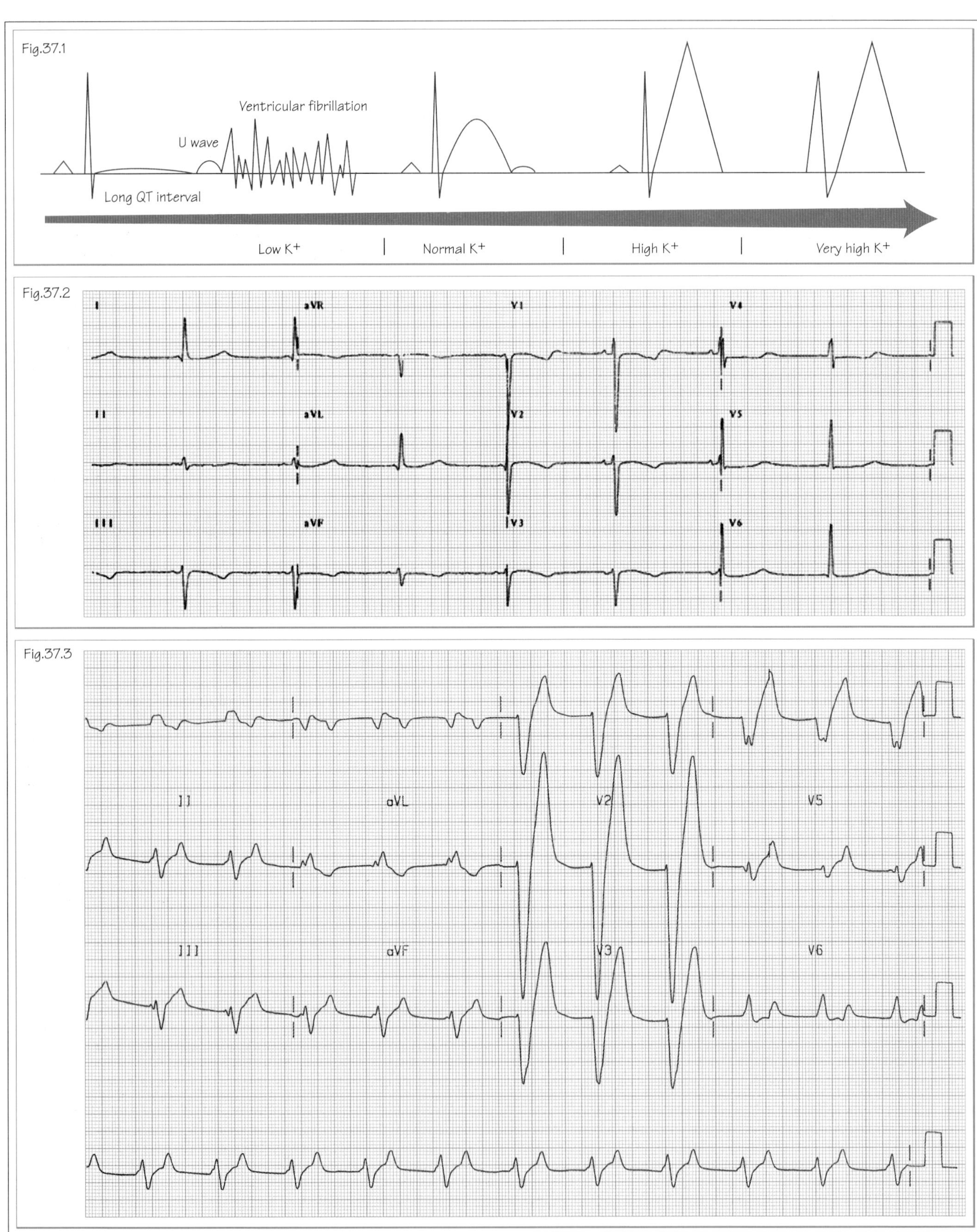

Electrolytes and the ECG

The ECG manifestations of hypokalaemia (Figs 37.1 and 37.2) are:

- Flattened ST/T waves.
- Prominent U waves.
- QT interval prolongation, particularly if the QT is already prolonged, e.g. in those with left ventricular dysfunction. K^+ supplementation in such patients shortens the QT interval.
- Low serum K^+ levels can provoke atrial fibrillation.
- Ventricular arrhythmias: in some patients low K^+ levels are critical in promoting dangerous ventricular arrhythmias. Those at risk include: (i) those with structural heart disease, especially those forms themselves associated with QT interval prolongation (mainly those with heart failure); (ii) drugs that prolong the QT interval (often by blocking the *human ether-a-go-go* (*HERG*)-related repolarizing K^+ channel), or are otherwise pro-arrhythmic, e.g. non-sedating anti-histamines, macrolide antibiotics, anti-psychotic drugs amongst others, especially if in combination with drugs that block cytochrome P450; (iii) bradycardia (unless due to beta-blockers, where the anti-arrhythmic anti-adrenergic effect outweighs the pro-arrhythmic bradycardic effect); (iv) elderly; (v) female; (vi) renal failure; (vii) occult hereditary long QT mutations (present in 5–10% with torsade-de-pointes [TDP]). The more risk factors present the greater the chance that low K^+ levels promote ventricular arrhythmias, especially TDP-type ventricular tachycardia. The typical patient therefore with TDP is an elderly female with renal failure (leading to accumulation of QT prolonging drugs) given a QT prolonging drug (e.g. macrolide antibiotic). For these reasons low K^+ may be a proximate cause of many cases of sudden cardiac death. It may be that co-existing low Mg^{2+} levels magnifies the risk of TDP.

Hyperkalaemia leads to the reverse of these findings (Fig. 37.3):

- Increased size of the T waves.
- Broadening of the QRS complex.

These changes can lead to the ECG taking the appearance of a sine wave – this is an extremely worrying ECG, as often the sine wave is often shortly followed by cardiac arrest, either due to ventricular fibrillation or, more characteristically, asystole (regardless of whether pre-existing cardiac disease is present or not – in contradistinction to hypokalaemia, which is rarely pro-arrhythmic in those with normal hearts, not on pro-arrhythmic drugs). A sine wave due to hyperkalaemia is an indication to immediately institute therapy that stabilises the heart, and lowers potassium (calcium chloride intravenously, insulin–dextrose mix, as a prelude to immediate dialysis).

Endocrinological disease

Thyroid disease can have important ECG manifestations. Thyrotoxicosis commonly leads to:

Table 37.1 Risk factors for atrial fibrillation (AF) in thyrotoxicosis.

Age (years)	% with AF Female	Male
40–49	6	12
50–59	5	14
60–69	17	38
70–79	16	42

- Sinus tachycardia, almost invariable with significant thyrotoxicosis, and (except in the elderly) a good marker of the severity of the thyrotoxicosis and its response to treatment.
- Atrial fibrillation, the risk of which depends on age and sex (Table 37.1).

Heart failure can occur with thyrotoxicosis, in which case, in addition to atrial fibrillation, diffuse ST segment flattening and prolongation of the QT interval occur.

Hypothyroidism has numerous cardiac manifestations, including: sinus bradycardia (a fairly reliable sign), profound prolongation of the QT interval (which is held not to be arrhythmogenic, unlike other conditions associated with long QT intervals). As both pericardial effusions and mucinous infiltrates of the myocardium itself are common, the QRST voltages can be quite substantially decreased. Prolonged hypothyroidism can lead to premature coronary disease, so all the manifestations of ischaemic heart disease can be superimposed on the basic pattern.

Diabetes

Diabetes, especially type II, is a profound risk factor for coronary disease, and hence all the manifestations of ischaemic heart disease can occur. Minor ECG changes (ST/T wave flattening etc.) are common; they may be manifestations of coronary disease, in that they tend to be associated with an increased mortality risk. In addition, independent of this, the QT interval is prolonged, and changes abnormally with changes in heart rate. The autonomic neuropathy common to diabetics leads to a reduced heart rate variability on 24-h ECG taping.

Cushing and Conn syndromes

These syndromes both lead to hypertension, which if prolonged provokes left ventricular hypertrophy (LVH), which may be manifest as ECG LVH. They also both lead to hypokalaemia (see above).

Fig. 37.1 The effects of potassium on the ECG. Low K^+ leads to prominent P waves, unchanged QRS complexes, very flat (indeed often non-existent) T waves and prominent U waves. The QT interval is prolonged, and in structural heart disease (e.g. post-myocardial infarction, heart failure) an increased risk of ventricular fibrillation (VF). As K^+ levels increase, the P wave decreases in size, the QRS is initially unchanged, though at very high levels broadens, and the T wave increase dramatically in size (the best clue to the presence of hyperkalaemia is finding a T wave larger than the preceding R wave). It is taught that cardiac asystole is the arrhythmia complicating hyperkalaemia, and this is certainly a risk, but the risk of VF also rises substantially. Cardioversion is usually successful in VF with hypokalaemia, rarely so with hyperkalaemia.

Fig. 37.2 An ECG in a patient with a K^+ of 2.2 mmol/L. Sinus bradycardia, heart rate 48 b/min. Unremarkable P wave and PR interval. QRS unremarkable. T waves are very flat throughout the ECG. The ECG returned to normal with correction of the K^+ level.

Fig. 37.3 A patient with a K^+ of 7.8 mmol/L. Regular rhythm, though the P waves cannot be seen. Broad QRS, looking rather like left bundle branch block. Very tall T waves, especially in leads V1–4, where they are 'peaked', and are the largest part of the waveform. The ECG returned to normal with correction of the K^+.

38 Psychological disease and its treatment

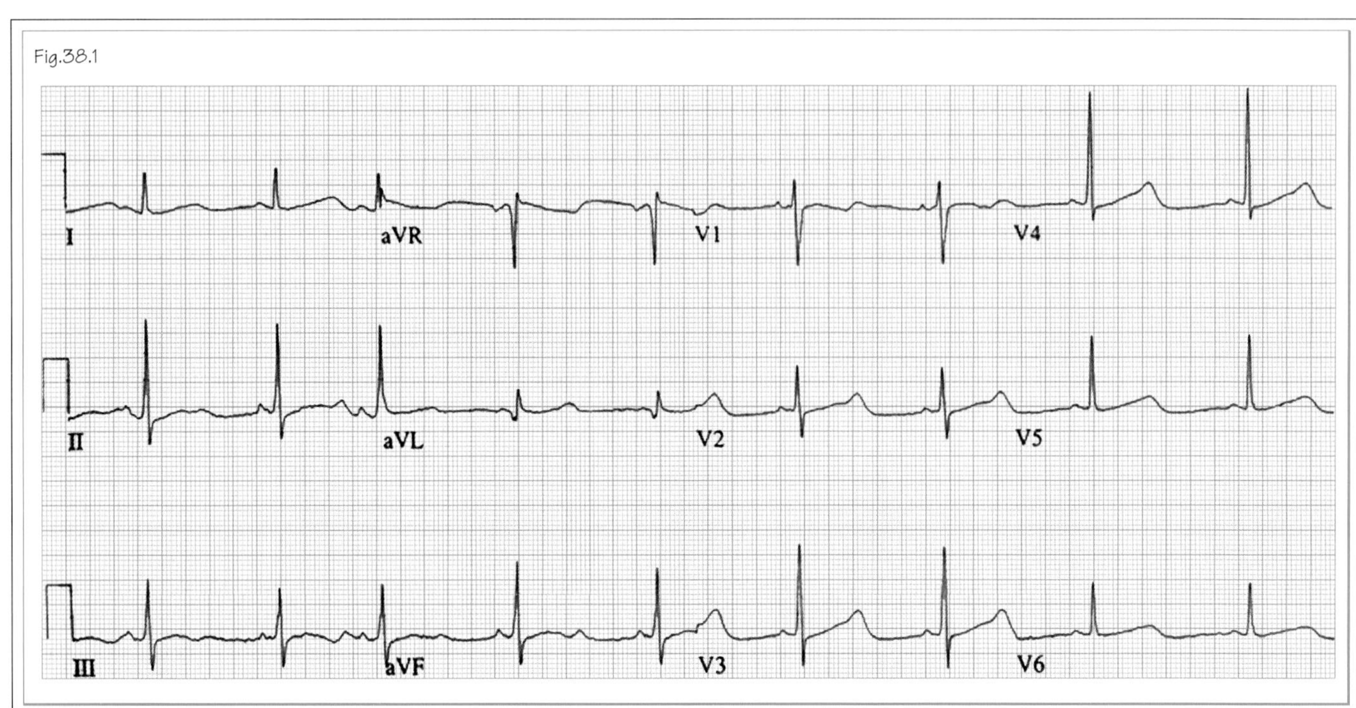

Fig.38.1

I
aVR
V1
V4
II
aVL
V2
V5
III
aVF
V3
V6

Fig.38.2

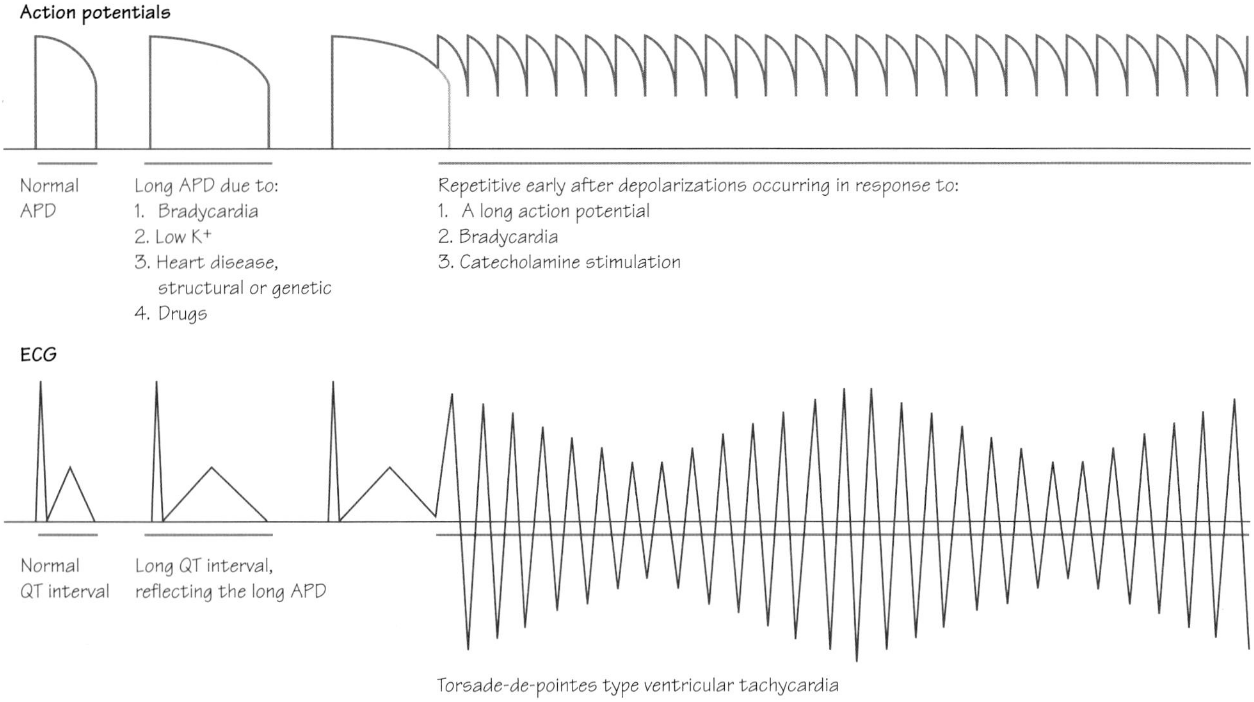

Action potentials
Normal APD
Long APD due to:
1. Bradycardia
2. Low K+
3. Heart disease, structural or genetic
4. Drugs
Repetitive early after depolarizations occurring in response to:
1. A long action potential
2. Bradycardia
3. Catecholamine stimulation
ECG
Normal QT interval
Long QT interval, reflecting the long APD
Torsade-de-pointes type ventricular tachycardia

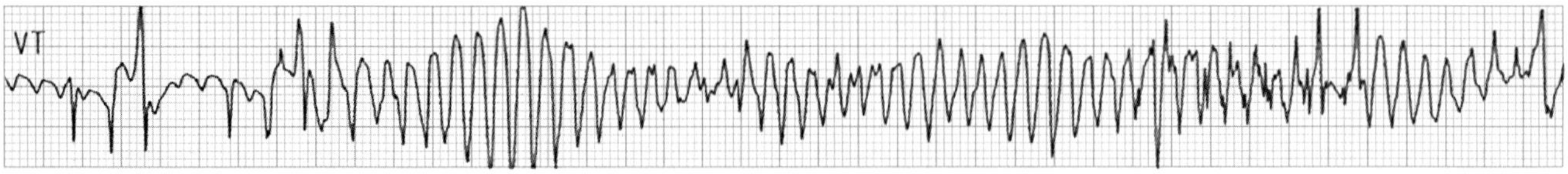

VT

Psychological disease and particularly its treatment can have a number of ECG manifestations.

Psychological stress

Stress, via numerous mechanisms, increases the risk of myocardial infarction (MI) (for ECG changes see Chapters 30 and 31), and treatment with selective serotonin reuptake inhibitors (SSRIs) appears to decrease the risk of MI either by ameliorating the effects of stress, or by inhibiting serotonin-induced platelet aggregation.

Anxiety

Anxiety, whether pathological or not, can lead to effects on the ECG. Tachycardia is very common, as is ST/T wave flattening. ST depression (see below with hyperventilation) can occur, though is not common.

Hyperventilation

Hyperventilation induces many metabolic changes, including low levels of carbon dioxide, alkalosis, and changes in autonomic outflow to the heart. It is therefore not surprising that the ECG should change in the face of vigorous hyperventilation. The changes seen with spontaneous hyperventilation include:

- T wave inversion in leads with previously upright T waves – this is the most frequently observed change.
- ST segment shift can also occur; however as it is in any individual not possible to say whether such ST shift relates to anxiety or coronary disease, when such ST depression is seen full work up for suspected coronary disease should take place.

In experimentally-induced hyperventilation ST depression may occur both in those known to have coronary disease and in those known not to have coronary disease.

Psychotropic drugs

Psychotropic drugs can have profound affects on the ECG. The most important abnormality seen is prolongation of the QT interval (Fig. 38.1), especially in those with pre-existing cardiac disease. This QT interval prolongation may predispose to ventricular arrhythmias (usually of the torsade-de-pointes type) (Figs 38.2 and 38.3), and so sudden cardiac death, the incidence of which is increased in elderly patients taking major anti-psychotic drugs (Fig. 38.2). T wave changes also occur with psychotropic drugs as can ST changes.

Antidepressants

In therapeutic doses tricyclic antidepressants (TCAs) increase heart rate, prolong the PR interval, increase the duration of the QRS complex and prolong the QT interval (Figs 38.1 and 38.2). It is unlikely that for the vast majority of patients these changes are of any clinical relevance. QT interval prolongation with TCA or other anti-psychotic drugs may occur via blockage of the rapidly activating subtype (IKr) of the *human ether-a-go-go* (*HERG*)-associated potassium repolarizing current, which is one of the main currents determining the length of the action potential (and so the QT interval). This current is very sensitive to external levels of K^+, explaining in part why low external K^+ prolongs the action potential [QT interval], and why raising K^+ shortens the action potential [QT interval].

Antidepressant overdose

In TCA and thioridazine overdoses, marked increases in heart rate occur, often to ≥ 120–140 b/min, as do increases in QRS duration, often to ≥ 120 ms, and QTc interval, sometimes to more than 500 ms. Torsade-de-pointes type ventricular tachycardia, resulting in cardiac arrest, occurs in a small proportion of TCA overdose cases. No ECG sign is predictive of this (i.e. neither increases in heart rate, nor of any of the ECG variables), though perhaps the ratio of the R wave to the S wave in lead aVR (i.e. ignoring the initial Q wave) is most predictive (a very subtle sign!). An R/S ratio ≥ 0.7 has a positive predictive accuracy of about 40%, negative predictive accuracy of 95%. Given the lack of any predictor for cardiac arrest, continuous ECG monitoring is recommended until the TCA overdose clears.

Selective serotonin reuptake inhibitors have very few effects on the ECG, both in therapeutic doses and in overdose. For this reason they are generally considered to be safer drugs than their predecessors.

Lithium

Lithium in therapeutic doses has few effects on the ECG. It can, rarely, unmask latent Brugada syndrome (see Chapter 39).

Fig. 38.1 QT interval prolongation due to psychotropic drugs. Patent admitted with syncope. Sinus rhythm, normal PR interval. Unremarkable QRS complex, and apparently normal T wave. However, when the QT interval is measured, this comes out as 596 ms, using Bazett correction, 570 ms. The prolonged QT interval is most easily visible to the naked eye in lead II. Syncope was presumed due to torsade-de-pointes type ventricular tachycardia. The QT interval normalized on discontinuing the psychotropic drug.

Fig. 38.2 Scheme of the mechanism of torsade-de-pointes (TDP) ventricular tachycardia. The top line represents cellular events, the bottom line those in the surface ECG. Many factors prolong the duration of the action potential (APD), some are listed, of which bradycardia on top of an already prolonged APD is important. Catecholamines don't prolong the APD, but are important in promoting TDP. Arrhythmic APD prolongation predisposes to repetitive early after depolarizations (EADs), which may be linked to Ca^{2+} overload. With EADs, repeated action potentials occur, starting towards the end of the pathologically prolonged APD. These are often much shorter in duration than the original AP, and fire from a higher membrane potential. They underlie many cases of TDP: whether the entire TDP sequence is driven from a cell or group of cells with repetitive EADs, or whether self-perpetuating re-entrant circuits occur in the ventricle is unclear (probably both mechanisms apply in different patients). A burst of TDP often starts with an underlying bradycardia (which prolongs the APD), then an ectopic (a short RR interval), which gives rise to a compensatory pause (a long RR interval), which further prolongs the APD, setting of the burst of TDP (with the interval from the last normal beat to the first TDP beat being short), i.e. there is a characteristic *short–long–short sequence* before many episodes of TDP. Suppressing the compensatory pause and its associated arrhythmogenic APD lengthening (e.g. with a pacemaker) can sometimes prevent episodes of TDP.

Fig. 38.3 Torsade-de-pointes type ventricular tachycardia, showing classical 'twisting of the points'.

39 Genetic pro-arrhythmic conditions

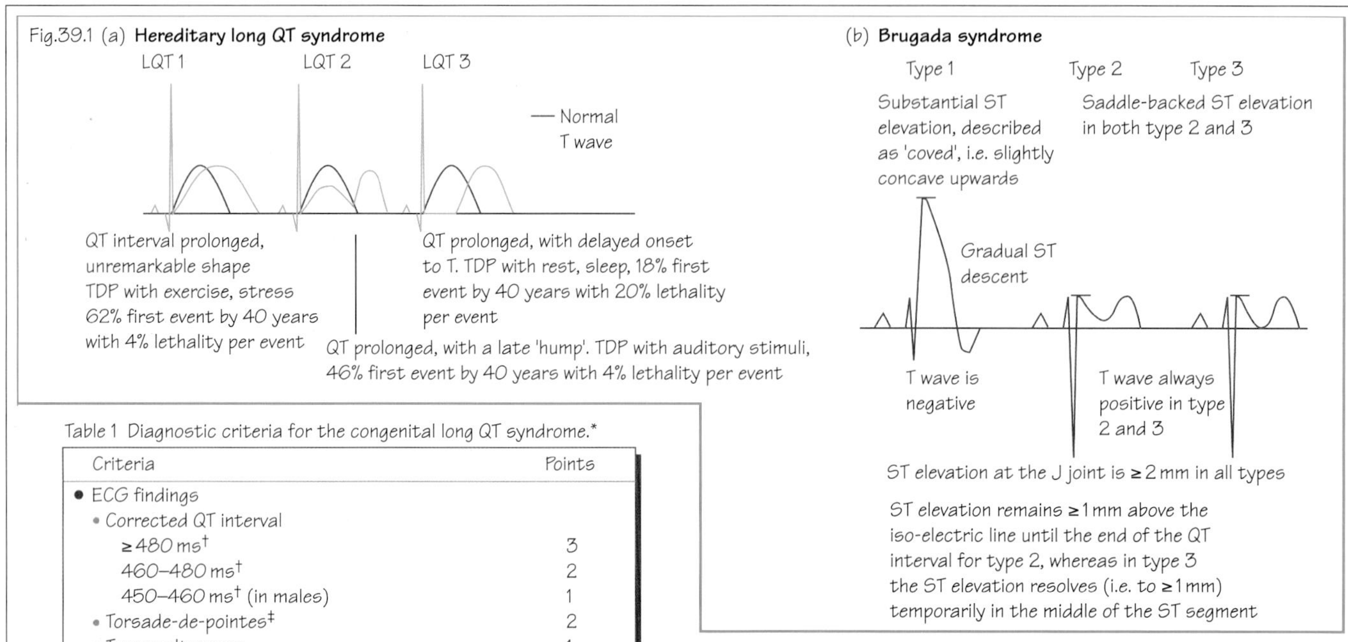

Fig.39.1 (a) Hereditary long QT syndrome
LQT 1
LQT 2
LQT 3
— Normal T wave
QT interval prolonged, unremarkable shape
TDP with exercise, stress
62% first event by 40 years with 4% lethality per event
QT prolonged, with delayed onset to T. TDP with rest, sleep, 18% first event by 40 years with 20% lethality per event
QT prolonged, with a late 'hump'. TDP with auditory stimuli, 46% first event by 40 years with 4% lethality per event
(b) Brugada syndrome
Type 1
Type 2
Type 3
Substantial ST elevation, described as 'coved', i.e. slightly concave upwards
Saddle-backed ST elevation in both type 2 and 3
Gradual ST descent
T wave is negative
T wave always positive in type 2 and 3
ST elevation at the J joint is ≥2 mm in all types
ST elevation remains ≥1 mm above the iso-electric line until the end of the QT interval for type 2, whereas in type 3 the ST elevation resolves (i.e. to ≥1 mm) temporarily in the middle of the ST segment

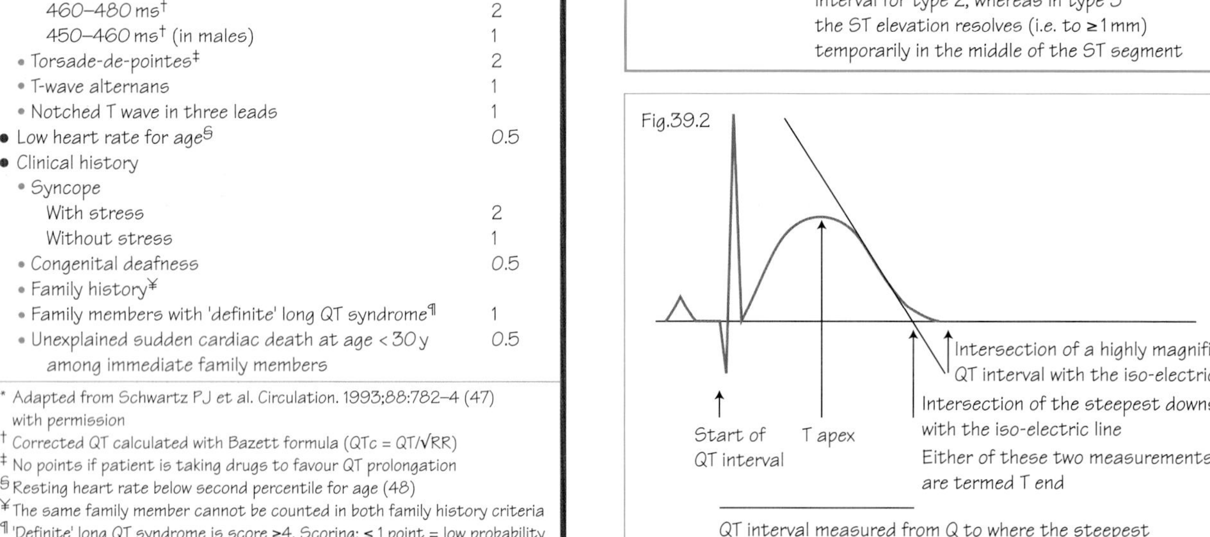

Table 1 Diagnostic criteria for the congenital long QT syndrome.*

Criteria	Points
• ECG findings	
◦ Corrected QT interval	
≥480 ms†	3
460–480 ms†	2
450–460 ms† (in males)	1
◦ Torsade-de-pointes‡	2
◦ T-wave alternans	1
◦ Notched T wave in three leads	1
• Low heart rate for age§	0.5
• Clinical history	
◦ Syncope	
With stress	2
Without stress	1
◦ Congenital deafness	0.5
◦ Family history¥	
◦ Family members with 'definite' long QT syndrome¶	1
◦ Unexplained sudden cardiac death at age < 30 y among immediate family members	0.5

* Adapted from Schwartz PJ et al. Circulation. 1993;88:782–4 (47) with permission
† Corrected QT calculated with Bazett formula (QTc = QT/√RR)
‡ No points if patient is taking drugs to favour QT prolongation
§ Resting heart rate below second percentile for age (48)
¥ The same family member cannot be counted in both family history criteria
¶ 'Definite' long QT syndrome is score ≥4. Scoring: ≤1 point = low probability of long QT syndrome; 2–3 points = intermediate probability

Fig.39.2
Start of QT interval
T apex
Intersection of a highly magnified QT interval with the iso-electric line
Intersection of the steepest downslope with the iso-electric line
Either of these two measurements are termed T end
QT interval measured from Q to where the steepest downslope of the T wave meets the iso-electric line

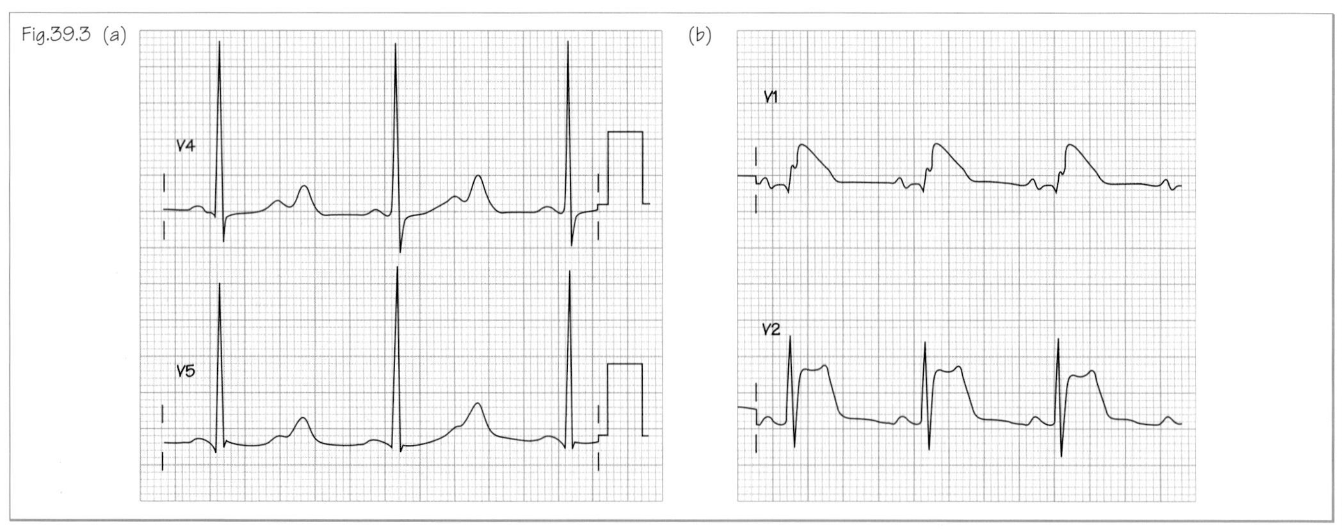

Fig.39.3 (a)
V4
V5
(b)
V1
V2

Hereditary long QT syndrome

Hereditary long QT syndrome (HLQTS) is rare (1 in 10 000) but accounts for 50% of sudden cardiac death (SCD) in infancy and childhood. It is usually autosomal dominant (autosomal recessive genes are associated with deafness), and occurs in different forms, termed *LQT1*, *2*, *3*, etc. (Fig. 39.1a). The mechanism of death is a long-QT associated torsade-de-pointes (TDP) type ventricular tachycardia degenerating into ventricular fibrillation. The pathophysiological basis is genetic prolongation of the action potential duration (APD) leading to early after depolarizations (EADs), which underlie TDP (see Fig. 38.2). Only 60% of patients have any TDP; however, 30–40% of patients die during their first TDP event, in others TDP episodes are self-terminating until the final non-self-terminating lethal one. Eighty-five per cent of TDP episodes relate to physical/emotional stress. The untreated life expectancy is substantially reduced. Treatment (beta-blockers ± implantable cardioverter defibrillator [ICD]) is fairly effective. The diagnosis can be extraordinarily easy or extremely difficult, in part as 5% of affected family members have normal QT intervals! A scoring system (Table 39.1) has been suggested. However, the key to diagnosis is to measure the QT interval accurately (Fig. 39.2) and to think of the diagnosis in syncope.

Acquired long QT syndromes

Acquired long QT syndromes are common and the complicating arrhythmias (TDP) is the same as in HLQTS, emphasizing the importance of QT interval measurement in all syncope, regardless of family history:

1 Those prone to drug pro-arrhythmia often have long baseline QT intervals, due to disease (e.g. heart failure), sex (women have longer QT intervals than men), or genetic variability (e.g. *human ether-a-go-go HERG* gene-related polymorphisms).

2 In drug-related acquired long QT syndromes drugs affect the *HERG* repolarizing K^+ channel, prolonging the QT interval, similar to the defective gene in *LQT2*.

3 Low K^+ promotes drug binding to the channel and decreases the action of the *HERG* repolarizing potassium channel, both prolonging the QT interval. Drug binding prevents channel function, prolongs the QT interval, leading to EADs/TDP.

Brugada syndrome

Brugada pattern ECG is a relatively common autosomal dominant condition (affecting 1–6 in 1000) due to mutations in the sodium channel *SCN5A* gene (the same gene mutated in *LQT3*). Affected individuals may experience episodes of polymorphic ventricular tachycardia/fibrillation (pVT/F), and syncope or death (patients are then described as having Brugada syndrome). The diagnostic hallmark is ST elevation in leads V1–3 in the resting ECG. Three types of ECG are described (Fig. 39.1b): in the absence of symptoms, only type 1 is diagnostic. Other ECG abnormalities include: QT interval prolongation, PR interval prolongation to ≥ 200 ms. The ECG abnormalities often only occur intermittently; fever, alcohol, a large meal of sticky rice (i.e. glucose and insulin load) brings them (and pVT/F) out, as do cardiac Na^+ channel blockers (so these drugs are used to diagnose those suspected of Brugada pattern ECGs with non-diagnostic ECGs). Alpha-channel blockers, Li^+, tricyclic antidepressants and cocaine have similar effects.

The arrhythmia in Brugada syndrome is pVT/F, usually at night. Most patients with pVT/F are male (though the condition is not sex-linked). The outlook depends on the necessity of drug challenge for diagnosis (i.e. absence of spontaneous Brugada pattern ECG – if high doses of sodium channel blockers are needed then outlook is very good). Asymptomatic individuals, especially with type 2 and 3 ECGs, have a good outlook. Those presenting with syncope have high rates of SCD, and those with failed SCD very high rates of recurrence. Implantable cardioverter defibrillators (ICDs) are the only effective treatment.

Other diseases

Hypertrophic cardiomyopathy, familial dilated cardiomyopathy, arrhythmogenic right ventricular dysplasia, familial atrial fibrillation, catecholamine-induced ventricular tachycardia and atrioventricular block can have a genetic basis. See Chapter 34 for ECG findings.

Fig. 39.1 Different forms of hereditary long QT and Brugada syndrome. (a) Hereditary long QT syndrome. Though many have rather diffusely abnormal ST/T waves, many do not; the diagnosis rests on thinking of the diagnosis, then measuring the QT interval. LQT, long QT syndrome; TDP, torsade-de-pointes; (b) Different forms of Brugada syndrome.

Fig. 39.2 Measurement of the QT interval. It is usual to measure the QT interval in lead II (the T wave is often very well defined). The QT interval is measured from the start of the QRS complex to the end of the T wave, where it meets the iso-electric line. The start of the QRS complex is easily determined, whereas the end of the T wave can be difficult. If difficulty is encountered, then the extrapolation of the steepest downslope of the T wave to the iso-electric line is used. Computer measurement of the QT interval is much more accurate than hand measurement; different programs measure different intervals (average QT interval across all the leads for some, in others the longest QT interval).

Fig. 39.3 (a) Hereditary long QT syndrome type 2 pattern ECG. Sinus rhythm, normal PR interval. QRS normal. T wave shows a late curious hump, especially lead V4. The QT interval here is 600 ms; the heart rate is 60 b/min; no heart rate correction is needed (see Chapter 17). (b) ECG from Brugada type 1. Normal P wave, PR interval, QRS complex. ST elevation in leads V1–3; lead V1 most convincing for type 1 Brugada, though T wave remains positive.

40 Distinguishing supraventricular from ventricular tachycardia

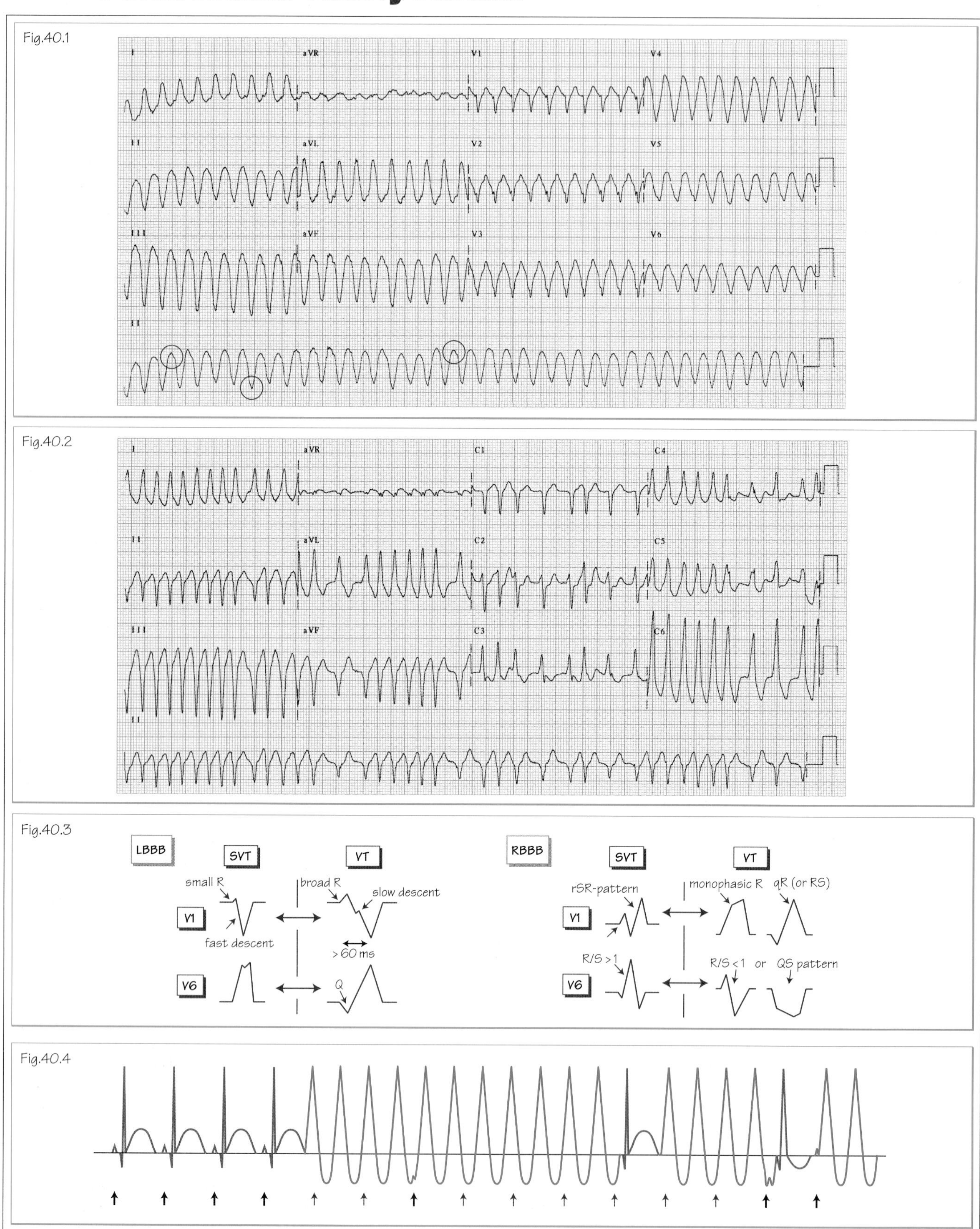

A key question in managing sustained arrhythmias is to determine the origin/mechanism of the electrical disturbance. How can this be done?

Narrow complex tachycardias

Tachycardias where the QRS complex is narrow (≤ 120 ms) are universally of supraventricular origin. The common arrhythmias are:

- atrial flutter (see Chapter 44).
- atrial fibrillation (AF) (see Chapter 43).
- atrial tachycardia (see Chapter 44).
- atrioventricular nodal re-entrant tachycardia (AVNRT) (see Chapter 45).
- atrioventricular re-entrant tachycardia (AVRT) (see Chapter 46).

Broad complex tachycardias

Broad complex tachycardias can be either supraventricular or ventricular. **All broad complex tachycardias should be considered to be ventricular tachycardia (VT) unless proven otherwise!** How can these two diagnoses be distinguished?

- The clinical situation offers clues; cardiac disease (e.g. post-myocardial infarction, known left ventricular dysfunction from another cause) increases the chance of VT (Fig. 40.1).
- Physical examination; haemodynamic collapse/near collapse (i.e. cool sweaty, low blood pressure) increases the chance of VT, but does not rule out a supraventricular origin. Absence of haemodynamic disturbance does not alter the probability one way or another.
- *Intermittent* 'cannon' waves in the neck (the atria contracting against a closed atrioventricular [AV] valve) or varying intensity of the first heart sound greatly increase the chance of VT. The 'cannon' waves are intermittent as the atria, beating independently of the ventricle, occasionally contract just when the AV valve closes. A 'cannon' wave *with each and every beat* (seen as very frequent large pulsations in the neck veins) usually indicates an arrhythmia starting in the AV node, i.e. an AVNRT.

Though the above are useful pointers, the exact pattern of ECG changes is very helpful. As in all tachycardias, the key to the diagnosis is determining the relationship between the QRS complex and the P waves, best done by carefully examining lead II/V1. If independent atrial activity is seen, then the diagnosis is VT (Fig. 40.1). Other pointers are:

- Irregularly irregular QRS rate = AF (Fig. 40.2). The broad QRS complex then either arises from conducting tissue disease (Fig. 40.3) or from Wolff–Parkinson–White syndrome.
- Capture or fusion beats are diagnostic of VT (Fig. 40.4). These are the consequence of ongoing sinus node activity continually bombarding the AV node. Usually these impulses are blocked by ventricular activity. Occasionally the supraventricular beat arrives at a critical moment in the ventricular rhythm and manages to either partially or completely capture the ventricle, resulting in a fusion or capture beat.
- The broader the QRS complex, the more likely is VT especially if the QRS ≥ 160 ms.
- If praecordial (leads V1–6) beats are either all positive or negative (praecordial concordance) then VT is likely.
- If the beats look similar to ventricular premature contractions, VT is likely.
- If the beats look exactly like right or left bundle branch block, then supraventricular origin with aberrancy is likely.

Often (not always) supraventricular arrhythmias that possess the AV node as an obligatory part of their re-entrant circuit (i.e. not pre-excited AF, which uses the accessory pathway) can be terminated (or slowed) by intravenous adenosine (a very short acting drug that induces AV block) whereas most VT is unaffected by adenosine. This is a useful diagnostic test to differentiate VT from supraventricular tachycardia (Fig. 41.3).

If doubt exists, and there is time, it may be possible to position electrodes to clearly record atrial and ventricular activity, to determine the relationship between P waves and QRS complex, to establish whether they are operating independently (when the diagnosis is VT).

Fig. 40.1 Broad complex tachycardia. Experienced readers will immediately diagnose ventricular tachycardia (VT). Why? There are three good reasons. This is a broad complex tachycardia, with very broad QRS complexes (point 1) – the broader the QRS complex the more likely is VT. The rhythm strip probably shows independent P waves (red circles), as a subtle variation in the morphology of the QRS complexes (point 2) – independent P wave activity indicates VT. The QRS complexes in the chest leads are all negative (i.e. the QRSs are all greater below rather than above the iso-electric line), another sign of VT (praecordial concordance, point 3).

Fig. 40.2 Pre-excited atrial fibrillation (AF). Tachycardia. No visible P waves. QRS duration varies between leads; the maximum being 130 ms. The key diagnostic clues are: (i) QRS complexes occur very irregularly (see rhythm strip), indicating that the rhythm must be AF (ventricular tachycardia is fairly if not completely regular); (ii) the upstroke of the QRS complex is 'slurred', especially laterally – the delta wave of Wolff–Parkinson–White; most QRS complexes are activated via the accessory pathway.

Fig. 40.3 Ventricular tachycardia (VT). This diagram illustrates how one can often distinguish VT from SVT with aberrancy (that is, SVT with either right- or left bundle branch block (R/LBBB)) mainly using leads V1 and 6, and looking at the exact pattern of the ECG in these leads. In SVT with LBBB, the V6 appearance is of a slurred *M*, with the first upstroke being smaller than the second, the QRS complex always remaining positive (i.e. above the iso-electric line). If the complex deviates below the line, then the diagnosis is likely to be VT. In SVT with RBBB, the QRS appearance in lead V1 is of an rsR′ appearance, that is, a small positive deflection, a slightly larger negative deflection, then a very large late positive deflection. In VT with a right bundle branch block appearance, either the complex is always positive, often with the first deflection much more positive than the later deflection, or the complex starts with a negative deflection, an S wave, not an R wave or aberrancy? LBBB, left bundle branch block; RBBB, right bundle branch block; SVT, supraventricular tachycardia.

Fig. 40.4 Capture and fusion beats in ventricular tachycardia (VT). Sinus rhythm giving way to a broad complex tachycardia. P waves are arrowed, bold ones = P waves visible on the ECG, lighter arrows P waves 'swallowed' by the QRS complex. P waves are most easily visible on the top or bottom of a QRS complex. There is no relationship between the P waves and the QRS complex – the diagnosis is therefore VT. The trace shows a 'capture' beat, where the timing of the P wave allows penetration of the atrioventricular node, then into the normal conducting tissue and the ventricular myocardium, at the precise moment the VT circuit has passed, the ventricle has repolarized and the refractory period is over. As the basic VT circuit persists, the VT starts immediately afterwards. Later on a beat occurs, comprising partly a ventricular beat activated by the P wave and the normal conducting tissue, and partly by the VT circuit beat – a fusion beat. Fusion and capture beats are pathognomonic of VT.

The electrode used to record the atrial activity can be positioned in the oesophagus, immediately behind the left atrium ('oesophageal electrode'), or a transvenous pacemaker electrode positioned in the right atrium.

It is usually best, if the diagnosis is not clear-cut, to treat the rhythm disturbance as ventricular; this may mean that the initial treatment should be DC cardioversion.

DC cardioversion

DC cardioversion terminates most but not all arrhythmias. The principle of DC cardioversion is that a strong uniform depolarizing current is applied throughout the heart simultaneously; this breaks almost all re-entrant arrhythmias, as the uniform depolarization prevents the onward march of the depolarizing wavefront. The heart then uniformly repolarizes, allowing the normal supraventricular pacemaker, the sinus node, to take over. However, arrhythmias due to an automatic focus within the heart are often not terminated by DC cardioversion. This is because while the entire heart is depolarized by the applied current, which in most hearts allows the sinus node to take over, the automatic focus itself is often either unaffected by the cardioversion current, or only affected briefly, and takes over the heart following cardioversion

- Examples of re-entrant arrhythmias usually terminated by DC cardioversion include: AF, atrial flutter, AVNRT, AVRT, scar-related VT.
- Automatic arrhythmias that may not be terminated by DC cardioversion include atrial tachycardias, automatic arrhythmias relating to digoxin toxicity, and some forms of VT.

Practical aspects of cardioversion

The patient should be connected to a defibrillator with a paper print out, so allowing the moment of cardioversion to be recorded. As cardioversion is painful, the procedure is usually carried out under general anaesthesia. However, if the patient is very unwell (for example VT with haemodynamic collapse, very fast atrial fibrillation in Wolf–Parkinson–White syndrome, etc), it is quite acceptable to carry this procedure out under heavy sedation, particularly using amnesic drugs such as medazolan. Once asleep/heavily sedated, the procedure itself is carried out:

- Energy can be delivered either via the defibrillator paddles applied to the chest wall (activated via buttons on the paddles), or through adhesive pads (remotely activated through buttons on the defibrillator itself)
- The paddles/pads are usually place anterior-apex, that is to say, one pad is placed at the apex of the heart (i.e. over the 5/6th intercostal space, mid to anterior axillary line on the left chest), and another just below the right clavicle. An alternative position for the pads, said by some to be more effective, though also logistically more difficult is the 'anterior-posterior' position, in which one pad is placed over the left lower chest, the other in the middle of the back, between the scapula.
- Ensure the defibrillator is set to deliver a 'synchronized' shock. This means that the defibrillating current, which is of very brief duration, is synchronized so that it does not occur during cardiac repolarization (i.e. during the T wave). If it were to occur at this time, it may well induce ventricular fibrillation.
- Set the power output (measured in joules) at the appropriate level. How do you determine this? Some arrhythmias are reputed to terminate easily at low power (atrial flutter, which often needs only 25 or 50 J), whereas others may need much more power (e.g. VT, which often needs 150 J or more). The larger the patient, particularly the larger the chest, the more power needs to be applied to the chest wall to ensure an adequate current penetrates to the heart. It is elegant to try and use the minimum amount of power that is required, though better to use the fewest shocks possible.
- Note that monophasic defibrillators (an old fashioned form of defibrillator) need to be set to approximately twice the power setting as biphasic defibrillators to deliver the same amount of energy to the heart.
- Shock the patient; always ensure that no-one is touching the bed, and confirm with the anaesthetist that the patient is satisfactorily sedated.
- If your first shock is unsuccessful, double the power, and then double again if required. The maximum power is 360 J (monophasic), 200 J (biphasic); give two shocks at this level if needed.
- If cardioversion remains unsuccessful with the paddles in anterior–apex position, consider switching to the anterior–posterior position.
- If external cardioversion remains unsuccessful, then in selected cases internal cardioversion can be undertaken. Here a complex electrode is inserted transvenously into the left pulmonary artery. The catheter has a distal defibrillation array, and another one sited more proximally in the atria, between which the defibrillation energy is passed. As energy is delivered within the heart, energy delivery is more effective at much lower energies, and overall success rate is higher.
- Warfarin (see below) must be continued for at least 1 month following cardioversion, as while co-ordinated electrical activity can be restored immediately within the atria, mechanical activity may take several weeks to return.

Complications of cardioversion

- Failure to terminate the arrhythmia.
- Appearance of another arrhythmia e.g. VF, if the defibrillator has not been synchonized.
- Anaesthetic issues.
- Stroke: this is the most worrying complication, and occurs when patients with an atrial arrhythmia (atrial flutter, AF, etc.) ejects a preformed thrombus out of the left atrium (often the left atrial appendage) into the arterial circulation. This can usually be prevented either by ensuring that the arrhythmia has not gone on long enough to generate a thrombus (it is held that 2 days of AF are required), or anti-coagulating with warfarin (ensure INR is always > 2) for a month beforehand. If it considered necessary to cardiovert a patient in chronic AF without warfarin, a transoesphageal echo (TOE) may identify whether thrombus is present in the left atria. Unfortunately, a normal TOE, though reducing the chance of stroke, does not remove it.

41 Narrow complex tachycardia

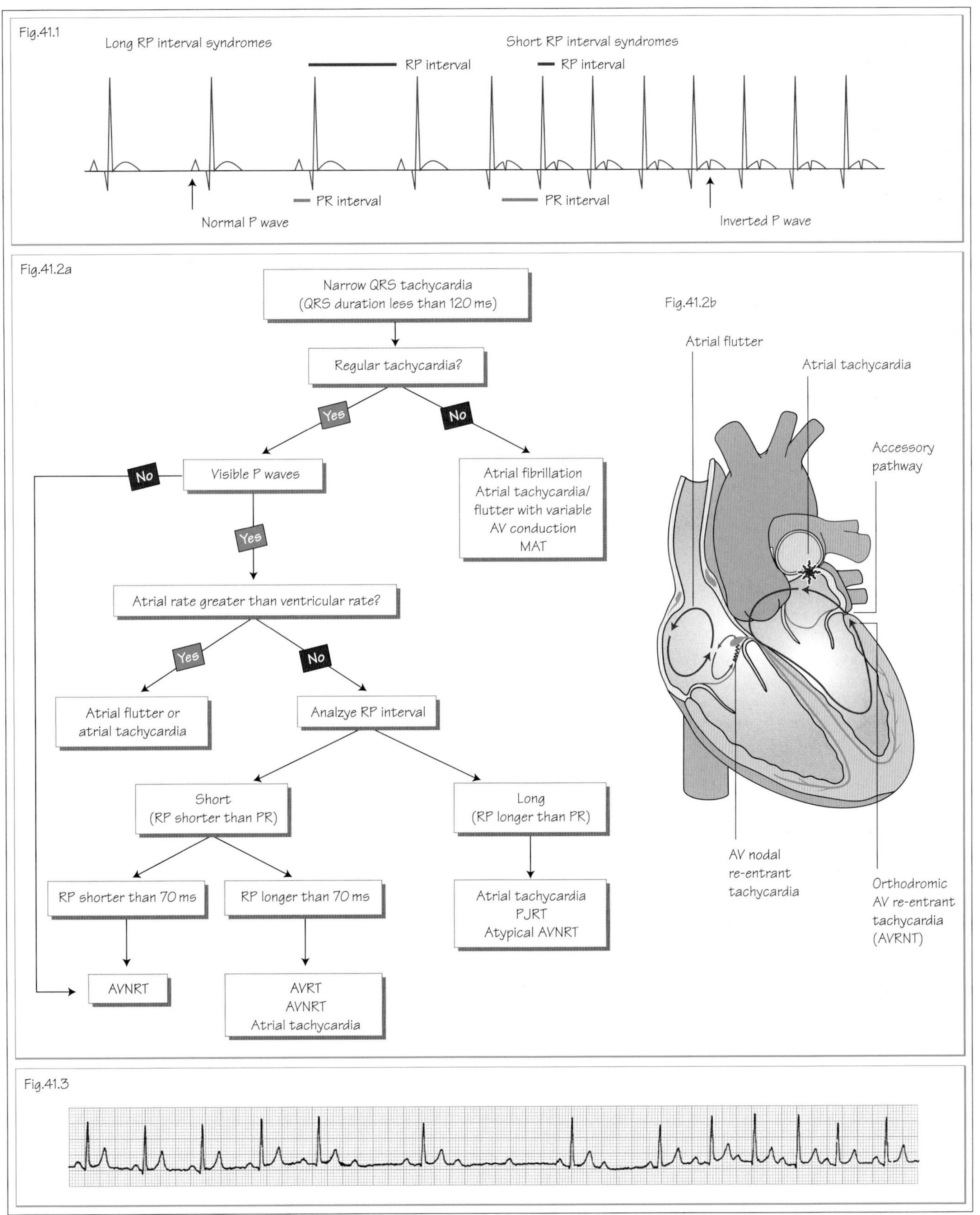

Fig.41.1
Long RP interval syndromes
Short RP interval syndromes
RP interval
RP interval
PR interval
PR interval
Normal P wave
Inverted P wave
Fig.41.2a
Narrow QRS tachycardia (QRS duration less than 120 ms)
Regular tachycardia?
Yes
No
Visible P waves
Atrial fibrillation
Atrial tachycardia/ flutter with variable AV conduction
MAT
No
Yes
Atrial rate greater than ventricular rate?
Yes
No
Atrial flutter or atrial tachycardia
Analzye RP interval
Short (RP shorter than PR)
Long (RP longer than PR)
RP shorter than 70 ms
RP longer than 70 ms
Atrial tachycardia
PJRT
Atypical AVNRT
AVNRT
AVRT
AVNRT
Atrial tachycardia
Fig.41.2b
Atrial flutter
Atrial tachycardia
Accessory pathway
AV nodal re-entrant tachycardia
Orthodromic AV re-entrant tachycardia (AVRNT)
Fig.41.3

In diagnosing narrow complex tachycardias, the first objective is to decide whether the rhythm is sinus or a tachyarrhythmia (Table 41.1). The key to this, as in any arrhythmia, is to determine the relationship of the P wave to the QRS complex. In particular:

- How many P waves to each QRS complex?
- If there are more P waves than there are QRS complexes (and provided the QRS rate is fast, i.e. this is not pathological heart block), then the diagnosis is an atrial arrhythmia with a degree of 'physiological block'. What is this? Many atrial arrhythmias beat at rates of 200–300 per minute, and the normal AV node cannot repolarize fast enough to allow this number of impulses to the ventricle. The AV node will then often let every second or third beat through, resulting in the QRS rate being half or one third of the atrial rate. This is physiological block, a finding that does not imply any pathological damage to the conducting tissue of the heart. Arrhythmias with organized atrial beats, and so similar shaped P waves, include atrial flutter, and atrial tachycardia.
- If the ratio of P waves to QRS complexes is 1 to 1, next ascertain whether the P wave precedes or follows the QRS? If the P wave precedes the QRS complex (i.e. the PR interval is short, and conversely the RP interval is long), then the diagnosis is usually sinus tachycardia (Table 41.2). If the P wave closely follows the QRS complex (i.e. the RP interval is short, and conversely the PR interval is long), then the diagnosis is usually an arrhythmia (very rarely sinus rhythm with a very long PR interval gives rise to this pattern). If the P wave follows very close indeed to the QRS complex (Figs 45.2c and d), then the diagnosis is usually atrioventricular nodal re-entrant tachycardia (AVNRT); if the P wave is quite distinct, and occurs within the T wave, usually the diagnosis is atrioventricular re-entrant tachycardia (AVRT).
- If the P waves cannot clearly be seen, either the rhythm is sinus, and the heart rate is so high that the P waves of one beat are buried in the T wave of the preceding beat, or, more likely, the P wave occurs simultaneously with the QRS complex, so hiding its appearance, as in most cases of AVNRT.

The accurate determination of this relationship allows one to diagnose whether an arrhythmia is present and its nature.

Sinus tachycardia

The key features pointing to sinus tachycardia are:

- The P waves are usually clearly visible; their shape is the same as normal rhythm.
- Usually there is an obvious illness (sepsis, hypovolaemia, thyrotoxicosis, drugs, etc.). If not, and the P wave is normally shaped, consider: (a) inappropriate sinus tachycardia due to sick sinus syndrome; (b) postural orthostatic tachycardia (PAT) syndrome; or (c) sinus node re-entrant tachycardia (very rare).
- PR interval << RP interval, a 'long RP' tachycardia; most, not all, long RP tachycardias are sinus (Table 41.2 & Fig. 41.2). If the PR interval > RP interval then the diagnosis is usually an arrhythmia.
- If the heart rate is very fast, say ≥ 150 b/min, it can be difficult to separate the P wave of one beat from the T wave of the preceding beat. This leads to a problem: is this a sinus tachycardia or an arrhythmia? To clarify the diagnosis, note; (i) in sinus rhythm the heart rate usually varies continuously, increasing and decreasing by many beats per minute over very short time periods, whereas in most arrhythmias, the heart rate is fixed and rarely varies by much (except atrial fibrillation, where the heart rate increases and decreases rapidly, but the diagnosis is so obvious from the QRS irregularity as to prevent any doubt over the diagnosis). This variation in heart rate can be diagnosed from an ECG monitor or a 24-hour ECG. (ii) Patients with sinus tachycardia of this degree usually have an underlying illness making them very ill, whereas many patients with an arrhythmia of this rate are fairly well. (iii) If doubt remains, intravenous adenosine (Table 41.3, and below) clarifies the diagnosis.

P wave morphology

If the focus for atrial depolarization starts other than in the sinus node, the direction and sequence of the wave of atrial depolarization is altered, changing P wave shape, e.g. atrial tachycardia or the retrograde P waves of AVNRT (where atrial depolarization starts at the AV node, rather than finishing there) or AVRT.

Table 41.1 Features of sinus tachycardia.

Sinus tachycardia	Arrhythmia
P wave shape normal	P wave shape abnormal
PR < RP interval	PR > or < than RP interval
Heart rate varies substantially	Heart rate usually fairly fixed
Underlying illness (sepsis, hypovolaemia, etc.) obvious	Often no underlying illness (occasionally known heart disease)
Adenosine; temporary slowing of P waves, with transient AV block	Either arrhythmia terminates, or AV block allows nature of the underlying atrial arrhythmia to be diagnosed. If no AV block, either too little adenosine used, or VT.

AV, atrioventricular; VT, ventricular tachycardia.

Fig. 41.1 Sinus rhythm giving way to short RP tachycardia. This cartoon starts with sinus rhythm, and demonstrates the long RP interval. Atrioventricular nodal re-entrant tachycardia (AVNRT) starts in the middle of the strip, so (i) the QRS rate speed up (ii) retrograde P waves, with a different shape from normal sinus rhythm occur (iii) resulting in a RP interval now being shorter than the PR interval.

Fig. 41.2 (a) Approach to diagnosing narrow complex tachycardias. (b) Pathways taken by common supraventricular tachycardias.

Fig. 41.3 Intravenous (IV) adenosine inducing transient atrioventricular (AV) block. A bolus (2–18 mg) of IV adenosine has been given. Sinus rhythm is present for 5 beats, then a P wave occurs without a QRS complex – heart block has occurred, initially 2:1, then 3:1, then 2:1. After a few seconds the adenosine wears off, and sinus rhythm (often slightly faster than before, as here) is re-established. When giving adenosine, start at a low dose, 3 mg, then work up to a high dose (18–24 mg). Stop when AV block has been induced, the arrhythmia terminated, or side-effects (flushing, breathlessness, chest pain) become troublesome.

Short RP tachycardia

If RP interval < PR interval, then the diagnosis is short RP tachycardia, which has a differential diagnosis; most commonly this is an arrhythmia (Table 41.2), where the P wave is abnormal. Very rarely short RP tachycardias are due to sinus rhythm with a long PR interval from conducting tissue disease (P wave normal shape).

Diagnostic tests to differentiate tachycardias

In diagnostic doubt, intravenous adenosine clarifies the diagnosis. Adenosine slows the sinus node and causes transient atrioventricular (AV) block.

- Adenosine breaks all arrhythmias using the AV node as part of the re-entrant circuit (AVRT and AVNRT).
- If the circuit sustaining the arrhythmia is 'contained' within the atria (e.g. atrial flutter, atrial tachycardia, atrial fibrillation) then the AV block induced by adenosine will reveal the true nature of the arrhythmia. After the adenosine-induced AV block has gone, the heart rate usually returns to the pre-adenosine one (Table 41.3). Frustratingly adenosine terminates (and not just slows) 10–15% of atrial tachycardias/flutter, leading to confusion with AVNRT.
- Ventricular tachycardia is unaffected by adenosine.

Heart rate

- If the heart rate is exactly 150 b/min and does not vary, the likely diagnosis is atrial flutter with 2 to 1 heart block.
- If the rhythm looks sinus (see above, normal shape P wave, PR interval), but does not vary, the diagnosis may be the extraordinarily rare sinus node re-entrant tachycardia: here the arrhythmic re-entrant circuit involves the SA node and its borders, so the wave of electricity depolarizes the atria using the normal pathway, so the P wave shape is normal, the heart rate is 'fixed' and does not vary over time.

Table 41.2 Differentiation between long and short RP tachycardias.

Long RP tachycardia	P wave shape	Short RP tachycardia – *all have abnormally shaped P waves*
Common		
Sinus tachycardia (ST)*	Normal	Typical AVNRT (fast retrograde limb to circuit)†
Atrial tachycardia	Abnormal	AVRT (fast retrograde conduction)
Uncommon		
Permanent form of junctional reciprocating tachycardia††	Abnormal	Junctional ectopic tachycardia§ (JET) (also called focal junctional tachycardia)
Sinus nodal re-entrant tachycardia (SNRT)*	Normal	Non-paroxysmal junctional tachycardia (NPJT)**
Atypical AVNRT†	Abnormal	
AVRT (slow retrograde conduction)	Abnormal	

* Sinus tachycardia and SNRT can be distinguished by whether the heart rate varies (ST) or is fixed (SNRT) on a 24-h ECG.
† Typical AVNRT is much commoner than the rare atypical AVNRT.
†† Very rare tachycardia that involves a slowly conducting, concealed, usually postero-septal (infero-septal) accessory pathway, characterized by an incessant supraventricular tachycardia.
§ JET, extremely rare (common in children with congenital heart disease post-cardiac surgery), ECG features of AVNRT, but not based on a re-entrant circuit (i.e. does not convert with single extra-stimulus or more complex electrophysiology (EP) stimuli, or to cardioversion). It probably relates to an automatic focus or area of triggered activity (explaining why it can occur with digoxin toxicity).
** Enhanced automaticity within a high junctional focus, often due to digitalis toxicity, ischaemia or cardiac surgery.
AVNRT, atrioventricular nodal re-entrant tachycardia; AVRT, atrioventricular re-entrant tachycardia.

Table 41.3 Impact of adenosine on arrhythmias.

Rhythm	Effect of adenosine	Post-adenosine
Sinus	Slowing of sinus activity (fewer P waves); transient AV block	Unchanged from pre-adenosine ECG
Atrial flutter	Transient AV block, revealing 'saw tooth baseline'	Unchanged from pre-adenosine ECG
Atrial tachycardia	Transient AV block, revealing frequent regular abnormally shaped P waves, with separating iso-electric line	Unchanged from pre-adenosine ECG
Atrial fibrillation	Slowing of the QRS rate, revealing underlying *f* waves	Unchanged from pre-adenosine ECG
AVNRT	AV block	Sinus rhythm
AVRT*	AV block	Sinus rhythm
VT	No impact	No impact

* Do *not* use adenosine for pre-excited atrial fibrillation – the AV block may encourage all impulses to go down the accessory pathway, resulting in a very fast ventricular responses and ventricular fibrillation.
AV, atrioventricular; AVNRT, atrioventricular nodal re-entrant tachycardia; AVRT, atrioventricular re-entrant tachycardia; VT, ventricular tachycardia.

42 Atrial ectopic beats

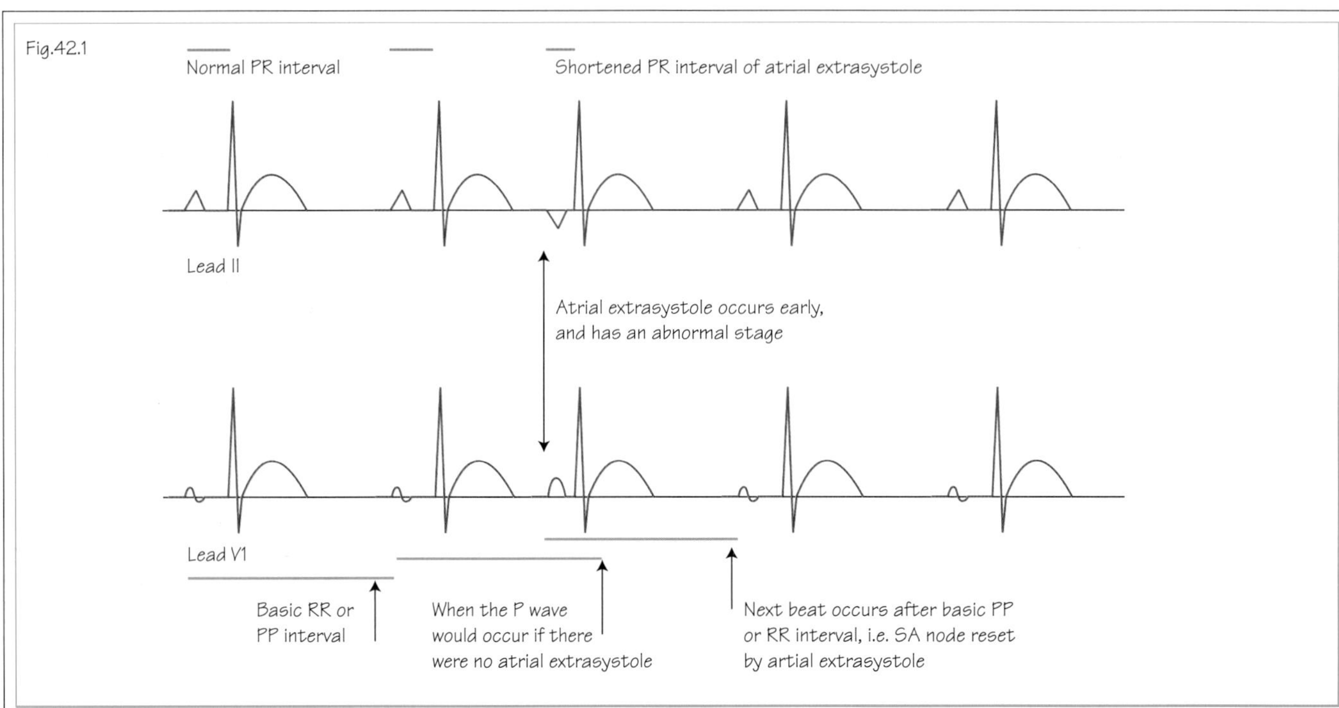

Fig.42.1
Normal PR interval
Shortened PR interval of atrial extrasystole
Lead II
Atrial extrasystole occurs early, and has an abnormal stage
Lead V1
Basic RR or PP interval
When the P wave would occur if there were no atrial extrasystole
Next beat occurs after basic PP or RR interval, i.e. SA node reset by artial extrasystole

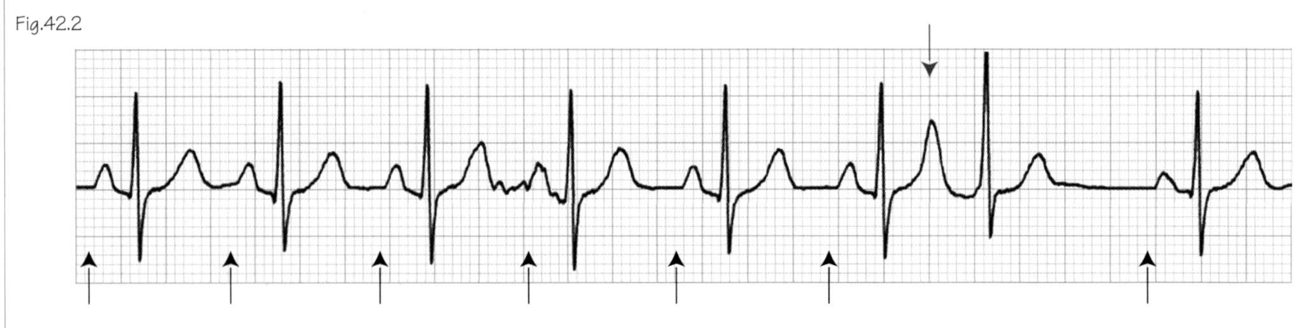

Fig.42.2

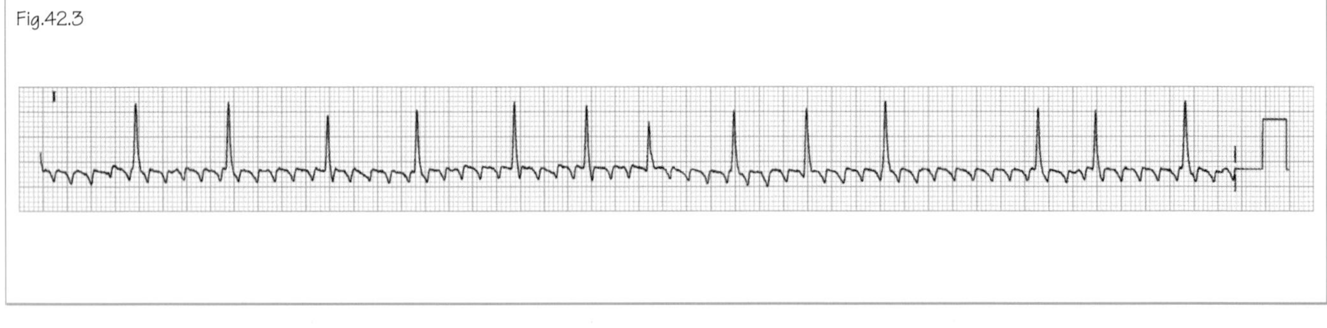

Fig.42.3

Atrial ectopic beats are extremely common. The features of atrial extrasystoles are:

• Atrial ectopic beats are beats initiated in the atria, at a site distant from the normal sinus node, and occurring earlier than the normal sinus beat. The mechanism of occurrence of atrial extrasystoles varies; some are due to atrial re-entry, others to atrial automaticity.

• The P wave occurs much earlier than expected. In normal sinus rhythm the PP (and thus the RR) intervals are roughly constant. There is some variation, due to the effects of the autonomic nervous system on the sinus node, the vagus nerve can cause the PP (and RR) interval to changes in succeeding beats by ≥ 50 ms. Nonetheless the PP interval normally does not change from one beat to the next by more than 60–80 ms, i.e. by less than two small squares. If the P wave is therefore much earlier than two small squares than anticipated, atrial ectopic activity should be suspected.

• The P wave has an abnormal shape, because the site of origin of the ectopic beat is different from the normal sinus node, so the spread of excitation over the atria is different from normal, and hence the surface manifestation of this, the P wave, has a different shape from normal.

• The PR interval following the atrial extrasystole is often but not always different from the normal PR interval for two contradictory reasons. Firstly, given that the atrial beat originates in a site different from the normal sino-atrial (SA) node, the time taken for the wave of depolarization initiated by the atrial extrasystole to reach the atrioventricular (AV) node and hence excite the ventricle, differs from the normal PR interval, and indeed may be shorter, if the focus is close to the AV node. Secondly, the AV node may still be partially refractory and so it takes longer to transmit this impulse to the ventricle.

• The QRS is of a normal, or at least its usual, shape.

• The PP interval following the atrial extrasystole is usually about the length of the normal PP interval. In other words, there is no compensatory pause, as there is with many ventricular extrasystoles. This is due to the fact that atrial extrasystoles usually 'invade' and re-set the sinus node (Fig. 42.1).

Atrial extrasystoles can follow every second or third sinus beat, when they are known as atrial bigeminy or atrial trigeminy. There is usually a fixed coupling interval to the preceding normal P wave; the mechanism is therefore usually atrial re-entry.

Atrial extrasystoles may not be conducted to the ventricle if they occur particularly early. This is usually due to the fact that the normal AV node is still physiologically refractory; it does not necessarily imply any conducting tissue disease. Such beats should be referred to as non-conducted beats, rather than blocked beats. A corollary of this is that if the atrial extrasystole occurs early, and conduction through the AV is possible, it still may be that one or other of the bundle branches are still refractory, so that an abnormally shaped QRS complex (with a right or left bundle branch morphology) results (the 'Ashman' phenomena).

Junctional extrasystoles

Junctional extrasystoles arise from around the AV junction; in essence they are a variation of the more standard atrial extrasystoles. They have one key difference; whereas atrial extrasystoles usually reset the sinus node, so eliminating a compensatory pause following the beats, junctional extrasystoles often do not reset the sinus beat, so there is a compensatory pause (Fig. 42.2).

Significance of atrial extrasystoles

Usually, atrial extrasystoles have no significance. In a few patients they relate to structural disease of the atria (e.g. due to left or right ventricular disease, or valvar heart disease), to thyrotoxicosis, or to excess alcohol. The relationship to more sustained atrial arrhythmias (e.g. atrial flutter or fibrillation) is weak.

Ectopic atrial pacemaker

Sometimes a string of P waves distant from the sinus node occurs; they are recognized by having a P wave shape different from the normal one, and are called by different names according to their speed. If the P waves occur at roughly the normal heart rate, then it is termed an ectopic atrial pacemaker – if every beat has a slightly different shape from the preceding one (usually the PR interval varies as well) it is termed a wandering atrial pacemaker. If the rate is high, e.g. 140–180, then it is termed an ectopic atrial tachycardia, and if the rate is high and the P wave shape varies from beat to beat, it is termed a multifocal atrial tachycardia (Fig. 42.3). Only every second, third or fourth atrial beat is transmitted through to the ventricles – a physiological heart block.

Fig. 42.1 Atrial extrasystoles invading and resetting the sinus node. Most atrial extrasystoles: (i) have an different P wave shape when compared to the normal sinus beat P wave (as they arise in a different part of the atria, and so travel over the atria taking a different route from that taken by the sinus beat); (ii) invade the sinus node retrogradely, so resetting it, and altering the timing of the next sinus beat (unlike ventricular ectopic beats, which do not reset the sinus node, so are usually followed by a compensatory pause). SA node, sino-atrial node.

Fig. 42.2 An atrial extrasystole (red arrow), occurring on the top the T wave, resulting in an early QRST complex. Most atrial extrasystoles reset the sinus node, this does not happen here and the extrasystole is followed at the appropriate time by another P wave, the timing affected by the extrasystole.

Fig. 42.3 Ectopic atrial tachycardia; well defined frequent P waves, too fast to be sinus, with block, every 4–6 atrial beats gets through to activate the ventricle. These P waves are best seen in leads I, aVR, V1. Their shape is very different from a normal sinus rhythm P wave. In some leads, e.g. III, aVF, and the lateral chest leads, they appear irregular and of small voltage, and could easily be confused with atrial fibrillation. The QRS complexes are normal and there is lateral T wave flattening.

43 Atrial fibrillation

Fig.43.1

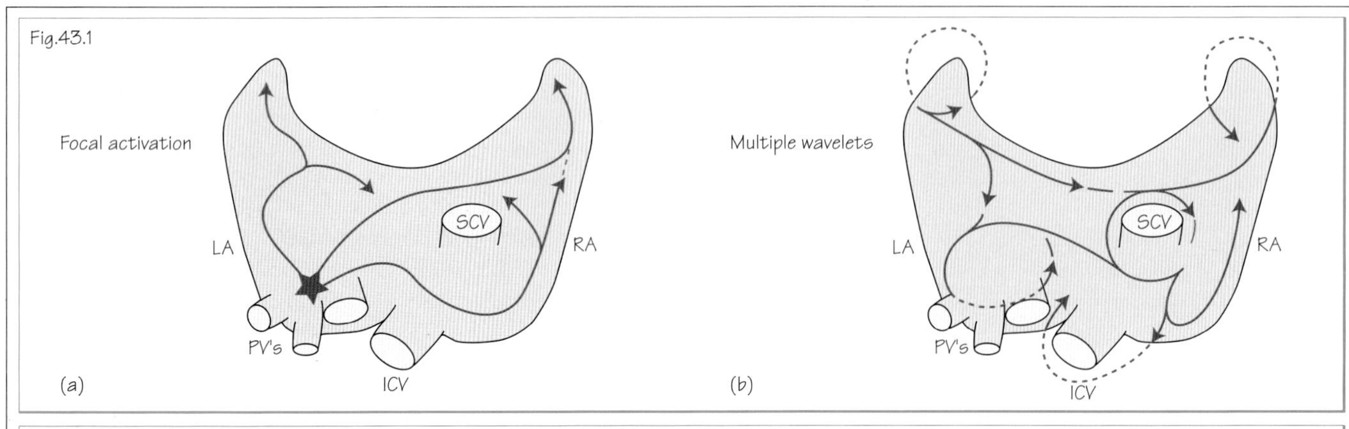

Fig.43.2

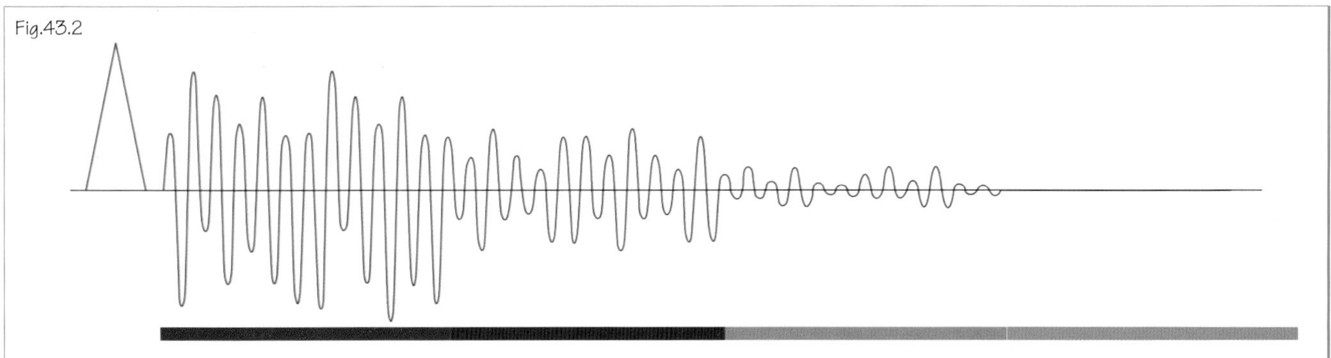

Fig.43.3

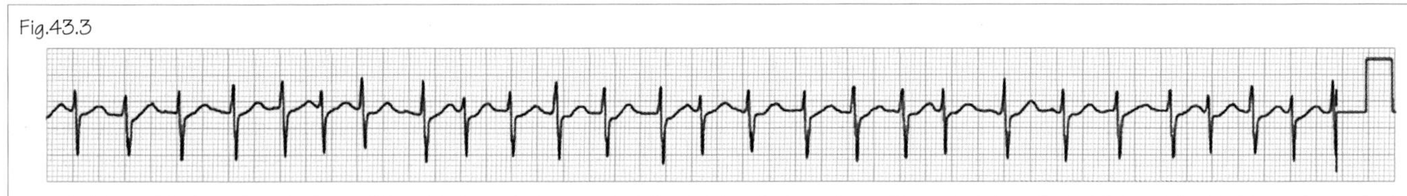

Fig.43.4

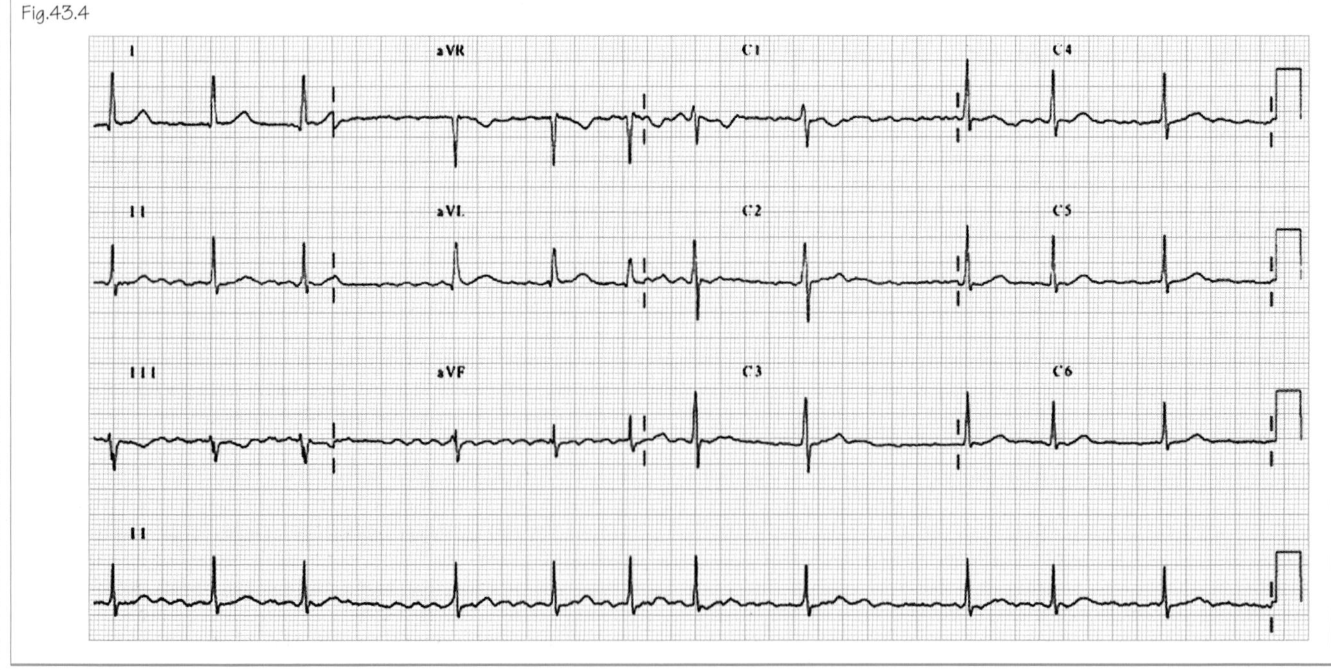

Atrial fibrillation (AF) is the commonest serious arrhythmia. Its incidence increases with age, and with certain diseases, which themselves cause symptoms: (i) thyroid disease; weight loss, irritability, diarrhoea, etc.; (ii) alcohol excess; (iii) left ventricular (LV) dysfunction; breathlessness, usually suddenly deteriorating when AF starts; (iv) angina, which can provoke AF, or result from AF; (v) other causes including pneumonia, pulmonary emboli and Wolff–Parkinson–White syndrome.

Atrial fibrillation results in characteristic symptoms irrespective of causation:

- Palpitations, sudden onset and offset, defined duration, fast and irregularly irregular.
- Breathlessness, in pre-existing LV dysfunction.
- In some, the first manifestation is, distressingly, a stroke, due to blood clot embolizing from the left atrium to the brain. Emboli to other parts of the body also occur (the gut, limbs, etc.).

Mechanism and substrate for AF

Atrial fibrillation is often triggered by ectopics/rapidly discharging focus (or, in a few, a re-entrant circuit) arising in the origin of a pulmonary vein (so pulmonary vein focus ablation/isolation is in some a successful treatment for recurrent AF – radiofrequency burns destroy the focus or produce an electrically inert scar separating the pulmonary vein from the atria, preventing transmission of pulmonary vein electricity into the main atria). Atrial fibrillation is sustained by a large left atrium, which allows multiple wavelets (≥ 7) to pass continually/randomly throughout the atria (accounting for the success of MAZE procedures in preventing AF – radiofrequency burns are made in the atria, reducing the electrical size of the atria, preventing re-entry) (Fig. 43.1a,b).

Atrial fibrillation is classified into:

- Paroxysmal AF (pAF); episodes terminate spontaneously, usually ≤ 24 h. Paroxysmal AF is sometimes divided into: (i) vagal AF, which starts when the vagal tone is high, e.g. at night; (ii) sympathetic pAF, starting with sympathetic stimulation, e.g. exercise. This classification is rarely useful.
- Persistent AF; episodes do not terminate spontaneously, but can be terminated by chemical or electrical cardioversion.
- Permanent; episodes of AF resistant to cardioversion, or where cardioversion is not appropriate, and not attempted.

The signs of AF are a tachycardia (Fig. 43.3), especially on exercise, and an irregularly irregular pulse. The '*a*' wave of the venous pressure disappears: in a few patients, signs of heart failure occur. The ECG shows:

- A continuously active baseline composed of varying amplitude fibrillatory or '*f*' waves, reflecting the continual electrical activity in the atria. As time passes, the magnitude of the '*f*' waves declines (Fig. 43.2).
- At the onset of AF there is often a high QRS rate (≥ 150 b/min) as the sympathetic nervous system is often activated, allowing for 'slick' atrioventricular (AV) conduction (Fig. 43.3) – if there is an unremarkable QRS rate in the absence of AV nodal blocking drugs, then intrinsic AV nodal disease should be suspected. Equally however the QRS rate becomes much slower in long-standing AF.
- The RR intervals occur at completely irregularly irregular intervals, as the AV node is bombarded completely randomly by impulses from the atria (Fig. 43.4). Indeed the finding that the RR interval is not fixed (i.e. the heart rate is 'irregularly irregular') is a key method of determining whether a broad complex tachycardia is ventricular in origin or supraventricular. If there is a broad complex tachycardia in AF, especially if the heart rate is high, consider whether an accessory pathway (see Chapters 12 and 46), due to Wolff–Parkinson–White syndrome underlies the AF.
- Non-specific ST segment changes. In those with coronary disease, or LV hypertrophy, ST depression may occur.

Sinus node disease and AF

In a few patients, sinus node disease underlies AF. The mechanism is probably sinus bradycardia allowing parts of the atria to prolong their refractory period more than others (i.e. increased dispersion of atrial refractoriness). This allows a re-entrant atrial arrhythmia to form, which then breaks up, resulting in AF. When the AF terminates, the sinus node, which should start firing immediately, can in sinus node disease take 3–5 s to start up, during which time cardiac output is lost and the patient may blackout. The risk of AF can be reduced, and syncope prevented, by pacing the atria (AAI pacing – see Chapter 59).

Fig. 43.1 Pathophysiology of atrial fibrillation (a,b). The commonest substrate is multiple re-entrant wavelets passing continuously through both atria (b). Trigger mechanisms include: (i) repetitively discharging focus in the left atrium near one of the pulmonary veins; (ii) a single re-entrant circuit.

Fig. 43.2 The amplitude of the fibrillatory waves in atrial fibrillation (AF). As a generalization, at the onset of AF, the *f* waves are of large amplitude (red); after days–weeks, the amplitude declines (blue), becoming quite small after weeks–months (orange). In long standing AF the baseline is often quite flat (green) – the clue to the presence of AF is not so much the *f* waves, as the regularity or otherwise of the QRS complexes. In AF the QRS complexes occur irregularly, as there is no pattern to the electrical bombardment of the atrioventricular (AV) node, whereas in sinus rhythm and arrhythmias other than AF the RR interval is usually fairly constant.

Fig. 43.3 At the onset of atrial fibrillation the heart rate is high, and can sometimes, as in this example, be surprisingly regular (giving rise to symptoms of regular rather than irregular palpitations). However, careful inspection (for example, by mapping out the RR intervals on a piece of paper) shows that the RR intervals vary continuously – a key clue as the fibrillatory '*f*' waves are so fine as to hardly be visible.

Fig. 43.4 Atrial fibrillation (AF). The clue that the rhythm is AF is not the fibrillatory waves – they are rather small – but the irregularly irregular heart rate. The heart rate is very well controlled, due to: (i) possibly intrinsic disease of the atrioventricular (AV) node; (ii) drugs, such as a beta-blocker (digoxin is unlikely here as there are no ST/T waves changes); (iii) AF being long standing. The QRST complexes are normal.

44 Atrial flutter and atrial tachycardia

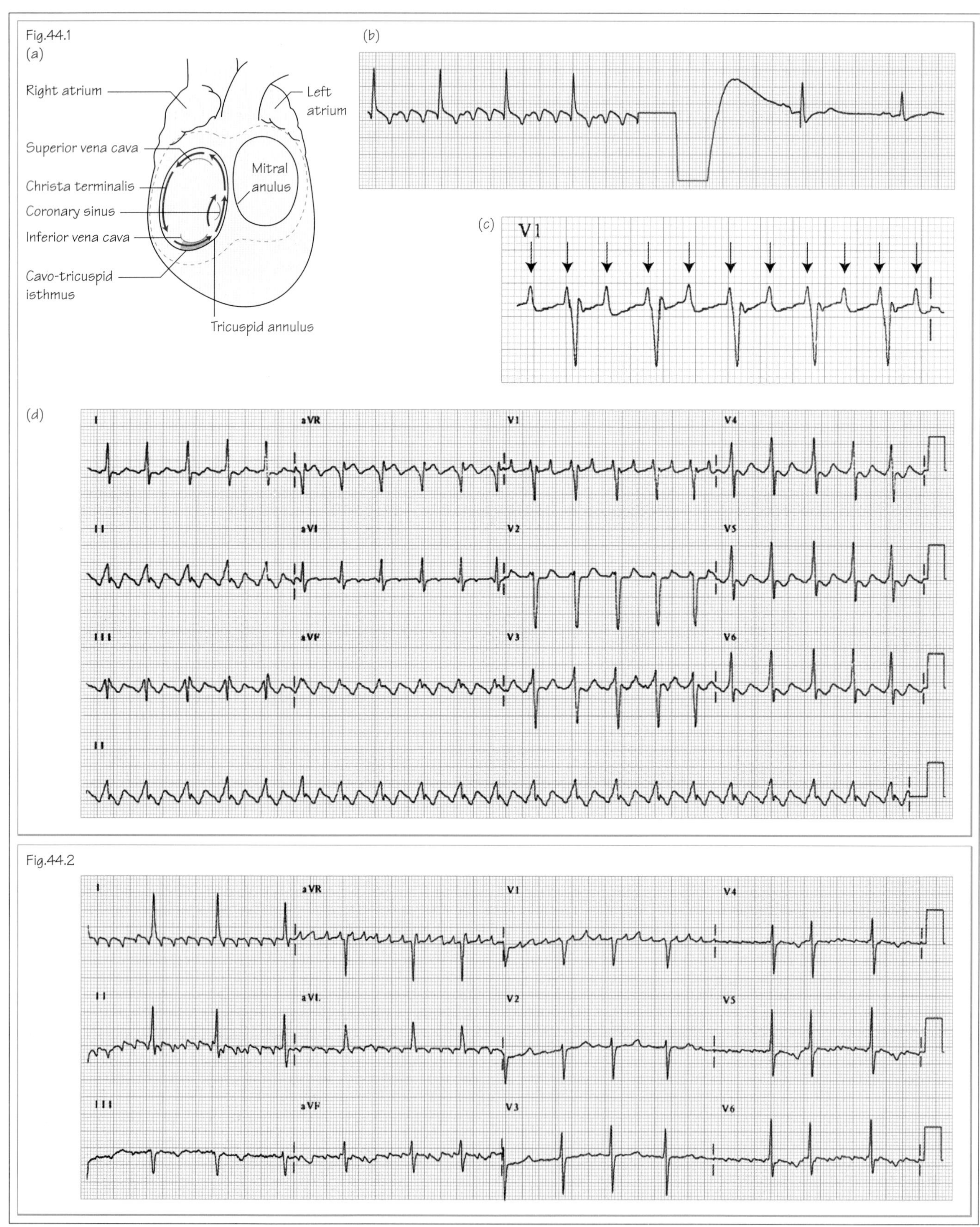

Atrial flutter is a common arrhythmia, especially in men (perhaps as they have larger hearts) (Table 44.1). It is due to a macro re-entrant circuit in the right atrium (Fig. 44.1a–d) and results in a highly characteristic ECG appearance, with continual electrical activity best seen in the inferior leads. The 'sawtooth' baseline typically has a slow downstroke and a rapid upstroke. P wave activity is often reasonably well seen in lead V1, when it is predominantly positive. Occasionally the P waves in lead V1 are not well developed.

The right atrial circuit is usually of such a length that 300 circuits occur per minute. This is too fast for the atrioventricular (AV) physiologically to allow for 1 to 1 conduction down to the ventricles, and usually a fixed proportion of beats get through, often one in two, giving a QRS (and hence heart) rate of 150 b/min. This has led to an aphorism in arrhythmology; whenever a tachycardia is seen with a heart rate of exactly 150 b/min, the rhythm disturbance is atrial flutter until proved otherwise. Sometimes the conduction is 1 in 3 or 4, giving a QRS rate respectively of 100 and 75 b/min. If the rate of transmission is (in the absence of anti-arrhythmic drugs) less than this, say 1 in 5 or 1 in 6, then there is a high probability that there is also intrinsic conducting tissue disease.

Sometimes anti-arrhythmic drugs (such as propafenone) can slow the atrial rate, say to 250 b/min, sufficient for the AV node to allow 1 to 1 conduction. Thus paradoxically, some drugs used to slow the heart rate may in fact end up increasing it! This can have dangerous consequences.

Atypical atrial flutter (Table 44.1) is a rare rhythm disturbance, recognized when the deflections in the inferior leads are positive (probably as the circuit proceeds in a clockwise rotation, rather than the anti-clockwise motion of typical atrial flutter). The P wave in lead V1 is usually negative. The rate can be 300 b/min, less or more (the latter in truly atypical atrial flutter).

Prognosis of atrial flutter

Prognosis is usually that of any associated disease (chronic obstructive pulmonary disease [COPD], ischaemic heart disease [IDD], mitral/tricuspid valve disease). A high proportion of patients go on to develop atrial fibrillation. If the heart rate remains too high in untreated atrial flutter, a 'rate-related' cardiomyopathy can develop (with decreased left ventricular systolic function) usually reversible on rigorously controlling the heart rate.

Treatment of atrial flutter

Treatment should slow the heart rate from the usual 150 b/min to a more physiological level (beta-blockers, rate slowing Ca^{2+} blockers, amiodarone), possibly anticoagulation, DC cardioversion. If troublesome, atrial flutter circuit ablation is a reasonably successful procedure.

Atrial tachycardia

Atrial tachycardia is due to a rapid firing ectopic focus in the atria, either due to automaticity or due to a micro-re-entrant circuit. It is recognized by there being an iso-electric line in all the leads between each P wave, which itself has an abnormal morphology (Fig. 44.2). Like atrial flutter, the AV node cannot physiologically transmit all the impulses, and a degree of physiological block occurs, often 2 or 3 to 1. Treatment involves drugs to increase the degree of AV block to slow the QRS heart rate, cardioversion (with anticoagulant cover) and, occasionally, ablation of the abnormal focus.

Table 44.1 Characteristics and ECG findings in regular atrial arrhythmias. Atrial fibriallation is distinguished from these arrhythmias by finding an irregular QRS rate, while these arrhythmias usually have a regular QRS rate.

	Typical atrial flutter	Atypical atrial flutter	Atrial tachycardia
Incidence	Common	Rare	Intermediate
Inferior lead deflection	Negative	Positive	Positive or negative
Continual electrical activity in inferior leads	Yes	Yes	No
V1 deflection	+ve	–ve	+ve or –ve
Atrial rate	300 b/min	Often 300 b/min, occasionally slower or quicker	Variable – often 200–250 b/min
QRS rate	Often 150 or 100 b/min	Often 150 or 100 b/min	Integer divisor of atrial rate

Fig. 44.1 (a) Mechanism of typical atrial flutter. Atrial flutter is due to a macro re-entrant circuit contained within the right atrium. If part of the circuit is destroyed by radiofrequency catheter ablation, the arrhythmia is prevented. The narrowest part of the circuit is bordered by the inferior vena cava (IVC) and tricuspid valve, and this is the site targeted in ablation procedures. (b) DC shock converting atrial flutter to sinus rhythm. There are three flutter waves for each QRS prior to the shock, then sinus rhythm with a rather wide bifid P wave. (c) Magnified lead V1, illustrating two P waves to every QRS complex; one P wave is well hidden close to the QRS complex. (d) Typical atrial flutter: the baseline shows typical sawtooth flutter waves in the inferior leads (II, III, aVF). In lead V1, though it is not easy to see, there are two sharply defined P waves for each QRS complex, i.e. there is 2 to 1 heart block. The QRS complexes look normal, and it is difficult to interpret the T waves, as they are distorted by the sawtooth baseline.

Fig. 44.2 Atrial tachycardia. This can be a challenging ECG to read. Start from first principles. *Look at leads II and V1 to determine the rhythm.* Lead II shows movement artefact, and in this ECG it is better to use lead I and V1. There are very frequent abnormally shaped P waves – a little less than a square separates them, so their rate is just over 300 b/min. Note: (i) the absence of an inferior lead sawtooth appearance; (ii) that in all leads there is at least some flat iso-electric lines between each beat. This cannot be atrial flutter, but is an atrial tachycardia. A variable number of P waves are conducted through to fire the ventricles, usually around 7 to 1. This is physiological, not pathological atrioventricular block. The underlying QRS complex appears unremarkable; the inferior and lateral lead T waves are flat. This ECG came from an elderly man not known to have heart disease other than atrial tachycardia.

45 Atrioventricular nodal re-entrant tachycardia

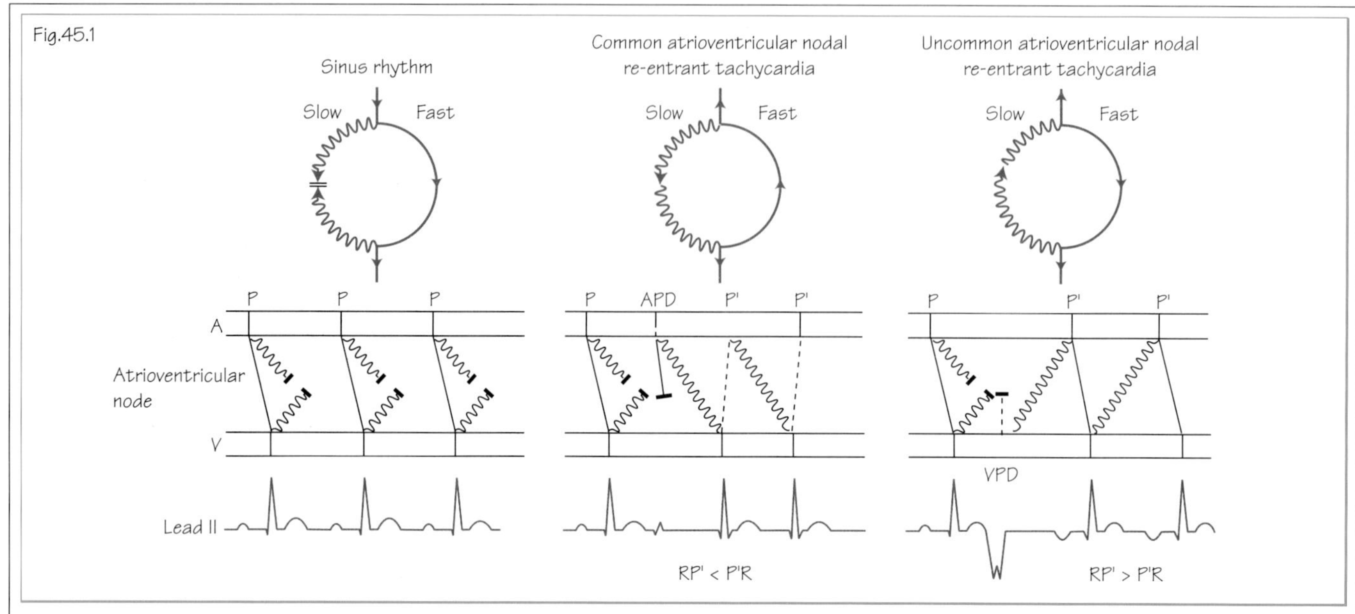

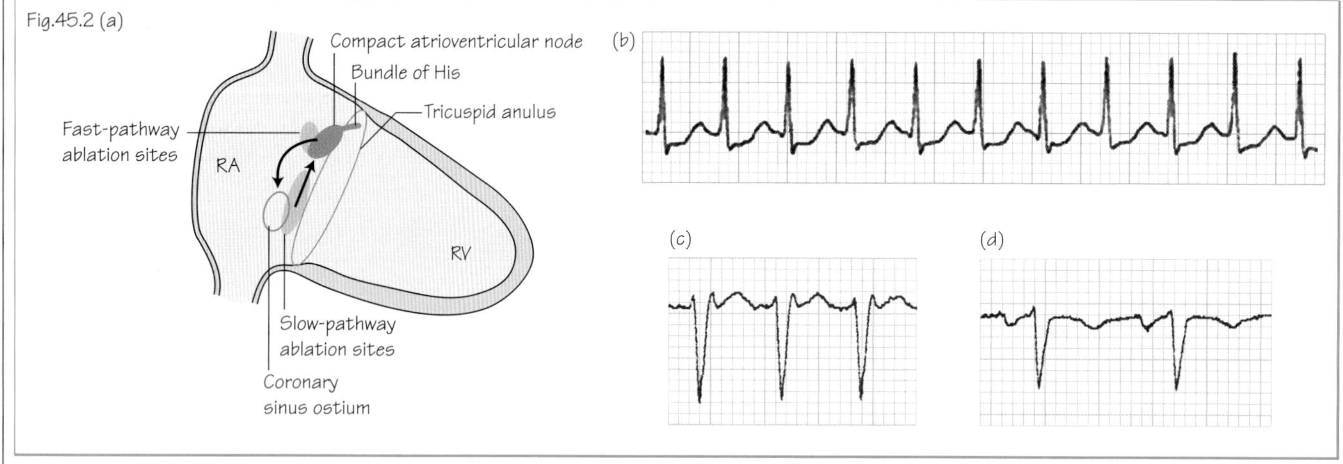

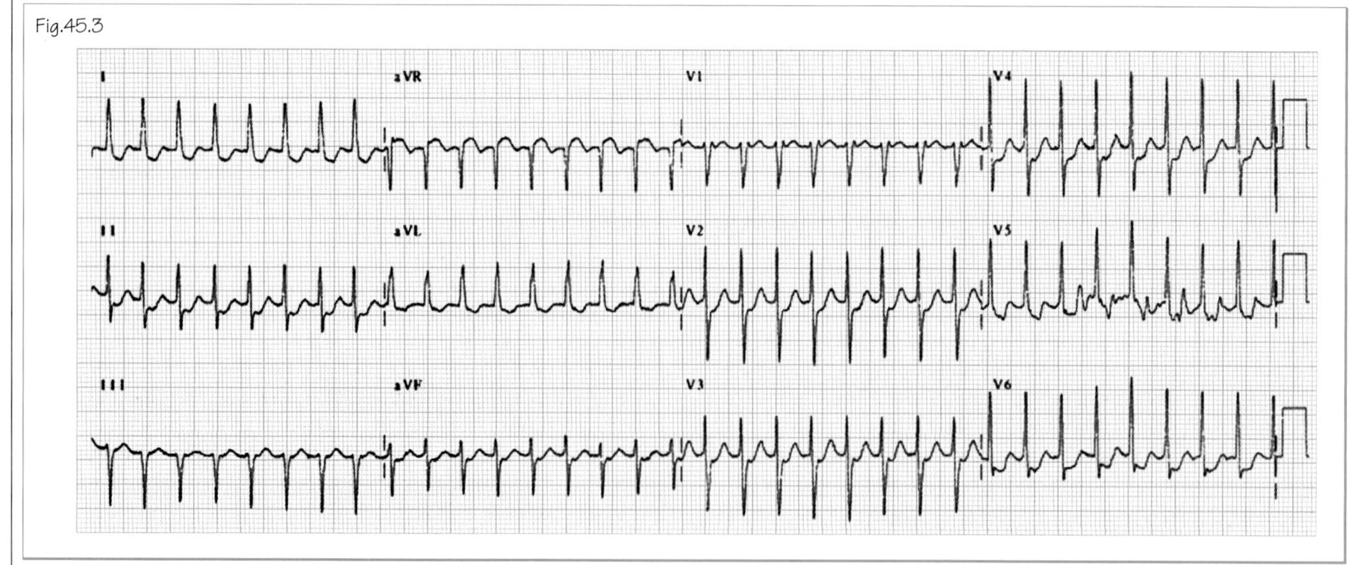

Atrioventricular nodal re-entrant tachycardia (AVNRT) is common. Seventy per cent of patients are female; medical help is most commonly sought in those 30–50 years old. In AVNRT an abnormal extra pathway, congenital in origin, near or within the atrioventricular (AV) node allows, from time to time, the depolarizing wave to become trapped within structures local to the AV node, describing a continuous circular re-entrant pattern (Fig. 45.1). Each time the depolarizing wave passes round the circuit, it fires off the ventricle and then the atria. Due to this basic pathophysiology, the ECG features of AVNRT are:

- A narrow-complex tachycardia, as the ventricles are excited by the normal route via the AV node (Fig. 45.2a,b). The QRS complex can be broad due to pre-existing bundle branch block, or rate-dependent bundle branch block, though this is rare and most AVNRTs are narrow complex.
- The QRS rate is usually 140–240 b/min.
- The P wave is abnormally shaped, as the atria are activated retrogradely from the AV node. The P wave is often not visible, as it is buried in the QRS complex. In some the retrograde P wave appears as a late small R wave in lead V1 (i.e. an rSR′ pattern, not present in sinus rhythm) or an S wave in the inferior leads (also disappearing in sinus rhythm).
- ST depression is common at high heart rates, even in the absence of coronary artery disease.

The symptoms of AVNRT are:

- Sudden onset fast regular palpitations of defined duration.
- Sometimes a regular pounding in the neck (as the atria contract onto a closed AV valve, blood is pushed retrogradely up into the jugular veins). The neck veins can pulsate very prominently, which observers may comment on.
- As a consequence of atrial stretch, atrial natriuretic peptide is released; this can lead to a diuresis following the tachycardia (post-event polyuria).
- Rarely, syncope can be due to AVNRT, the usual mechanism being co-existing sinus node disease; continual bombardment of the sinus node during tachycardia suppresses its function. When tachycardia ceases the sinus node takes several seconds to restart, during which time there is cardiac standstill leading to near or actual syncope.

Treatment

Treatment is termination of the acute attack, and suppression of further attacks:

- Vagal manoeuvres or intravenous adenosine are standard therapies (replacing intravenous verapamil or beta-blocker). These work by inducing temporary AV block or altering the electrophysiology of the AV node sufficiently that the circus movement ceases and the sinus node can depolarize the atria and invade the AV node in the normal manner.
- Any drug that slows conduction through the AV node can suppress attacks: beta-blockers, Ca^{2+} channel blockers (verapamil or diltiazam) and digoxin. Theoretically (not practically due to side-effects) there is a role for class I or III agents. If drugs fail, ablation of the slow pathway can be a satisfactory option (with a 1% chance of inadvertently damaging the fast pathway, leading to complete heart block, necessitating a permanent pacemaker).

Extraordinarily rare related arrhythmias involving the AV node

Non-paroxysmal junctional tachycardia is a very rare arrhythmia in adults, and relates to a focus near the AV node continually firing (due to one of several mechanisms, not however re-entry), and may result from inflammation to this part of the heart (e.g. after mitral valve surgery, myocardial infarction) or digoxin toxicity. A narrow complex tachycardia occurs, either with 1 to 1 retrograde P wave activation or, bizarrely, AV dissociation.

Fig. 45.1 Mechanism of atrioventricular nodal re-entrant tachycardia (AVNRT). The top panels represent the atrioventricular (AV) node with dual pathways, a fast conducting/slowly repolarizing one to the right and a slow conducting/fast repolarizing one to the left. The middle panels represent the passage of electricity through the heart (a 'Lewis' diagram) diagrammatically as a ladder (sometimes known as a 'ladder' diagram). Solid lines are anterograde AV nodal conduction, broken lines retrograde conduction, straight lines conduction through the fast pathway, and wavy lines through the slow pathway. In sinus rhythm the slow pathway does not transmit impulses, as the depolarization exciting the fast pathway anterogradely turns round at the far end and invades the slow pathway retrogradely meeting the slow pathway anterograde conduction head on, so eliminating it. An atrial premature depolarization (APD) can occur with the right timing such that it can pass down the slow pathway (as it repolarizes quickly) but not into the fast pathway (which takes longer to repolarize). At the far end of the AV node, the impulse transmitted from the slow pathway, in addition to firing the ventricles, can turn into the fast pathway, passing retrogradely. When the impulse reaches the proximal end, in addition to firing the atria retrogradely, the impulse can re-enter the slow pathway (as this has now repolarized) so setting up a circus movement. Atria and ventricles are excited almost simultaneously – there is a slight delay between QRS complexes and the inverted retrograde P′ wave, which can sometimes be seen in the inferior leads as an apparent (or pseudo) S wave. In atypical AVNRT the retrograde limb is the slow pathway. This means the atria are excited some time after the ventricles resulting in a late negative P′ wave.

Fig. 45.2 (a) Atrioventricular nodal re-entrant tachycardia (AVNRT) ablation sites. (b) Atrioventricular nodal re-entrant tachycardia: (b′) rhythm strip; (c) lead V1 showing rSR′ deflection during tachycardia; (d) not present during sinus rhythm.

Fig. 45.3 Supraventricular tachycardia (SVT) due to atrioventricular nodal re-entrant tachycardia (AVNRT). Tachycardia, rate about 210 b/min. No P waves before the QRS complex, lead V1 shows R′ (see Fig. 45.2c,d)), a hallmark of AVNRT. The QRS complexes are otherwise normal, but there is widespread ST depression anterolaterally. The heart rate is so high that the ST depression does not necessarily indicate coronary disease. The arrhythmia terminated with adenosine.

46 Atrioventricular re-entrant tachycardia

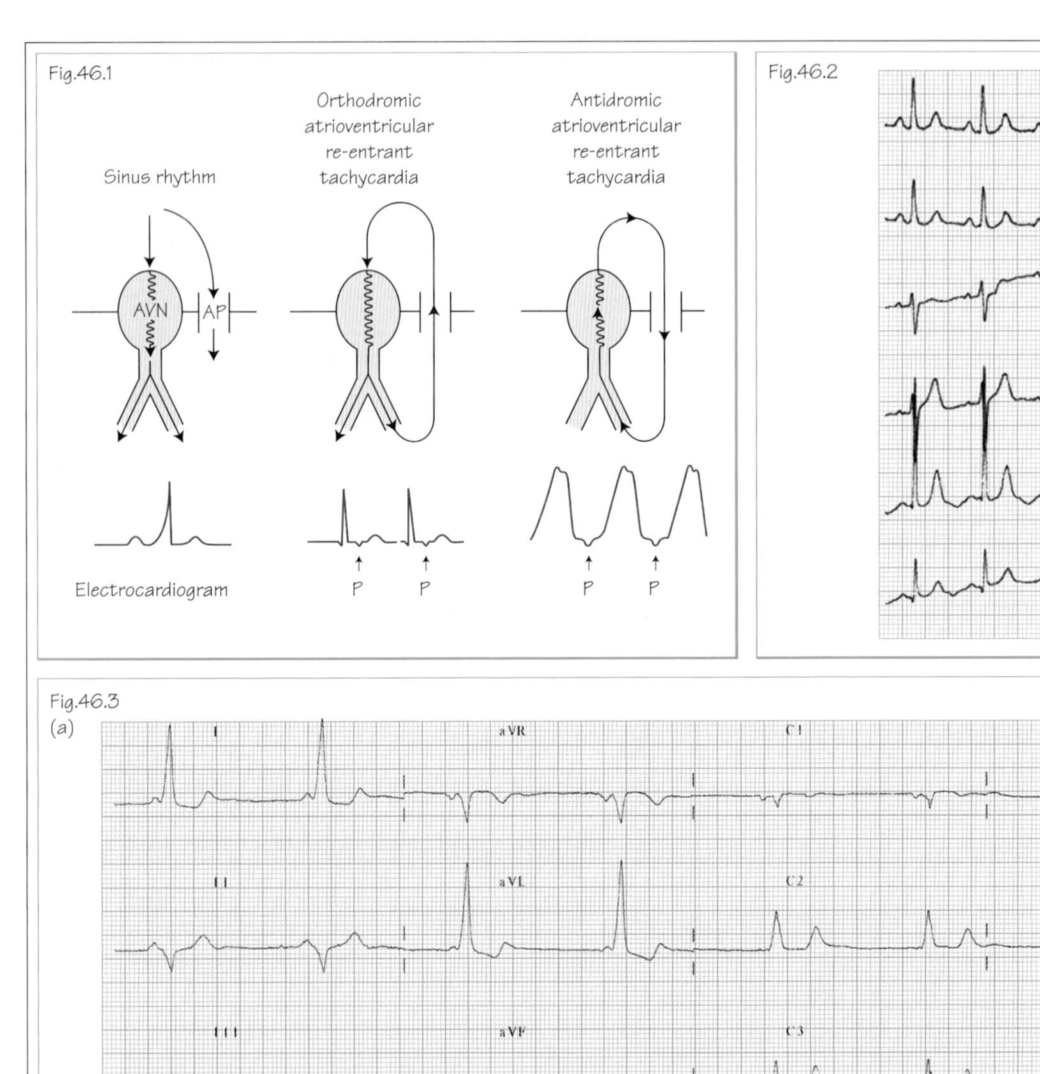

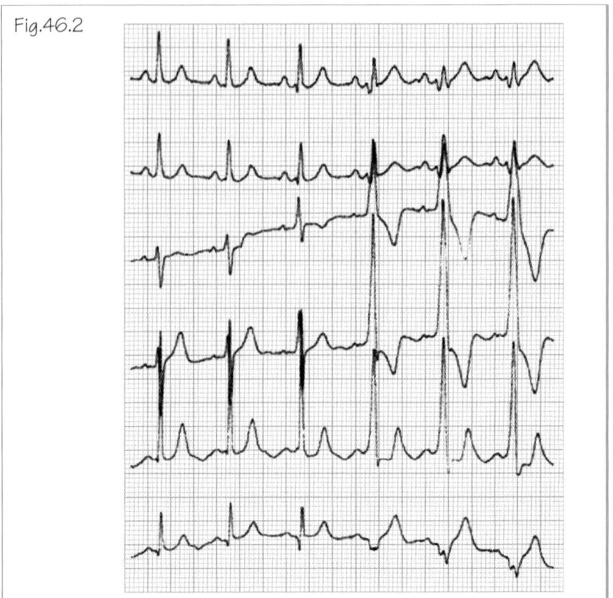

Fig.46.3

(a)

I aVR C1 C4

II aVL C2 C5

III aVF C3 C6

(b)

I aVR C1 C4

II aVL C2 C5

III aVF C3 C6

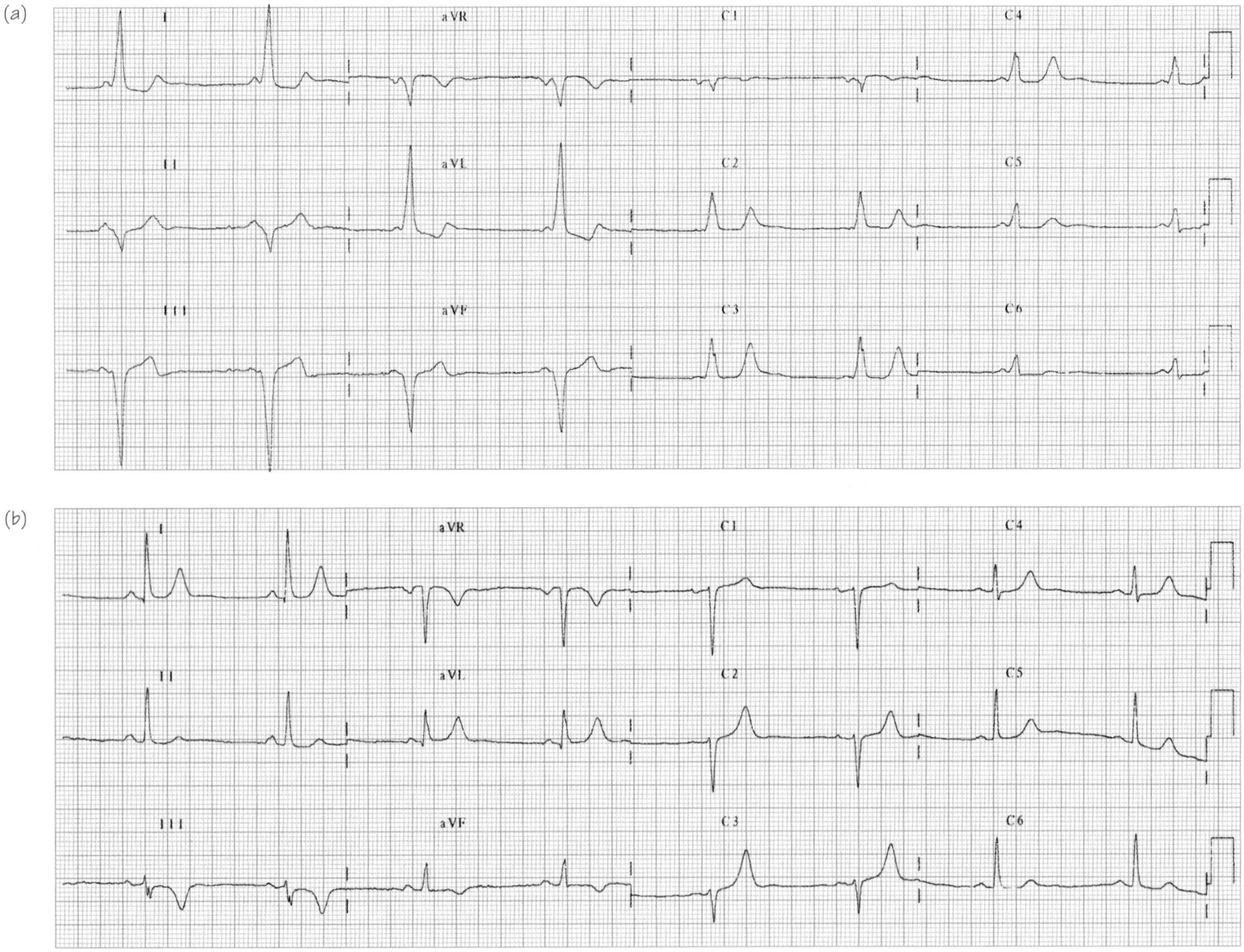

Wolff–Parkinson–White (WPW) syndrome affects 0.1–0.3% of the population, and is one substrate for atrioventricular re-entrant tachycardia (AVRT) (Figs. 46.1 and 46.2). In WPW syndrome there is an additional electrical connection between the atria and the ventricles, an 'accessory pathway', present throughout life, seen as a delta wave, which may not produce symptoms until mid or late adulthood or indeed never. This accessory pathway forms the basis for a re-entrant circuit and tachyarrhythmias.

Accessory pathways and their variation

The accessory pathway results in a delta wave, which may be always present on the inter-attack ECG, sometimes, or never (due to distance from the normal electrical path, or to the pathway only conducting retrogradely; Fig. 46.2). Only accessory pathways with visible delta waves are termed WPW syndrome. The delta wave morphology reflects the anatomical location of the pathway (see Chapter 12).

Arrhythmias associated with accessory pathways

- Orthodromic AVRT is the common tachyarrhythmia and results in a narrow complex tachycardia. In sinus rhythm the depolarization passing via the normal route and the accessory pathway into the ventricle meet and neutralize each other such that neither can pass up the other pathway. A ventricular ectopic occurring at just the right moment passes unopposed retrogradely up the accessory pathway, across the atria, into the atrioventricular (AV) node, through the ventricle, then back up the accessory pathway, setting up a 'circus' movement type tachyarrhythmia (Fig. 46.1). As the circuit uses the normal AV node and specialized conducting tissue the QRS complex is narrow (unless there is co-existing conducting tissue disease). An abnormally shaped (retrograde or P′ wave) P wave occurs after the QRS complex, as the atria are activated after the ventricles (Fig. 46.1).
- Antidromic AVRT results in a broad complex tachycardia (Fig. 46.1) and mechanistically is the reverse of orthodromic tachycardia. An abnormally early atrial impulse passes down the accessory pathway, through the ventricle, up the AV node, across the atria, and down the pathway again. As the ventricle is activated via the accessory pathway and consequent slow myocyte-to-myocyte transmission the QRS complex during tachycardia is broad. This is a very rare tachycardia.
- Atrial fibrillation (AF) occurs in 20% of WPW patients and is initiated when the electrical impulse from a ventricular ectopic passes up the accessory pathway retrogradely into the atria, breaks up and causes multiple re-entering wavelets – atrial fibrillation. In AF both the AV node and the accessory pathway are bombarded continually by atrial electricity. Those impulses passing successfully down the AV node result in narrow QRS complexes, whereas those transmitted down the accessory pathway result in a broad QRS complex. In patients without an accessory pathway, the AV node acts as a filter, transmitting not more than 150–180 impulses per minute into the ventricles. Accessory pathways do not have similar filtering properties, as their refractory period can be short. In some patients a very high heart rate can result (Fig. 40.2), so high that the heart does not have time to fill, so cardiac output and coronary perfusion fall, myocardial ischaemia develops and ventricular fibrillation (VF) occurs. Sudden cardiac death (SCD) affects 0.15% of untreated WPW patients per annum, i.e. most patients do not have a pathway that can conduct AF at rates so high as to be dangerous. At risk patients have: (i) symptoms from their accessory pathway (asymptomatic patients have very low rates of SCD); (ii) a minimum RR interval during spontaneous AF of < 220–250 ms) pathways capable of transmitting impulses at very high heart rates during invasive electrophysiological studies. Those at risk of SCD (or with unacceptable symptoms) should have radiofrequency catheter ablation of the accessory pathway (Fig. 46.3a,b).

Fig. 46.1 Supraventricular arrhythmias in Wolff–Parkinson–White syndrome. Left: sinus rhythm, dual impulses from the atria pass down via the atrioventricular node (AVN) and the accessory pathway (AP), resulting in a short PR interval, slurred QRS upstroke (the delta wave). Middle: orthodromic atrioventricular re-entrant tachycardia (AVRT), the current passes down the atrioventricular (AV) node, exciting the ventricles (narrow complex), across the ventricles, then up the AP, so exciting the atria, resulting in a late retrograde P wave. Right: antidromic AVRT, the reverse of orthodromic AVRT resulting in a broad complex tachycardia, with a P wave just preceding the QRS complex. Drugs that interrupt AV conduction, e.g. adenosine terminate the arrhythmia.

Fig. 46.2 Adenosine revealing Wolff–Parkinson–White (WPW). Suspected WPW syndrome, but non-diagnostic ECG. Intravenous adenosine given, which blocks all conduction down the atrioventricular (AV) node for 2–6 s – if there is no accessory pathway, complete heart block occurs (i.e. P waves with no following QRS complexes). In WPW syndrome, all conduction to the ventricle passes down the accessory pathway, resulting in a very broad slurred QRS complex. Here the moment of transition is shown between ventricular activation via the normal AV node and the accessory pathway. The QRS complexes become broad, slurred and (best seen in leads V2/4, second and third from the bottom) show a very short PR interval.

Fig. 46.3 ECGs pre- and post-accessory pathway ablation. (a) A large delta wave, which implies that a lot of the ventricular myocardium is activated via the accessory pathway. PR interval very short, QRS upstroke slurred. 'Pseudo-infarction' pattern in the inferior leads (i.e. Q waves in leads II, III aVF). This patient has not had an inferior wall infarct; the Q waves reflect the very abnormal ventricular activation from the accessory pathway (a right posterior-septal pathway – see Chapter 12). (b) ECG after accessory pathway ablation. The ECG is virtually normal, except for the deep T wave inversion in lead III. Good sized inferior lead R waves, confirming the absence of inferior infarction. T wave inversion ('T wave memory') is common following catheter ablation (though does not occur with pathways which conduct only retrogradely), and usually resolves over time. Here, the inferior lead T wave inversion remained present many years later, for unknown reasons.

47 Ventricular ectopics

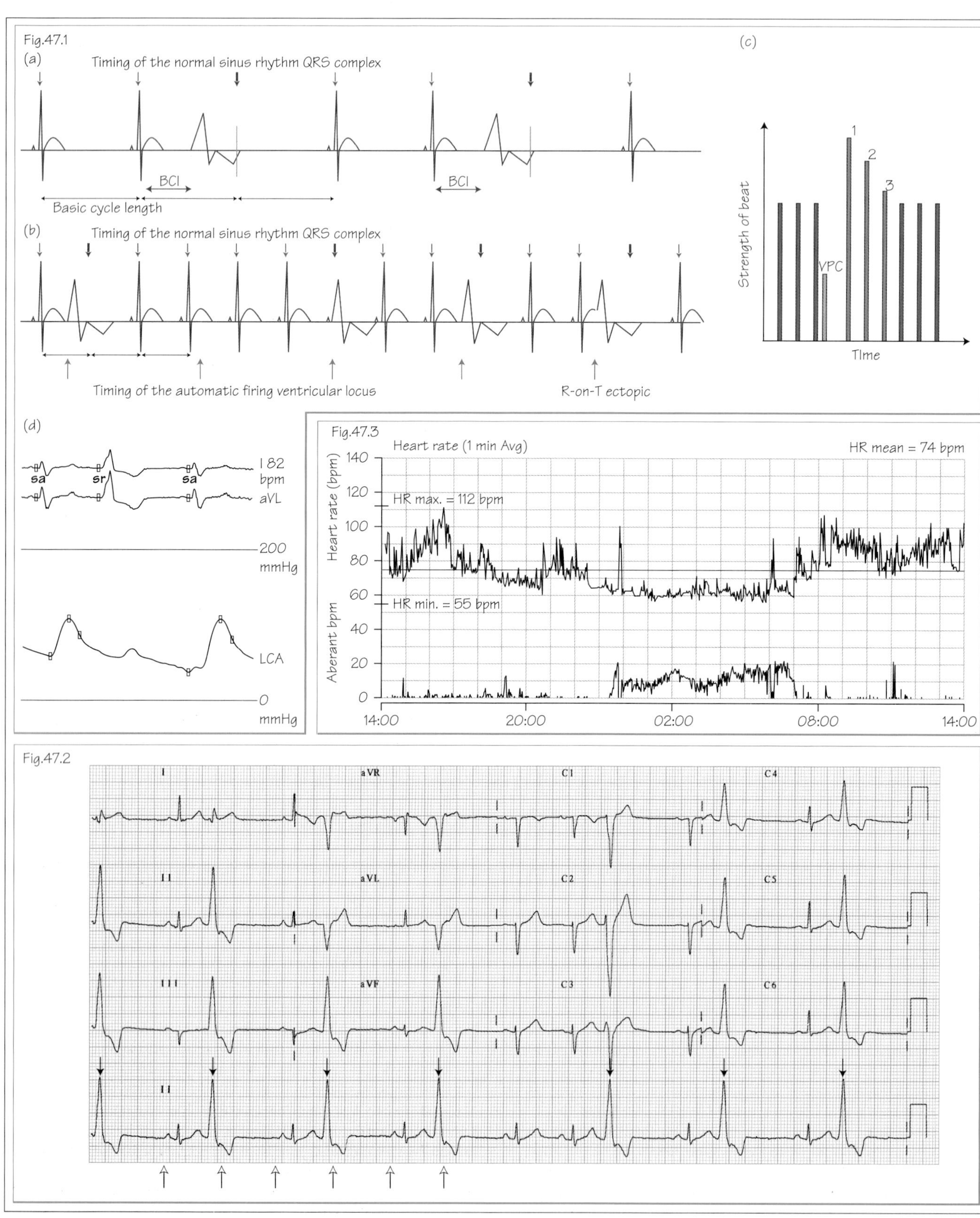

Fig.47.1
(a)
Timing of the normal sinus rhythm QRS complex
BCI
BCI
Basic cycle length
(b)
Timing of the normal sinus rhythm QRS complex
Timing of the automatic firing ventricular locus
R-on-T ectopic
(c)
Strength of beat
VPC
1
2
3
Time
(d)
sa
sr
sa
182 bpm
aVL
200 mmHg
LCA
0 mmHg
Fig.47.3
Heart rate (1 min Avg)
HR mean = 74 bpm
HR max. = 112 bpm
HR min. = 55 bpm
Heart rate (bpm)
Aberant bpm
140
120
100
80
60
40
20
0
14:00
20:00
02:00
08:00
14:00
Fig.47.2
I
aVR
C1
C4
II
aVL
C2
C5
III
aVF
C3
C6
II

Ventricular ectopic beats (also termed ventricular premature contractions [VPCs], ventricular premature beats [VPBs], ventricular extrasystoles [VEs]) are common and produce symptoms from:

- The extra-beat: irregular palpitations, differentiated from atrial fibrillation (AF) by heart rate (high in AF, normal with VPCs).
- The beats following the extrasystole. The VPC is weaker than normal and the few beats following are of increased strength (Fig. 47.1a–d). Patients often feel 'as if the heart stops' and then 'restarts' with a 'thud' or a 'bang'.

ECG appearance

Ventricular premature contractions arise within the ventricle and do not use the specialized conducting system, rather spreading slowly throughout the ventricle using myocyte-to-myocyte transmission, giving rise to a broad QRS complex, the shape of which reflects their site of origin:

- Left ventricular (LV) origin beats arrive last at the right ventricle (RV); delayed RV activation results in a right bundle branch block (RBBB) pattern.
- Beats arising from the right ventricle have a left bundle branch block (LBBB) pattern (Fig. 47.2).
- The T wave is almost always inverted, as the sequence of repolarization is usually quite different from normal.

Ventricular premature contractions arising from the superior part of the heart have an inferior axis and vice versa. During a myocardial infarction (MI), LV-pattern (RBBB appearance) VPCs are more strongly associated with ventricular fibrillation (VF) than RV-pattern (LBBB appearance) VPCs.

The VPC usually does not invade and reset the sinus node, so the P waves march through (Fig. 47.2). Rarely retrograde P wave activation occurs, usually without sinus node invasion and resetting. The first anticipated QRS complex following the VPC does not occur, as the ventricle is still refractory to excitation when the P wave occurs, the next QRS happens at the expected time (Fig. 47.1a–d). The relationship of VPCs to the preceding beat allows determination of their mechanism (Fig. 47.1a–d). Ventricular premature contractions are caused by:

- Idiopathic (most patients).
- Left ventricular hypertrophy.
- Left ventricle damage, rare in patients presenting solely with symptoms from VPCs, though VPCs are frequent in those with LV damage. Post-MI there is a weak relationship between VPC frequency and sudden cardiac death from ventricular arrhythmias.
- Right ventricle damage (e.g. cardiomyopathy).
- Long QT interval (see Chapter 17), including drug induced/exacerbated.
- Hypokalaemia, especially in heart failure.

Ventricular premature contractions, emotion and the diurnal rhythm

Ventricular premature contraction timing can be explained by understanding that VPCs are promoted by:

- Long QT intervals (which occurs with low heart rates and at night). Symptoms, therefore, often arise when patients are lying quietly in bed (Fig. 47.3).
- Catecholamines, which alter myocyte currents to promote extrasystoles from early and delayed after-depolarizations. Accordingly, emotions (stress, fear, anxiety) can provoke VPCs in those predisposed, especially when the QT interval is already long (e.g. at night, when resting).

Ventricular premature contractions are suppressed by:

- Manoeuvres that shorten the QT interval: exercise (increases heart rate, releases catecholamines) shortens the QT Interval and suppresses VPCs.
- Potassium supplementation: heart failure lengthens the QT interval, especially in the potassium depleted (e.g. by diuretics). Supplemental potassium shortens the QT interval, so supressing arrhythmias here.
- Drugs blocking/modifying cardiac adrenergic influence (beta-blockers/angiotensin-converting enzyme [ACE] inhibitors/angiotensin-receptor blockers [ARBs]). Digoxin increases cardiac vagal tone and reciprocally lessens adrenergic outflow, so suppressing VPCs.

Grading of VPCs

Previously ventricular arrhythmias were graded (Table 47.1) on the belief that complexity/frequency related to ventricular tachycardia (VT)/VF risk. However, the relationship between Lown grading and sustained ventricular arrhythmias is weak, and rarely useful.

Fig. 47.1 Ventricular premature contraction (VPC) timing and mechanism. (a) Triggered VPCs: both VPCs (third and sixth beats) have the same time interval to the previous sinus beat, i.e. they are triggered by this beat (early after depolarizations [EADs] or local re-entry). (b) Automatic-focus VPCs: no relationship between the preceding QRS complex and the VPCs, which march through. These VPCs relate to an automatic focus in the ventricle and are not triggered. In both traces from time-to-time VPCs suppress normal QRS complexes (bold arrow) when the ventricle is still refractory. In both, the time between the sinus beat before and after the VPC is exactly twice the basic cycle length. (c) Graph showing that the VPC is weak, and the first post-extrasystolic (PES) beat and the next few, are stronger (PES potentiation [PESP]). (d) Ventricular premature contractions and blood pressure (BP): ECG at the top; the second beat is a VPC. Blood pressure at the bottom; there is scarcely any BP increment with the VPC. Here there was no PESP.

Fig. 47.2 Left bundle branch block (LBBB) pattern ventricular premature contractions (VPCs). Rhythm strip (bottom) shows some beats clearly sinus (P waves, illustrated by open arrows from below, followed by narrow complex QRS), others (large bold arrow above) occur early, starting before the previous sinus beats have finished, have no preceding P wave, are broad, and have inverted T waves. These are VPCs. They have a fixed relationship to the preceding sinus beat, i.e. are triggered by that beat. The VPCs have a LBBB pattern, i.e. they arise from the right ventricle, high up as the VPC axis is directed towards lead III – i.e. from the RV outflow tract, usually idiopathic, but if there is a family history of sudden death/cardiomyopathy, or history of syncope, consider arrhythmogenic right ventricular dysplasia, a rare serious condition. The P waves march through at a regular rate (small arrows below), appearing on the downslope of the VPC T wave as a small indentation. Ventricular premature contractions are followed by a full compensatory pause. The underlying ECG is normal.

Fig. 47.3 Twenty-four hour Holter monitor. Top heart rate. The patient falls asleep when the heart rate falls, between 10 and 11 PM, and wakes around 7 AM. During the day the heart rate is much higher than at night. The bottom trace shows ventricular premature contraction (VPC) frequency (right-hand scale); VPC rate is much higher at night, when the heart rate is low, than during the day. This is the common pattern, and reflects VPC dependency on long QT intervals.

48 Non-sustained ventricular tachycardia

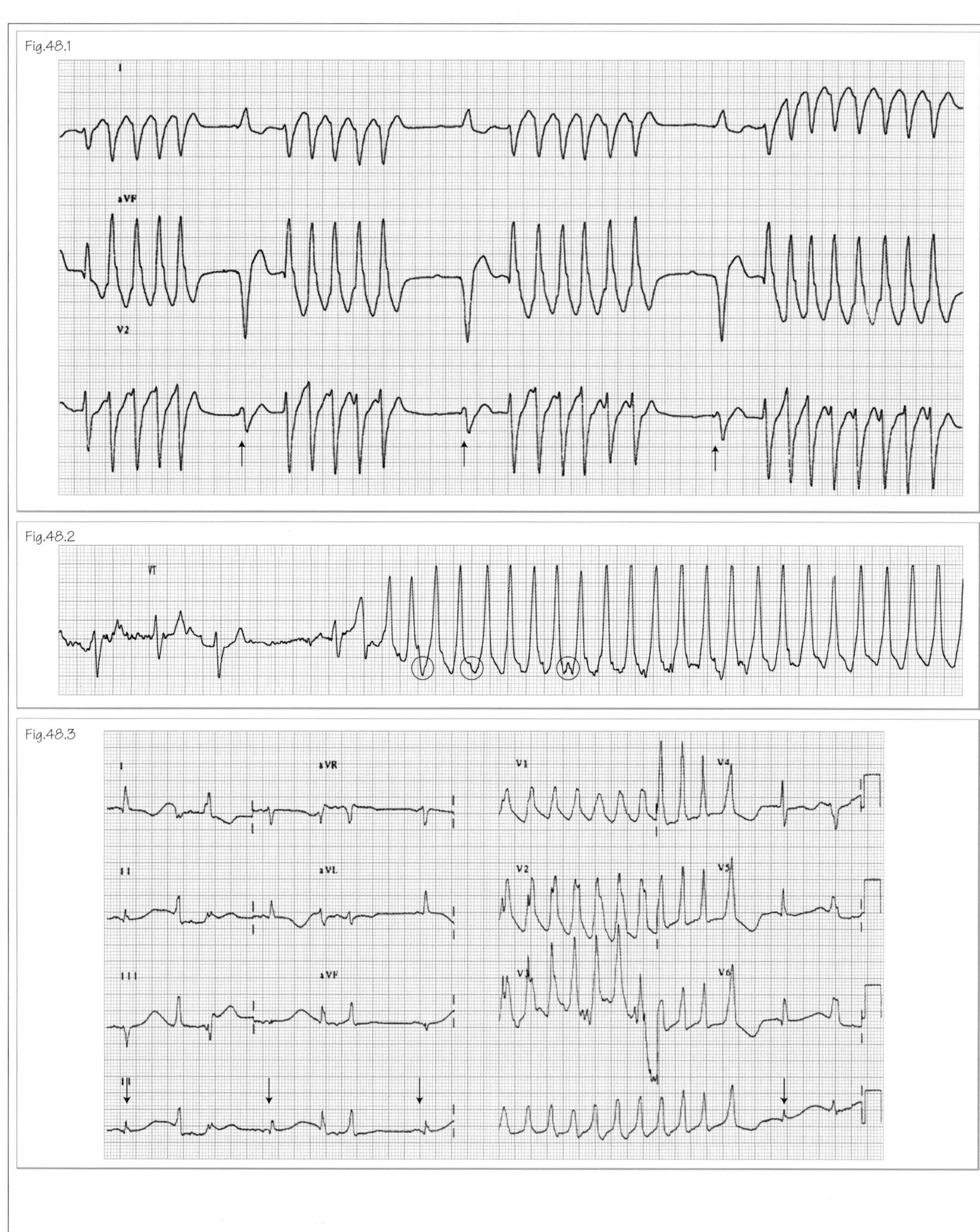

Non-sustained ventricular tachycardia (NSVT) is ventricular tachycardia (VT) (i.e. ≥ 3 ventricular beats strung together with no intervening supraventricular beat) that terminates spontaneously within 30 s (Table 48.1). It is a common and important rhythm disturbance; it may give rise to no symptoms, near or actual fainting and/or palpitations. It is associated with sustained VT and sudden cardiac death. The ECG appearance of NSVT is the same as sustained VT, except that it does not last as long!

- The heart rate is ≥ 100 beat/min (the definition of a tachycardia) and often but not always much faster (e.g. often > 150 b/min).
- The QRS complexes are broad, as the impulse travels by myocyte-to-myocyte transmission, not using the specialized conducting tissue of the heart.
- The axis is usually very different from that of the sinus beat.
- The QRS complexes usually do not look like either left or right bundle branch block. There are clues that the diagnosis is VT from the exact shape of the QRS complex in the different leads (see Chapter 49); the broader the QRS complexes, the less they look like left or right bundle branch block the more likely they are to be VT.
- There may be independent atrial activity (P waves marching through), capture or fusion beats (see Chapter 40).
- In monomorphic VT all the complexes look the same; in polymorphic VT the shape of the complexes changes continually. One variant of polymorphic VT is torsade-de-pointes (*French* 'twisting of the points', originally of the compass), where the complexes first increase in size (over 3–10 beats), then over 3–10 beats decrease in size. Torsade-de-pointes is a critically important and much misunderstood arrhythmia, responsible for much avoidable cardiac death (see Chapter 38).

The causes of monomorphic NSVT include:

- Normal heart – no underlying structural heart disease, when it is usually benign, unless class I drugs are used. These drugs transform benign into dangerous and potentially lethal VT. The absence of heart disease in NSVT may be difficult to prove, as NSVT may be the first manifestation of a very slowly progressive pathology (e.g. right ventricular cardiomyopathy); be suspicious of this if the VT complexes are left bundle branch block morphology, right axis deviation). Repeat assessment over several years is recommended to exclude such slow pathology.
- Hypertensive heart disease, where NSVT is commonly found, though rarely gives rise to symptoms. Its prognostic importance is uncertain.
- Post-myocardial infarction (i.e. ≥ 24 h), where NSVT is associated with subsequent sudden cardiac death, if the QRS is broad, ejection fraction low and monomorphic VT inducible at electrophysiology (EP) study (see Chapter 65). When these criteria are not met the importance of NSVT is uncertain.
- Hypertrophic cardiomyopathy; NSVT is one of several poor prognostic markers, particularly in the young, if repetitive, prolonged or associated with symptoms.
- Dilated cardiomyopathy (DCM), and other diseases causing left ventricular systolic dysfunction commonly give rise to NSVT. Their prognostic importance is unclear. In DCM the most powerful predictor is ejection fraction (EF) (increased relative risk 2.3-fold for each 10% decrease in EF). Non-sustained ventricular tachycardia may not add anything to prognosis beyond the EF data.
- Long QT interval syndromes (see Chapters 17 and 38).

The causes of polymorphic NSVT include

- The same as for monomorphic NSVT.
- Torsade-de-pointes type NSVT, which is a syndrome with: (i) typical ECG changes; (ii) underlying long QT interval (due to disease, genes and/or drugs – non-sedating anti-histamines, erythromycin, cisapride [now withdrawn], sotalol, etc); (iii) preceding bradycardia, which often occurs in elderly females (all of which prolong the QT interval).

Table 48.1 Definitions of ventricular tachycardia.

Non-sustained	> 3 beats, terminates ≤ 30 s
Sustained	Terminates ≥ 30 s, either spontaneously or with treatment
Self-terminating	Stops spontaneously
Monomorphic	All complexes one shape
Polymorphic	Complexes continually change shape

Management of NSVT

Define and treat any underlying heart disease (especially left ventricular dysfunction, ishaemic heart disease). Remove provoking drugs (e.g. class I anti-arrhythmics, QT interval prolonging drugs, etc) and hypokalaemia. Consider beta-blockers. Pace if bradycardia (and long QT syndromes) underlie the VT. Consider electrophysiological study (VT stimulation studies) if ischaemic heart disease is present, the EF is less than 0.35 and the QRS is broad.

Fig. 48.1 ECG of non-sustained ventricular tachycardia (NSVT). This ECG shows three leads (I, aVF. V2). Sinus beats are arrowed; the second and third sinus beat clearly has a preceding P wave, with a long PR interval, then a broad QRS complex. Following each sinus beat, there are bursts of ventricular tachycardia (VT) (five beats after the first arrow, then six, then eight), with a rate of about 170 b/min. These bursts of VT have a dramatic axis shift from the sinus beat (–ve not +ve in I, +ve not –ve in aVL); there may be small indentations on the VT suggesting independent P wave activity, though these are not unambiguous. This is NSVT in the setting of post-myocardial infarction left ventricular dysfunction.

Fig. 48.2 This monitoring strip shows four sinus beats initially, and then, after a pause prior to the succeeding sinus beat, a run of a very broad complex tachycardia, showing substantial axis shift from sinus rhythm, and clear-cut independent P wave activity (arrowed). Indisputably, this is ventricular tachycardia.

Fig. 48.3 Long QT interval dependent non-sustained ventricular tachycardia (NSVT). The arrowed beats (rhythm strip) are sinus. They have a very long QT interval, difficult to fully measure, as, before they fully finish, a ventricular ectopic arises or a run of 12 beats of NSVT. The sinus rhythm ECG looks diffusely abnormal (non-specific QRS broadening, T wave flattening) but it is difficult to be categorical, as not enough of the ECG is visualized. The patient had syncope, and was on psychotropic drugs; the diagnosis was long QT dependent ventricular tachycardia, induced by drugs.

49 Monomorphic ventricular tachycardia

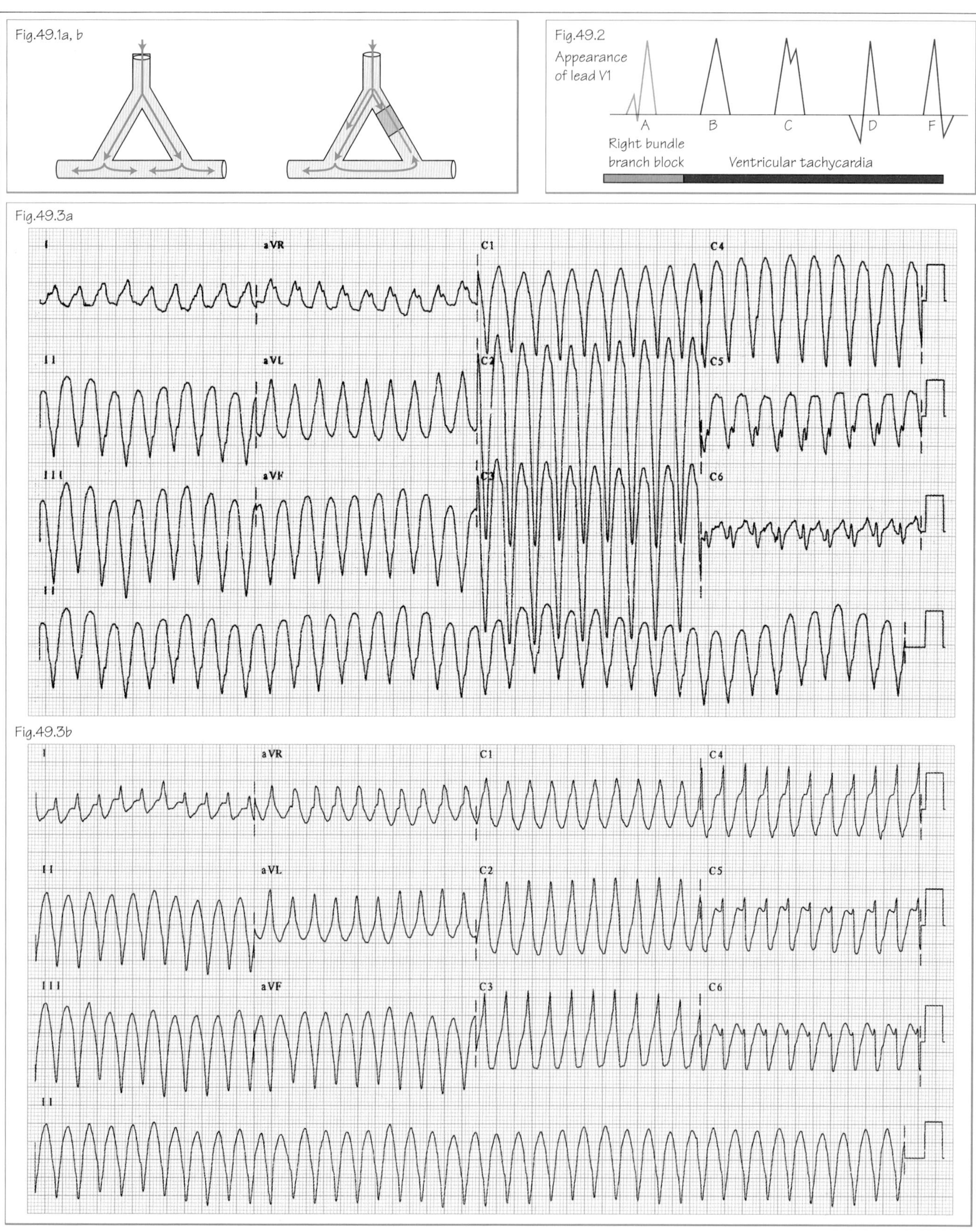

Monomorphic ('one shape') ventricular tachycardia (VT) is common, serious and has many causes (Table 49.1), most often a scar allowing 're-entry' (Fig. 49.1) and so the development of a 'circus movement' tachycardia (a re-entrant arrhythmia), the electrophysiological characteristics of which are:

- Initiated and terminated by an appropriately timed (paced) ventricular beat.
- Terminated by over-drive and/or under-drive pacing.
- Terminated by DC shock.

Monomorphic VT results in a broad complex tachycardia, in which:

- The atria usually beat independently and slower than the ventricles resulting in 'atrioventricular (AV) dissociation'. The P waves occur less frequently than, and are unrelated to, the QRS complexes. Usually the P waves do not capture the ventricles, as the self-sustaining ventricular rhythm sweeps so frequently past the bundle of His and distal conducting tissues that whenever an atrial impulse reaches this area the ventricular tissue is refractory, preventing further impulse propagation. Occasionally the timing of the atrial impulse is such that it reaches the tissue beyond the AV node just when the refractory period is over, so it is now able to capture all or part of the ventricle. This results in a beat either looking like the normal sinus rhythm one if the whole ventricle has been captured (a 'capture beat'), or if only part of the ventricle is captured, a beat halfway between a normal one and the VT beat, a 'fusion beat'.
- Very occasionally there is retrograde activation of the atria from the ventricles, i.e. a 1 to 1 relationship between the QRS complexes and the P waves, with the P waves following very closely to the QRS complex (i.e. a short RP′ tachycardia).
- All the complexes look (nearly) identical – the definition of monomorphic.
- There is hardly any/no heart rate variability, unlike atrial fibrillation (AF).
- The complexes are broad – the broader they are the more likely is VT.
- Usually the complexes do not look like right or left bundle branch block (RBBB or LBBB).
- If they look like RBBB, then, unlike true RBBB, the first upward deflection (R) is larger than the second (R′) (Fig. 49.2).
- The QRS axis is often very unusual, showing extreme right/left or an indeterminate axis.
- All the QRS complexes in the chest leads are positive or negative ('praecordial concordance').

Not all of the above are present in all cases; some 'clinch' the diagnosis ('AV dissociation') others make it highly likely (broad QRS, chest lead concordance). The key principle in approaching broad complex tachycardias is that 'if you don't know the diagnosis, treat as if it is VT' as by chance alone you are likely to be right. Eighty per cent of all regular broad complex tachycardias are VT, 95% if the patient has a remote myocardial infarction (MI). While the treatment for VT does no harm if the diagnosis is supraventricular tachycardia (SVT), the treatment for SVT can do considerable harm if the diagnosis is VT.

Table 49.1 Cardiac diseases associated with monomorphic ventricular tachycardia.

Disease	Frequency of VT due to this disease
Previous MI (new ischaemia must be considered)	++++
LV hypertrophy	+++
Dilated cardiomyopathy	++
Hypertrophic cardiomyopathy	+
Right ventricular cardiomyopathy	+
Normal heart VT	+
Congenital heart disease in adults	±

LV, left ventricular; MI, myocardial infarction; VT, ventricular tachycardia.

Other ECG findings in patients prone to VT

- Post-MI monomorphic VT is associated with an 'arrhythmogenic' scar, seen as a small delay at the end of the QRS complex, a 'late-potential' (see Chapter 28).
- Patients with low heart rate variability have an increased risk of VT (see Chapter 63).
- A long QT interval predisposes both to polymorphic and monomorphic VT.
- A broad QRS when in sinus rhythm in ishaemic heart disease with low ejection fraction increases the chance of VT.

Fig. 49.1 Circus movements in arrhythmogenesis. (a) Central obstruction (e.g. dead heart) around which current flows; depolarization proceeds down both limbs, and meets below, each cancelling the other impulse out. (b) There is now an area of damage (shaded in red), caused by ischaemia etc that greatly slows, or blocks, forward conduction, with normal retrograde conduction. The impulse from the opposite limb is now no longer cancelled out, and is able to pass retrogradely up the limb with the damage. When it reaches the proximal site of damage, the tissue there has already repolarized, allowing ongoing transmission back down the normal limb, across, back up the damaged limb, etc., setting up a 'circus movement' tachycardia.

Fig. 49.2 Differing ECG appearance in lead V1 indicating ventricular tachycardia (VT). Right bundle branch block (A) shows a rsR′ pattern; all the other patterns (B to F) suggest VT. A dominant QRS complex in lead V1 suggests that the VT is left ventricular in origin. If there is also left axis deviation, consider the rare diagnosis of fascicular tachycardia. (C) The V1 QRS complex is sometimes described as rabbit ears in VT (C), with the left (from behind) being larger than the right, the reverse of right bundle branch block (A).

Fig. 49.3 (a) Broad complex tachycardia. The rate is very fast, about 220 b/min. There are no clear cut P waves, but running your eye along the rhythm trace at the bottom, slight irregularities can be occasionally seen, which are likely to be P waves. The axis is extreme rightward (+ve aVR, aVL). The complexes are very broad. All the chest lead R waves are negative ('praecordial concordance'). On ECG grounds this clearly ventricular tachycardia (VT), of right ventricular origin (confirmed by knowing the patient had Fallot's tetralogy). (b) Broad complex tachycardia, rate 250 b/min, suggestive but no clear cut irregularities on the rhythm trace suggesting independent P wave activity. No praecordial concordance (QRS +ve in V1–3, –ve in V4–6), but QRS very broad (143 ms), QRS shape in lead V1 like (B) in Fig. 49.2, both strongly suggest VT. The diagnosis was post-myocardial infarction VT.

50 Polymorphic ventricular tachycardia

Fig.50.1

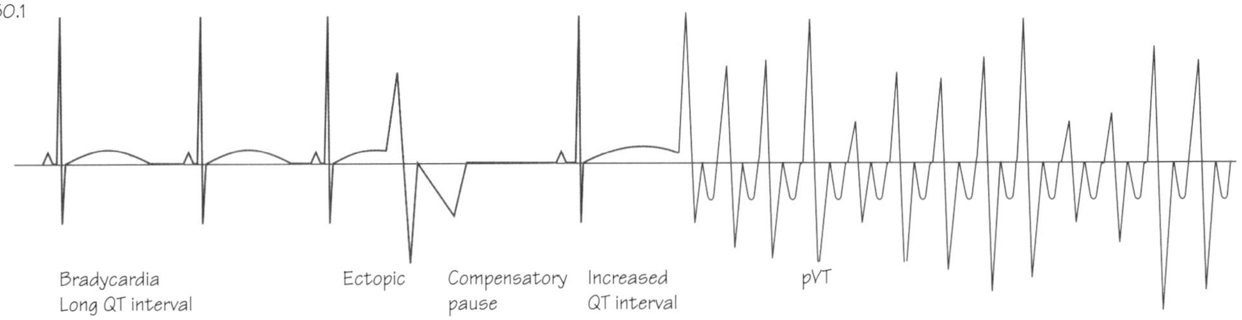

Bradycardia
Long QT interval

Ectopic

Compensatory
pause

Increased
QT interval

pVT

Fig.50.2

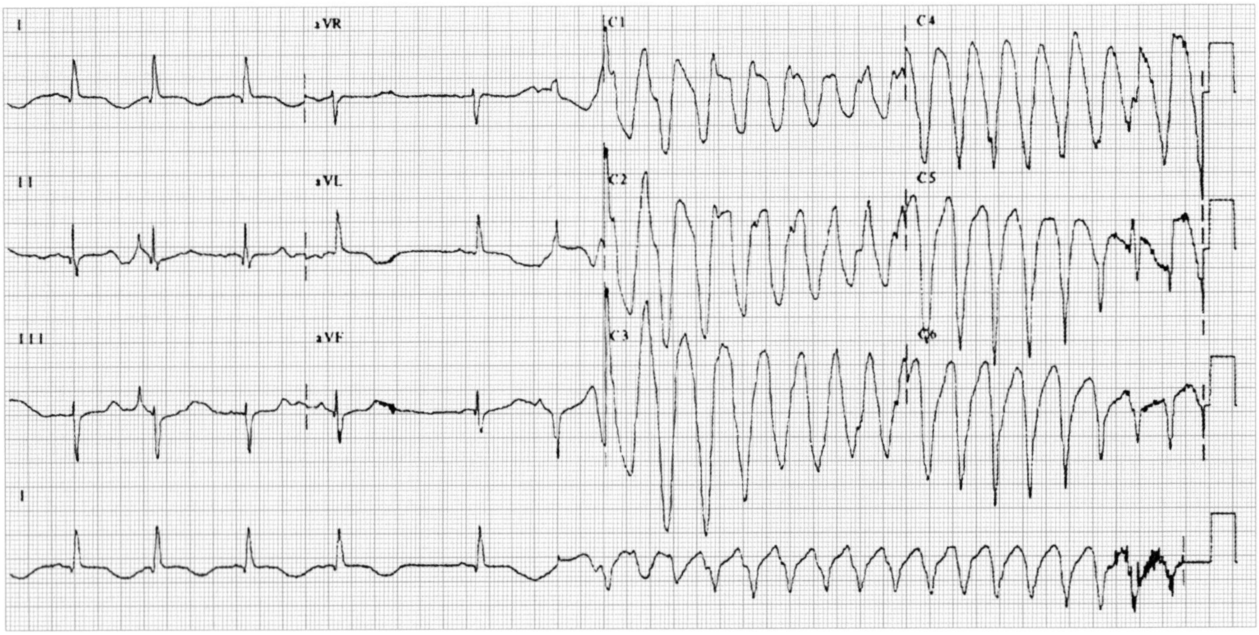

I aVR C1 C4
II aVL C2 C5
III aVF C3 C6
I

Fig.50.3

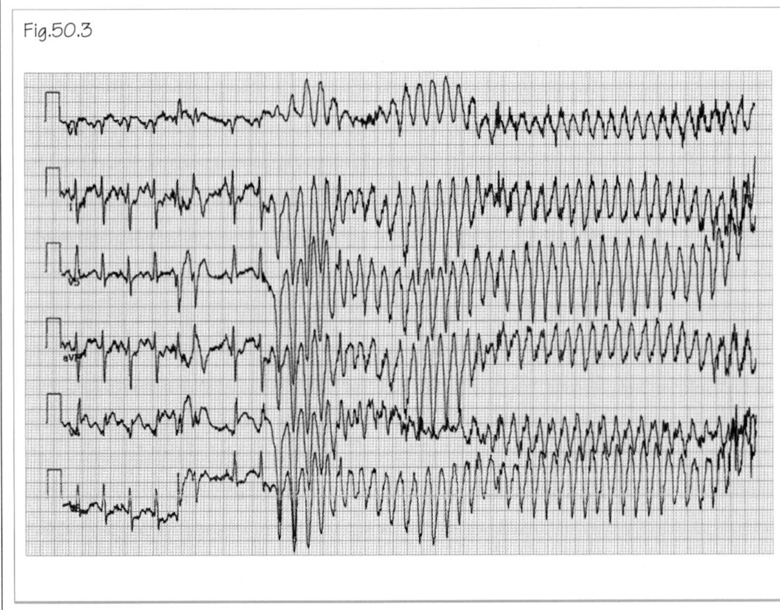

Fig.50.4

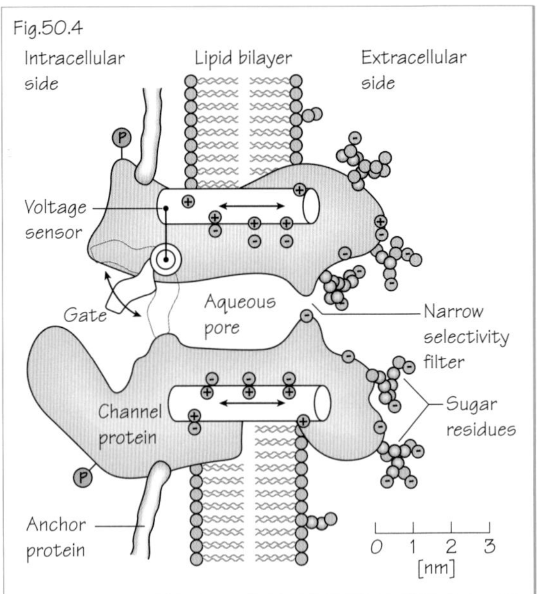

Polymorphic ('many shapes') ventricular tachycardia (pVT) is common. It is underdiagnosed, as either it progresses to ventricular fibrillation (VF), cardiac arrest and sudden cardiac death (so wiping out the evidence) or it terminates spontaneously, in which case presentation is with symptoms (syncopal or near syncopal episode) but an unremarkable heart rhythm at hospitalization (e.g. sinus, atrial fibrillation). Often (not always) the clue to the diagnosis is QT interval prolongation, which underlies many cases. Other clues include finding characteristic ECGs associated with genetic channelopathies.

Pathophysiology

In monomorphic VT the pattern of spread of each beat ('activation sequence') is the same, whereas in pVT the activation sequence differs randomly between beats. Monomorphic VT is often 'scar-related', whereas pVT more often relates to (genetic or acquired) channel disorders.

ECG findings in pVT

The ECG demonstrates a broad complex tachycardia, with a continuously and randomly changing pattern (Fig. 50.1). There is a spectrum of forms, varying from the very well formed, almost monomorphic, through forms in which repetitive patterns can be recognized (such as torsade-de-pointes [TDP]) ending up in the very disorganized patterns that are hard to distinguish from VF. The key aspects to the diagnosis are:

- The QRS complexes are very broad, often so broad that it is difficult to determine where the QRS finishes and the T wave starts.
- The rate is usually fairly to very fast (Fig. 50.2). The high heart rate in conjunction with the broad QRS means that the pattern is often like the serrated edge to a saw, a 'sawtooth' type pattern.
- The QRS complexes continually change shape, not in a predictable fashion. These random shapes change and affect the QRS height, duration and axis. The pattern can be so random as to lead to confusion with VF, from which it can be distinguished by: (i) Clearly visible discrete QRS complexes in pVT, whereas in VF this is not the case. (ii) In VF there is no cardiac output, and the heart along with the patient starts to die. All patients in VF are in cardiac arrest whereas many though not all are with sustained pVT. Given this, the QRS amplitude in VF declines very rapidly, certainly within a minute or two; whereas in pVT, as there is usually some cardiac output, the size of the complexes is often maintained, at least for a period of time. (iii) It is very rare indeed for VF to terminate spontaneously, whereas this is common with pVT.
- The differentiation from VF is probably not that important; if cardiac output declines seriously or is lost, the treatments are the same (DC cardioversion). Once over, the work up (for serious structural heart disease, metabolic disarray, and genetic disease) is often the same both for pVT as for VF.

Torsade-de-pointes ('twisting of the points') type pVT

This is a moderately well organized variant of pVT. Torsade-de-pointes usually occurs in self-terminating bursts, often 5–50 beats long. Characteristically, the QRS axis changes 180° in 10–12 beats, then back again over the same time period, so that in any one lead it looks as though the complex increase and then decrease in size. There is a greatly reduced cardiac output during the paroxysm, and syncope may result. Occasionally the rhythm changes to VF, clearly lethal unless promptly treated. There are numerous predisposing causes (Table 50.1). Many relate to acquired long QT syndromes, due to:

- Structural heart disease (especially left ventricular impairment, from any cause), but also ishaemic heart disease (Fig. 50.3).
- Drugs interfering with the *human ether a-go-go gene (HERG)*, so disrupting repolarizing potassium currents, prolonging the action potential and predisposing to repetitive early after depolarizations (Fig. 50.4). *HERG* polymorphisms may increase the risk of drug-induced VT.

Factors promoting TDP in those so predisposed include; bradycardia (common), hypokalaemia, renal failure (acts to retain QT prolonging drugs), hypomagnesaemia, and hypocalcaemia (rare). See also Table 50.1.

Treatment

Define the underlying cardiac disease, treat this if possible (e.g. revascularization for critical ischaemia), remove metabolic provocatants (e.g. hypokalaemia, drugs), prevent bradycardia if relevant to long QT dependent arrhythmias, once bradycardia treated/ruled out as relevant give beta-blockers, consider an implantable cardioverter defibrillator (ICD).

Table 50.1 Causes of torsade-de-pointes type ventricular tachycardia.

Underlying cause	Frequency
Post MI LV dysfunction	++++
Drugs	++++
Myocardial ischaemia	+++
Dilated cardiomyopathy	++
LV hypertrophy	++
Demographics – elderly female	++
Genetic polymorphisms, e.g. *HERG* etc. prolonging QT interval	++
Starvation syndromes (anorexia, gastric stapling, malnutrition)	++
Complete heart block	+
Hypothyroidism	+
Subarachnoid haemorrhage	+
Genetic illness (hereditary long QT syndrome, Brugada)	+/–

LV, left ventricular; MI, myocardial infarction.

Fig. 50.1 Scheme of polymorphic ventricular tachycardia (pVT). Sinus bradycardia, with a baseline long QT interval; an ectopic beat leads to a compensatory pause and further QT interval lengthening, at the end of which pVT starts.

Fig. 50.2 Example of long QT interval-associated pVT. Sinus rhythm, broad low voltage P wave seen in lead II (left atrial enlargement). Mild QRS broadening, bizarre ST segments/T waves (look at the unusual T wave inversion in leads I, aVL). Very long QT interval, best seen in the first beat in the second set of leads (aVR, aVL, aVF); a pause then occurs, with further QT lengthening in the next beat. Off this beat an ectopic occurs (look at the changed shape in aVF), then a fast broad complex tachycardia, with continually changing shape – this is pVT.

Fig. 50.3 Polymorphic ventricular tachycardia (pVT) starting during an exercise stress test. Sinus rhythm, then two ectopic beats, compensatory pause, one more sinus beat, then pVT starts, with continually changing axis (and QRS size).

Fig. 50.4 Ion channel, emphasizing the importance of drug-channel interactions in polymorphic ventricular tachycardia.

51 Ventricular fibrillation

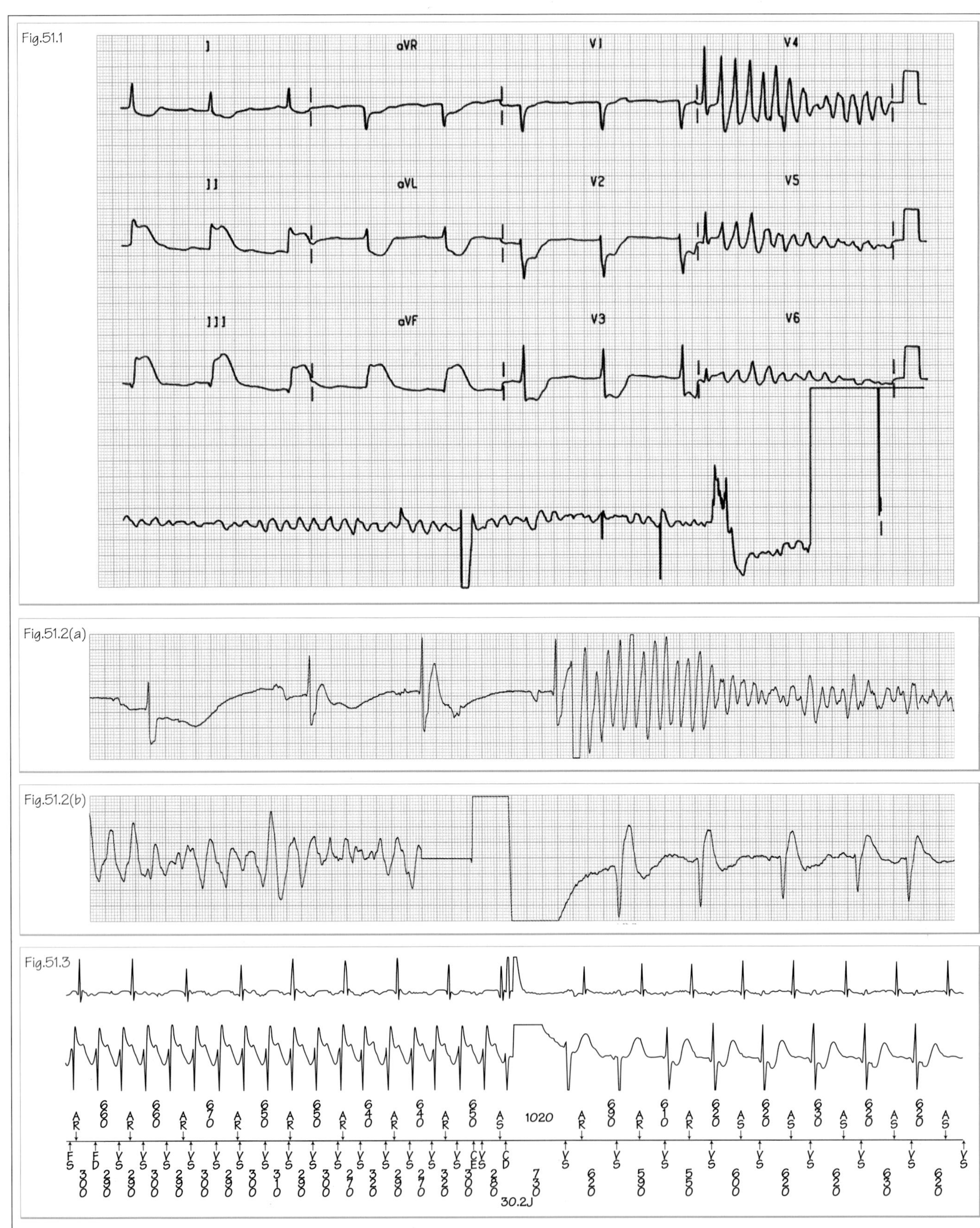

Much of cardiology is directed towards preventing death from ventricular fibrillation (VF). To do this one firstly needs to identify which patients are at risk of VF and then intervene to reduce this risk, and secondly to recognize and be able to treat the rhythm disturbance itself.

High-risk patients

Patients with pro-arrhythmic conditions in pro-arrhythmic situations comprise a high-risk population, and include those:

- In the acute phase of a myocardial infarction (MI), especially if left ventricular hypertrophy (LVH) is present. Ischaemia underlies most community sudden cardiac death.
- Post-MI, especially those with 'late-potentials' (see Chapter 28), which reflects an arrhythmic 'scar', and those with non-sustained ventricular tachycardia (VT).
- With left ventricular (LV) dysfunction, the more severe the higher the risk. Low heart rate variability when associated with a low ejection fraction is independently associated with ventricular arrhythmias.
- With LVH (see Chapter 8).
- With arrhythmogenic right ventricular dysplasia.
- With pro-arrhythmic genetic disease, including Brugada syndrome, hereditary long QT prolongation and hypertrophic cardiomyopathy (see Chapter 39).

Unfortunately most patients who develop VF are from a low-risk population – unfortunate as, though the individual risk is low, the overall numbers at risk is so large. This means that VF prevention, in a population sense, is problematic, except through reducing the risk of the coronary disease and intervening on standard risk factors.

High-risk situations include:

- Situations with high levels of catecholamines.
- Low heart rates, for arrhythmias depending on a long QT interval (torsade-de-pointes [TDP] type ventricular tachycardia, which easily degenerates into VF).
- Hypokalaemia, which promotes ventricular arrhythmias including TDP partly by prolonging the QT interval (especially in those with impaired LV function, which itself lengthens the QT interval) so promoting early after depolarizations.
- In the presence of pro-arrhythmic drugs, such as class I anti-arrhythmic agents, non-sedating anti-histamines, major tranquillizers and macrolide antibiotics amongst others.

Ventricular fibrillation

Sometimes VF occurs straight from sinus rhythm. Commonly however, another rhythm disturbance precedes VF:

- Ventricular tachycardia, monomorphic or polymorphic.
- Atrial fibrillation (AF), commonly in those with impaired LV function. Very rarely, 'pre-excited' AF (i.e. AF in those with an accessory pathway), can generate such high heart rates that VF occurs.
- Complete heart block can underlie polymorphic ventricular tachycardia (pVT) and so VF.

ECG recognition of VF

In VF electrical activity continually and randomly crosses the ventricle. This results in a totally disorganized surface ECG (Figs 51.1 & 51.2a,b). Initially the complexes are quite large; however, as the heart dies, the complexes become smaller and smaller, finally leading to a flat baseline. As there is no cardiac output during VF, the patient blacks out, and appears dead (i.e. pale, no capillary return, no pulses, no respiration) – this clearly distinguishes VF from other causes of a chaotic ECG (including a loose lead, and Parkinson's disease).

Treatment of VF

Immediate DC cardioversion is the only reliable treatment, though occasionally a thump to the chest ('thumpversion') converts VF to a rhythm compatible with life. DC shock may fail, either for technical reasons (paddles not applied firmly enough, energy setting too low – use at least 200–360 J monophasic or 100–150 J biphasic), for cardiac reasons (the heart pathology is too advanced, e.g. very severe LV dysfunction, critical widespread coronary disease such as left main occlusion, etc.) or metabolic reasons (potassium disturbance, hypomagnesaemia, etc). It is important to remember these factors if DC cardioversion is not working, as there may be specific available therapies that help.

Assessment following VF

As with all serious arrhythmias, management aims to define and treat the cardiac pathology and exclude other relevant conditions. Ventricular fibrillation occurring outside the acute phase (i.e. first 12–24 h) of an MI mandates a highly aggressive approach. Most cases relate to coronary disease (angiography is usually mandatory), a few to cardiomyopathy, and a very small number to genetic disease. Many patients who survive non-MI related VF require an implantable cardioverter defibrillator (ICD) (Fig. 51.3).

Fig. 51.1 Inferior ST segment elevation myocardial infarction (STEMI) complicated by ventricular fibrillation (VF). Sinus rhythm initially, gross inferior lead (II, III, aVF) ST segment elevation, with ST depression in leads I, aVL, V2 and V3. In other words, an inferior/posterior wall STEMI is underway. It is impossible to say what the lateral leads look like; at the start of the V4/5/6 recording, a grossly irregular, rapid arrhythmia starts. This then continues on the rhythm strip at the bottom, though the amplitude has declined markedly. These are classic appearances for VF. Right at the end of the trace is the artefact caused by DC cardioversion.

Fig. 51.2 (a) Sinus bradycardia degenerating into ventricular fibrillation (VF). To the left of the trace a slow sinus heart rate is seen (small P wave before each QRS complex), with a long PR interval (up to 440 ms). After a short period of bradycardia, a very fast tachycardia commences, which initially looks rather like torsade-de-pointes, but very rapidly degenerates into a completely chaotic arrhythmia. This is VF. (b) Successful cardioversion from VF (left of trace) to supraventricular rhythm (right of trace). It is not easy to see whether the supraventricular rhythm is sinus, or slow atrial fibrillation.

Fig. 51.3 Data from an implantable cardioverter defibrillator (ICD). Here ventricular fibrillation (VF) is terminated by DC shock into sinus rhythm. The top trace shows the intracardiac electrogram from the atrial electrode, the second trace the ventricular one, the final trace shows how beats are labelled and the RR intervals. To the left, the ventricular rate is seen to far exceed the atrial one – so the rhythm is ventricular tachycardia (VT) or VF. The defibrillator is programmed to call all ventricular arrhythmias higher than a certain rate VF and then apply an interval shock (30.2 J in this case). In the trace to the right sinus rhythm is seen, with each P wave being followed after a short interval by an R wave.

52 Sinus node disease

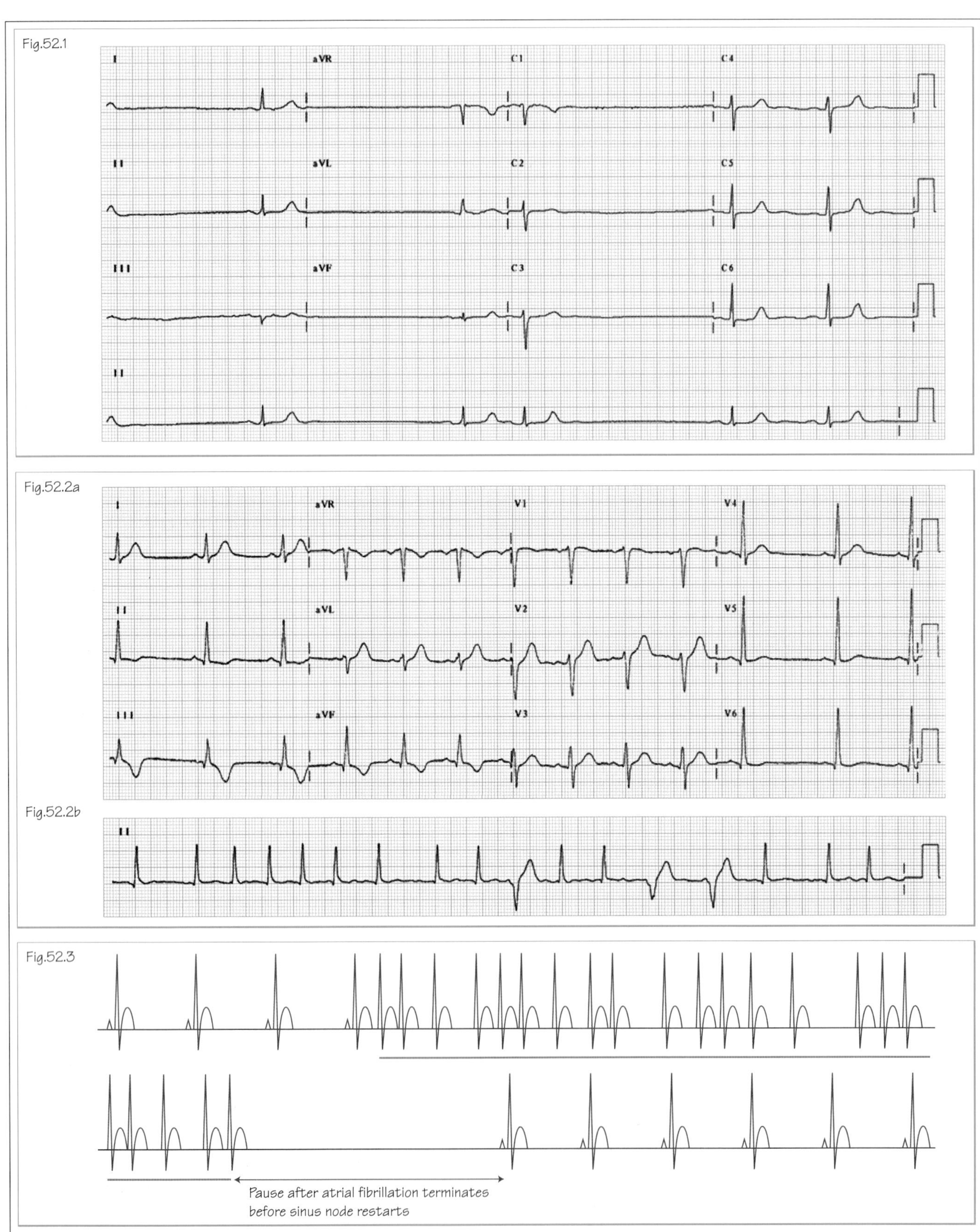

The sinus node beats at an intrinsic rate, modified by neural impulses to beat slower (sleep) or faster (exercise). The sinus node should therefore respond in a predictable way to neural impulses. On occasions, disease of the node ('sick sinus syndrome [SSS]') affects the intrinsic rate and/or the way in which the node responds to neural impulses. Several varieties of sinus node disease are recognized.

Overt SSS with inappropriate bradycardia

By far the commonest form of SSS; the resting heartbeat is unusually low (usually ≤ 40 b/min); the normal heart rate increase with exercise is greatly blunted or non-existent. This results in symptoms of tiredness, and effort intolerance, due to rather non-specific reasons. The heart rate can also intermittently be too low, e.g. intermittent pauses occur and syncope can result. It is difficult to be dogmatic about what pauses are significant – pauses > 2–3 s with symptoms are; without symptoms, especially at night, much longer pauses may not be relevant. Sick sinus syndrome is diagnosed from a 24-h ECG, corroborated by examining the heart rate increase during an exercise test. Intrinsic fibrosis is the commonest cause; amiodarone can underlie SSS. Beta-blockers can unmask mild forms. Sick sinus syndrome can be mimicked by hypothyroidism. Prognosis is a normal life expectancy in those without heart disease. SSS worsens the prognosis of any heart disease. Treatment is observation or pacing (AAI or DDD) for symptoms.

Overt SSS with inappropriate bradycardia and tachycardia

A rarer form of SSS; in addition to inappropriate bradycardia (resulting in tiredness, effort intolerance, and/or syncope), episodic inappropriate tachycardia occurs (both at rest and during effort). The tachycardia can cause symptoms of palpitations. A 24-h ECG is the best means of diagnosis. The differential diagnosis of symptoms which could indicate SSS with both bradycardia and tachycardia is wide, and includes arrhythmias, and many non-arrhythmic causes, including psychological distress. Treatment is often a pacemaker to prevent bradycardia and drugs (e.g. a beta-blocker) to suppress the tachycardia.

Overt SSS with inappropriate tachycardia

The rarest form of SSS; episodes of inappropriate sinus tachycardia occur, often only during the day, both at rest and during effort. The differential diagnosis of very high heart rates during low levels of exercise is: (i) unfitness, the commonest cause; (ii) sinus node tachycardia syndrome, mainly seen in young women; whether this reflects unfitness, anxiety or sinus node disease is unclear. Other illnesses which cause palpitations include: anxiety, thyrotoxicosis, and the very rare phaeochromocytoma. The treatment of SSS with inappropriate tachycardia is usually a beta-blocker.

Latent SSS

This is symptomatically silent during day-to-day activities, and is most commonly exposed when a supraventricular arrhythmia terminates. Normally, during tachyarrhythmia, either the sinus node continues to fire unimpeded (though the activity is not seen as atrial activity arises from the tachycardia focus) or, more usually, is suppressed by retrograde impulses entering from the right atrium. When tachycardia ceases, the sinus node normally fires after a delay of < 1 normal RR interval (i.e. ≤ 1 s), so firing the atria, atrioventricular (AV) node, etc. However, in SSS, when tachycardia ceases, the sinus node takes several (up to 5 or so) seconds to start firing. During this time there is no cardiac electrical activity and no cardiac output. Syncope can occur. The differential diagnosis of syncope is wide (see Chapter 23); the clue to the diagnosis of latent SSS is in the history (palpitations, then immediately, seconds after they stop, syncope) and the diagnosis confirmed by recording an ECG during symptoms (see Chapter 63). Treatment is to suppress the supraventricular tachycardia (SVT), rarely completely successful, or more commonly to implant an AAI pacemaker. Pacing (see below) may also prevent atrial fibrillation (AF).

Complications of bradycardic SSS

One important complication of bradycardic SSS is AF, which arises as the sinus bradycardia increases atrial refractory period dispersion so the atria do not repolarize synchronously. Asynchronous repolarization promotes atrial re-entry, which underlies some AF. The implications of this are: (i) it is important to look for SSS underlying AF; (ii) it is possible to prevent AF if the cause is bradycardic SSS by atrial pacing; (iii) some SSS is complicated by stroke, caused by clinically silent AF (so consider anticoagulation for AF complicating SSS).

Fig. 52.1 Profound sinus bradycardia. Sinus rhythm (each R wave preceded by a P wave, one P wave for each R wave). The heart rate is very slow – 2.5 s between beats, i.e. heart rate 24 b/min. The heart rate is not regular – as all the beats have similar shape P waves, the irregularity is not due to atrial extrasystoles. Though such a profound sinus bradycardia can be *reflex* in nature, i.e. due to a vasomotor syndrome, this was not the case here (the differentiation can be made by whether the bradycardia lasts a brief period of time, as in vasomotor syndromes, or whether it is more long lasting, as in sick sinus syndrome). The patient responded well to pacing.

Fig. 52.2 (a) Sick sinus syndrome (SSS). The rhythm is sinus (P wave before each QRS, no non-conducted P waves). The rate is far from regular, slow initially, then speeding up and then slowing down. These rate changes are too much to be explained by sinus arrhythmia, and indicate bradycardic SSS. The underlying ECG is unremarkable except for inferior lead (II, III, aVF) T wave inversion lead II, extending laterally to V6 as T wave flattening. This may indicate right coronary artery ischaemia; many cases of SSS are due to sinus node artery disease (a branch of the right coronary artery). (b) Rhythm strip from the patient in (a), later on. Atrial fibrillation (completely irregular baseline, fine fibrillatory wave, irregular QRS response). Three ventricular premature contractions occur later on.

Fig. 52.3 Cartoon showing sinus bradycardia due to sick sinus syndrome giving way to atrial fibrillation (AF) (no P waves, irregularly irregular QRS complexes). When the AF terminates, there is a prolonged pause before the sinus node starts firing again. During this pause patients may blackout.

53 Left bundle branch block

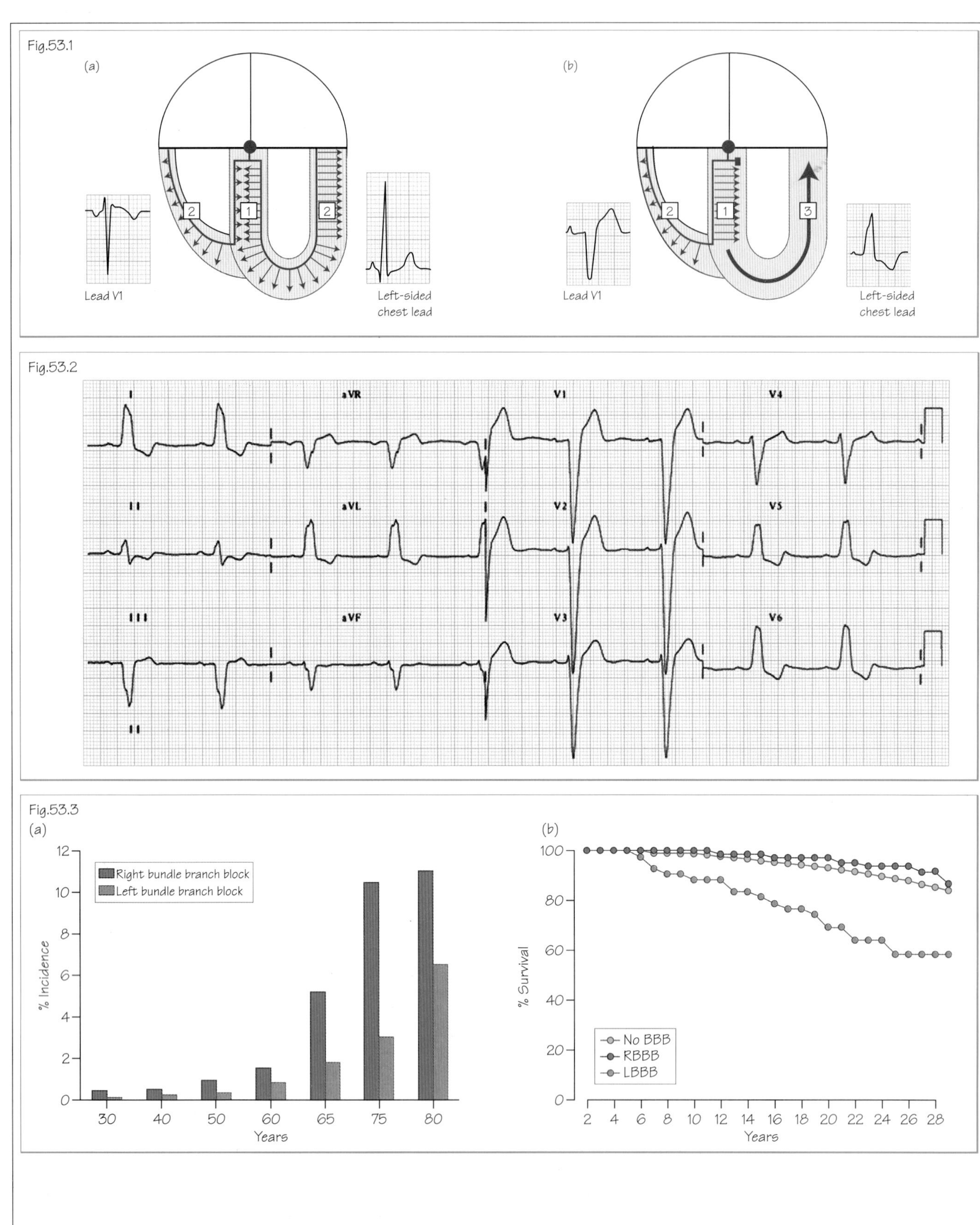

Fig.53.1
(a)
2
1
2
Lead V1
Left-sided chest lead
(b)
2
1
3
Lead V1
Left-sided chest lead
Fig.53.2
I
aVR
V1
V4
II
aVL
V2
V5
III
aVF
V3
V6
II
Fig.53.3
(a)
Right bundle branch block
Left bundle branch block
% Incidence
0
2
4
6
8
10
12
30
40
50
60
65
75
80
Years
(b)
% Survival
0
20
40
60
80
100
No BBB
RBBB
LBBB
2
4
6
8
10
12
14
16
18
20
22
24
26
28
Years

Left bundle branch block (LBBB) is a common conduction disturbance, with three distinct patterns of damage:

- Damage to one or other (but not both) of the two major subdivisions of the left bundle (see Chapter 10). Blockage results in QRS axis deviation without QRS broadening (left axis deviation with anterior hemi-fascicular block, right axis deviation with posterior hemi-fascicular block).
- Partial LBBB ('incomplete LBBB') has some but not all of the features of full LBBB, and is the consequence of partial rather than full interference with the function of the left bundle. The commonest finding is disappearance of the left side physiological septal Q waves with slight broadening of the QRS complex, which is still ≤ 120 ms. In time, this usually progresses to full LBBB.

Full LBBB

The ECG appearances of full LBBB are dominated by: (i) the reversal of the normal direction of septal depolarization; and (ii) delayed activation of the left ventricle (Fig. 53.1a,b). These result in:

- Broad QRS complex > 120 ms.
- Late positive deflections in the left-sided leads, reflecting late current flows towards the left-sided leads (Fig. 53.1a,b). These leads often have an M appearance (i.e. rR′).
- Broad negative deflections in the right-sided leads, as most current flows away from these electrodes.
- Inverted T waves over the left ventricle. As the conduction spreads slowly through the left ventricle, those areas activated last also repolarize last, unlike the normal situation where the epicardium, the last part of the heart activated physiologically, is the first to repolarize. The normal repolarization sequence away from the epicardium accounts for the normal upright T wave. In LBBB, the consequence of the slow activation and repolarization of the left ventricle is inversion of the left-sided T waves.
- The final sign of LBBB is the disappearance of the small physiological left-sided ECG lead Q waves; in health these are a consequence of septal depolarization passing from left to right. In LBBB the sequence of septal depolarization is reversed. The loss of left-sided physiological Q waves is one of the earliest signs of developing LBBB.

Variants of LBBB

When the heart is rotated anti-clockwise, the typical appearance can be modified, so that the QRS appears rather non-specifically broad. The key to the diagnosis is the loss of left-sided Q waves in the setting of a broadened QRS complex.

Symptoms

Depend on the integrity of the rest of the conducting tissue. If there is other conducting tissue disease, then complete heart block can occur, intermittently (resulting in syncope) or permanently (resulting in tiredness, effort intolerance, heart failure, death).

ECG consequences of LBBB

It is held that LBBB renders the ECG otherwise uninterpretable – this is largely true. It is very difficult to diagnose ST segment elevation myocardial infarction in the presence of LBBB (though complex rules have been proposed for this).

Diseases associated with LBBB

The incidence of LBBB increases with age (Fig. 53.3a,b). Many patients with LBBB have heart disease, including:

- Ischaemic heart disease.
- Disease damaging the left ventricle (e.g. myocarditis, cardiomyopathy, etc.). QRS duration is correlated to the severity of left ventricle damage. Broad QRS complexes in heart failure are usually of LBBB morphology. QRS broadening is independently associated with an adverse prognosis, and those who increase QRS duration fastest (regardless of the absolute duration) have a poorer outlook.
- Cardiac sarcoidosis results in conducting tissue disease, including LBBB.
- Some *asymptomatic* patients have no underlying structural heart disease, having only idiopathic isolated conducting tissue fibrosis.

Outlook in LBBB

The outlook in most patients with LBBB is of the underlying condition, the exception being heart failure, where prognosis is worsened (Fig. 53.3a,b).

Fig. 53.1 Left bundle branch block (LBBB). (a) Normal leads V1 and V6. The depolarization wave passes through the atrioventricular (AV) node and into the septum, down the left and right bundles. Most septal depolarization passes left to right (accounting for a small initial R wave in lead V1 and small physiological left-sided Q waves). After septal depolarization, right and left ventricles are depolarized simultaneously. The left ventricle is much larger than the right and dominates the ECG, so V1 sees a large current flow away and lead V6 a large current flow towards it. (b) ECG in LBBB. Septal depolarization is reversed, going right to left, accounting for the initial negative deflection in lead V1, and an early positive deflection in lead V6. The right ventricle is depolarized next, along with some left ventricle (though less than usual). The early left ventricular depolarization, though less than usual, still dominates over right ventricle depolarization, accounting for ongoing negative deflection in lead V1, and a slurred upstroke to lead V6. The final phase, going on after normal depolarization would have finished, is depolarization of the bulk and terminal portion of the left ventricle, unopposed by the right ventricle. The current flow away from lead V1 and towards lead V6 increases, accounting for a broad QRS with a prominent negative deflection in lead V1, positive deflection in lead V6.

Fig. 53.2 Left bundle branch block (LBBB). Sinus rhythm, normal P wave, PR interval. Broad QRS > 120 ms, broad negative deflection in lead V1, broad positive deflection with a slurred upstroke in lead V6. Deep S waves inferiorly, a consequence of LBBB. Inverted T waves laterally (I, aVL, V5, V6), a consequence of the very slow depolarization of the left ventricle reversing the normal repolarization sequence.

Fig. 53.3 (a) Age-specific incidence of bundle branch block (BBB). BBB increases with age, and at any age right bundle branch block (RBBB) is commoner than left (LBBB). (b) Prognosis of BBB.

54 Right bundle branch block

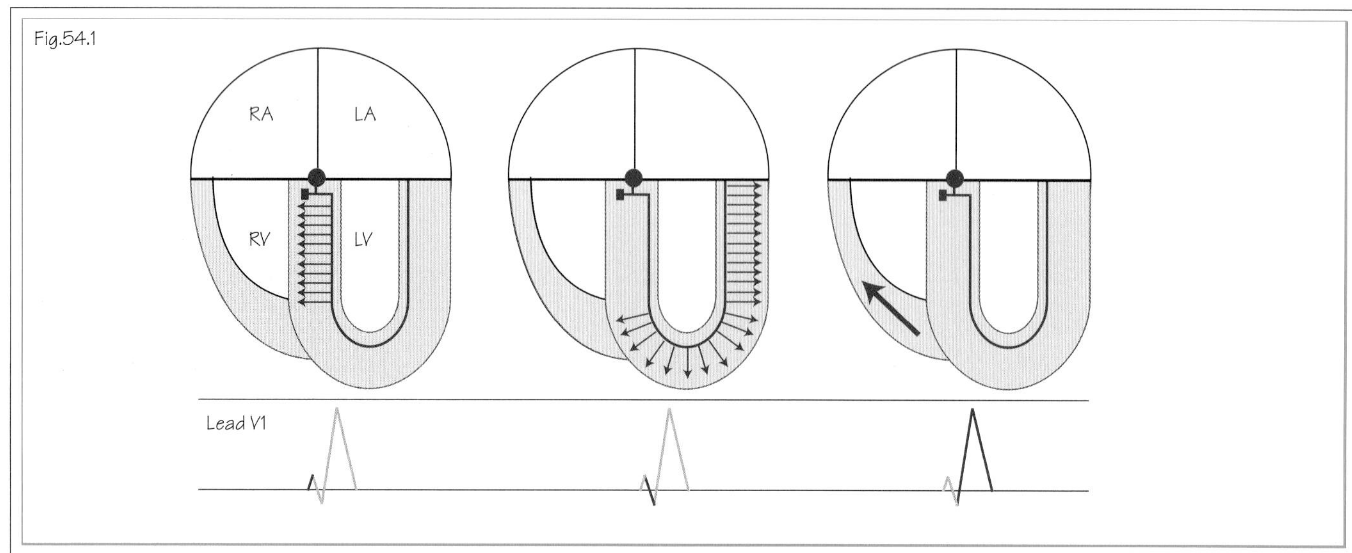

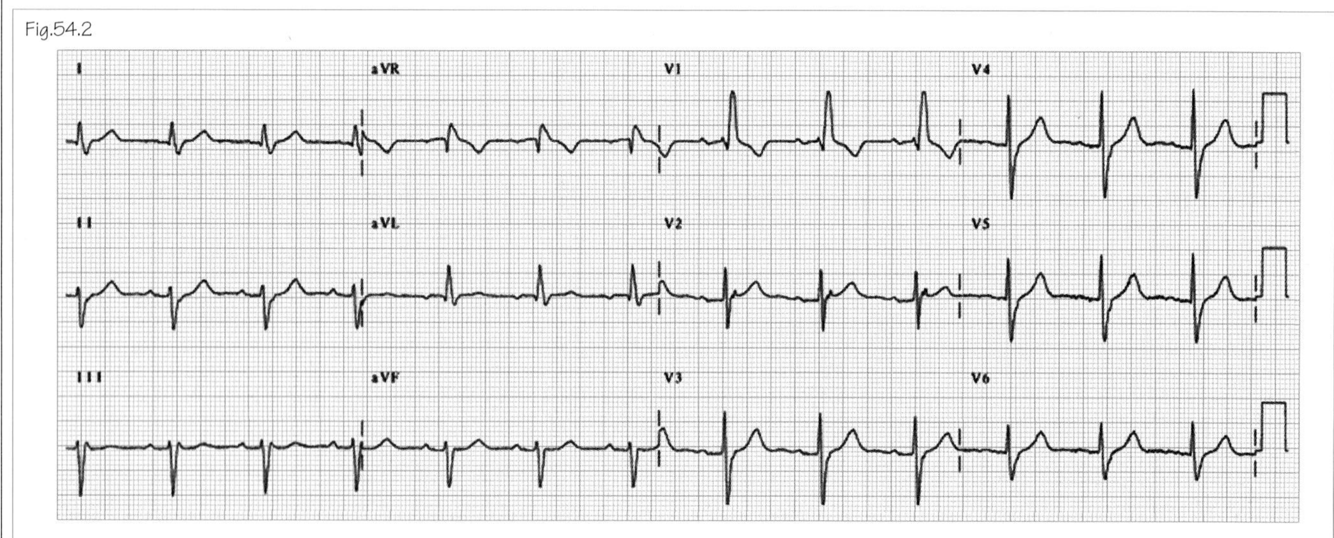

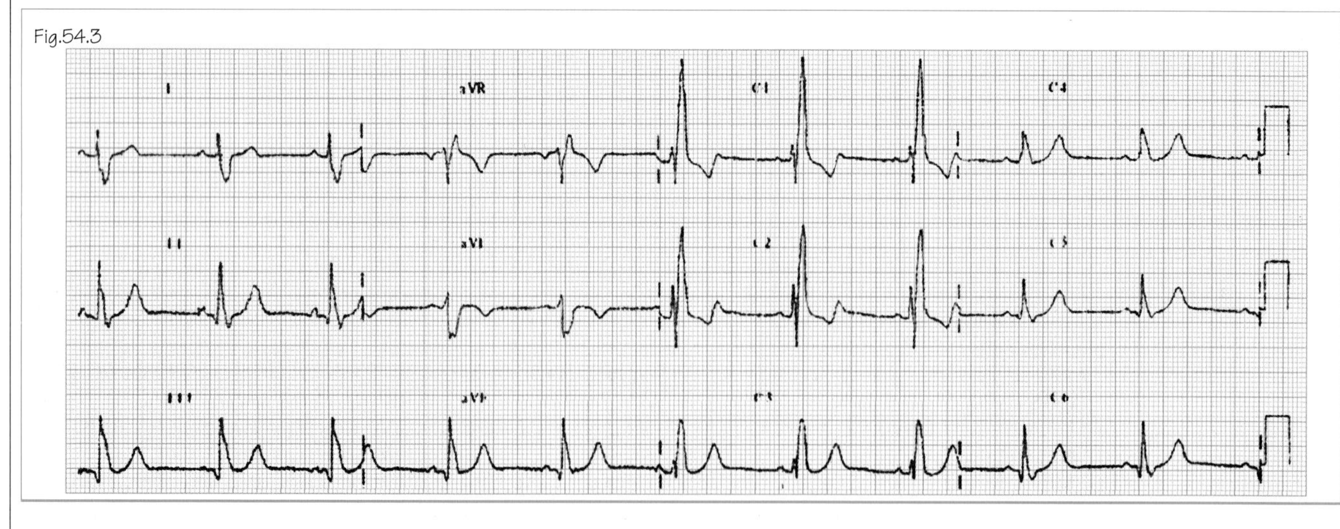

There are several forms of right bundle branch block (RBBB): partial, full and isolated, full and associated with disease elsewhere in the conducting tissue.

ECG appearances of isolated full RBBB

The ECG appearances of RBBB are dominated by the late activation of the right ventricle, leading to a late positive deflection in the right-sided leads, principally lead V1 (Fig. 54.1). This leads to the formal definition of full RBBB as: (i) QRS duration > 120 ms; (ii) PQ interval > 120 ms (i.e. no Wolff–Parkinson–White); (iii) rSR′ in lead V1 or V2; and (iv) S waves in lead I and either lead V5 or V6.

ECG findings in partial RBBB

Full RBBB is due to complete disruption of the function of the right bundle. However, partial disruption can occur. Here lead V1 looks normal (i.e. small initial R wave, followed by a reasonable size S wave) except that then a small R′ wave about the same size as the initial R wave follows the S wave (due to partially delayed activation of the right ventricle). QRS duration is normal. Partial RBBB is a very common finding, regarded as a variant of normal. Very rarely it is associated with an atrial septal defect.

Associated conducting tissue disease

In RBBB there may be associated disease in either the left bundle or the bundle of His or both:

- Associated disease in the left bundle results in an axis deviation (see Chapter 10). Left axis deviation occurs with block in the left anterior fascicle of the left bundle and right axis deviation with a block in the much larger posterior fascicle.
- Disease in the bundle of His may give rise to a long PR interval.

In those with RBBB, disease in one of the other parts of the conducting tissue system is referred to as bifascicular block (e.g. RBBB with either a long PR interval or an axis deviation), disease in both as trifascicular block (i.e. RBBB with both long PR interval and an axis deviation). Trifascicular block is actually a misnomer – as this would be complete heart block, and perhaps trifascicular conduction delay is a better way of expressing what is actually happening. Trifascicular block however has found its way into the medical language. Trifascicular block reflects the sort of conducting tissue disease that gives rise to complete heart block (and so syncope, etc.). Its presence is a reasonable guide that syncope relates to high-grade atrioventricular block (though remember that conducting tissue disease may relate to myocardial disease, which can cause ventricular tachycardia, especially in ishaemic heart disease [IHD]). The causes of RBBB are:

- Idiopathic.
- Disease only affecting the conducting tissues of the heart, the commonest being idiopathic fibrosis.
- Structural heart disease, the commonest being IHD in any of its phases. An occasional cause of RBBB (usually in young people) is an atrial septal defect.
- Pulmonary hypertension; chronic pulmonary hypertension tends to result in ECG evidence of right ventricular hypertrophy (RVH) (a narrow dominant R wave in lead V1), though it can lead to RBBB. Acute pulmonary hypertension, for example due to a massive pulmonary embolism, usually leads to RBBB, in association with right axis deviation to the QRS complex.

Outlook of RBBB

Right bundle branch block is less likely than LBBB to be associated with underlying structural heart disease. Isolated (i.e. no underlying cardiac disease) RBBB has a very good prognosis, is both unlikely to reflect underlying structural heart disease and is also unlikely to progress to extensive conducting tissue disease and a pacemaker.

Conditions that might be confused with RBBB

A dominant R wave in lead V1, *the key finding in RBBB*, is also found in a number of other conditions, and this can give rise to confusion. The common conditions causing such a dominant lead V1 R wave include:

- Right ventricular hypertrophy: the QRS complex in RVH is very narrow (i.e. << 120 ms), and the pattern tends to be just R, rather than the rSR′ found in RBBB.
- Old posterior wall myocardial infarction (MI). The QRS complex is also narrow; very often there is an associated Q wave inferior wall MI (i.e. leads II, III, aVF Q waves).
- Brugada syndrome (see Chapter 39).
- Skeletal myopathy (see Chapter 34).
- Ventricular tachycardia.

Fig. 54.1 Mechanism of right bundle branch block (RBBB). The major manifestation of RBBB is in lead V1. The initial left to right depolarization of the septum is not so different from normal, so the initial appearance of the QRS complex in lead V1 is unremarkable. The bulk of the left ventricle (LV) next depolarizes, without any right ventricle (RV) depolarization, accounting for the small S wave in lead V1. After LV depolarization has finished, the RV starts to depolarize, accounting for a late large positive deflection in lead V1.

Fig. 54.2 Right bundle branch block (RBBB). Sinus rhythm, normal P wave, PR interval, QRS shows left axis deviation (positive in lead I, negative in II, III). Lead V1 shows a rsR′ pattern with a very prominent late positive deflection, pathognomonic of full RBBB. The axis deviation here indicates blockage of the left anterior hemi-fasicles of the left bundle as well, i.e. this ECG shows bifascicular block.

Fig. 54.3 Sinus rhythm, normal P wave, PR interval, QRS shows right axis deviation, (+122°), full RBBB with rsR′ pattern in lead V1, very large late positive deflection in lead V1, suggesting in addition to RBBB, that right ventricular hypertrophy (RVH) is present. Inverted T's leads V1 and V2, due to RBBB. The QRS axis deviation is either due to RVH or to a block of the right posterior hemi-fascicular branch of the left bundle.

55 First degree atrioventricular block – long PR interval

Fig.55.1

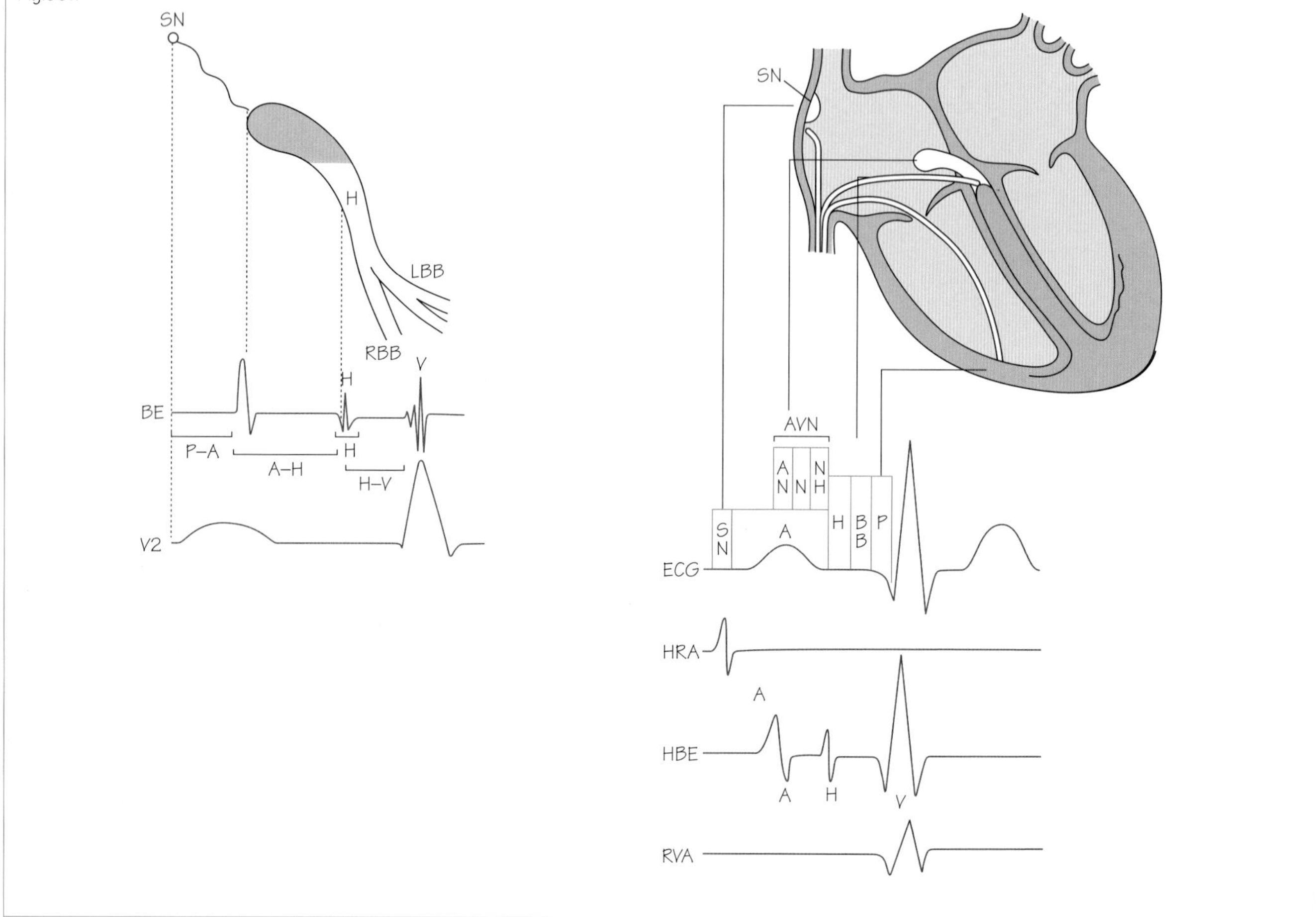

SN
H
LBB
RBB
H
V
BE
P–A
A–H
H
H–V
V2
SN
AVN
A N
N
N H
H
B B
P
S N
A
ECG
HRA
A
HBE
A
H
V
RVA

Fig.55.2

I
aVR
V1
V4
II
aVL
V2
V5
III
aVF
V3
V6

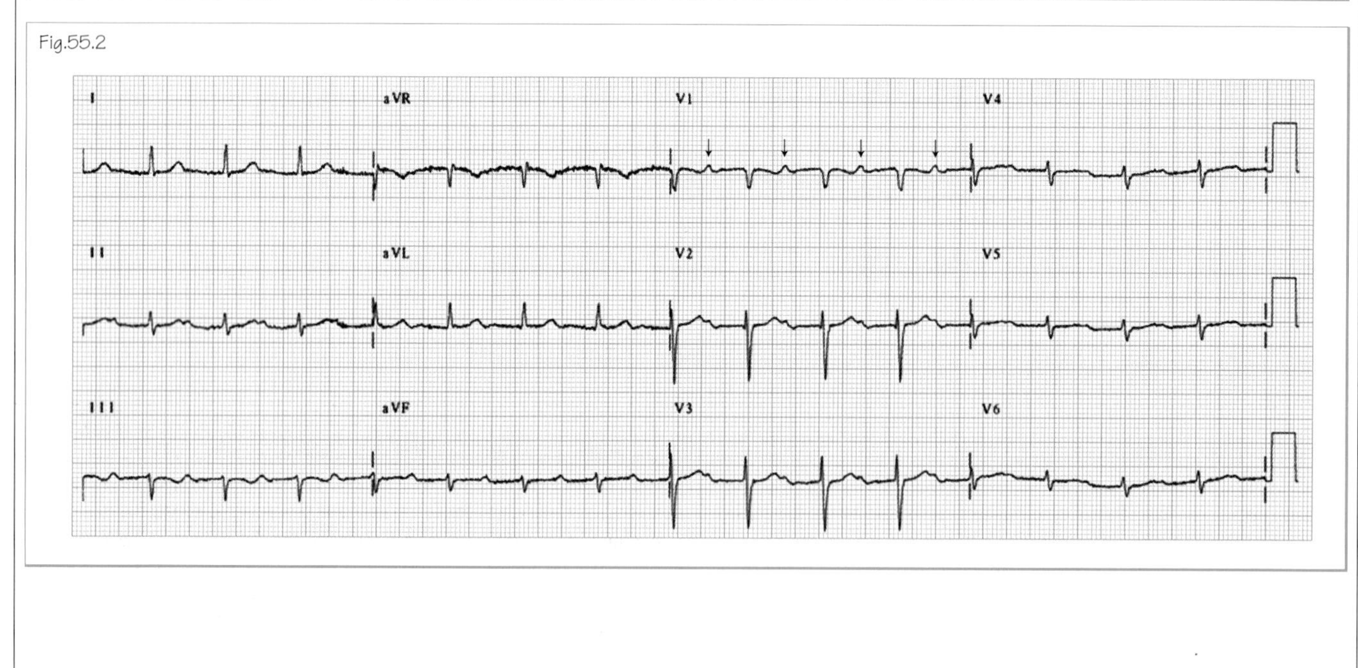

The PR interval reflects the time it takes for the depolarizing wave front to travel from the sinus node to the main body of the ventricle. It is made up of a number of constituent parts (Fig. 55.1): a long PR interval (also known as first degree heart block) can be due to disturbances in function in one (or more) of several sites. It is rather difficult non-invasively to diagnose where the problem is sited. Though knowledge of the site of the problem is often not of clinical significance, occasionally it is! For example, long PR interval due to disease of the atrioventricular (AV) node progresses only rarely to higher forms of AV block, whereas a long PR interval due to infra-Hissian disease not infrequently progresses to higher-grade heart block.

Physiological influences on the PR interval

The PR interval varies in health according to the state of the autonomic nervous system, and the heart rate. High sympathetic tone and low vagal tone shortens the PR interval, and vice-versa: these effects are mainly mediated by neurally mediated changes in AV node conductivity. High heart rate, by intrinsically altering the way the electrics of the heart work, also shortens the PR interval. Conversely, low heart rates, independent of any autonomic influences, results in a long PR interval. Physical fitness affects the PR interval: supremely fit subjects can have really quite long physiological prolongation of the PR interval, due to high vagal tone.

ECG findings in first degree heart block

It is usually fairly easy to diagnose prolongation of the PR interval. The time from the start of the P wave to the first deflection of the QRS complex is measured – in health this is less than five small squares or 200 ms – and if longer than this, PR interval prolongation diagnosed. If physiological influences (fitness, bradycardia, diurnal rhythm, i.e. night-time) do not account for PR interval prolongation, then it is likely to be pathological. There are several sites for diseases processes to result in a prolonged PR interval:

- Disease affecting the AV node.
- Disease affecting the bundle of His.
- Disease affecting simultaneously both bundle branches (if one alone were affected then right or left bundle branch block would result, but the PR interval would be normal).

It is usually not possible to diagnose the site of damage from the 12-lead ECG. If this is needed, then invasive studies are required (Fig. 55.1). The diseases resulting in PR interval prolongation include: idiopathic fibrosis, ischaemic heart disease, cardiomyopathies, myocarditis (including rheumatic fever) and sarcoidosis. Do not forget drugs (including digoxin, beta-blockers, calcium channel blockers and chronic amiodarone therapy) and metabolic conditions (e.g. hypothyroidism).

Complications

The major concern is that higher-grade heart block will result, such as second or third degree block, with their attendant risks. The risk of progression to higher-grade heart block depends on the site of damage (infra-Hissian sites are more likely to progress), and the disease process (and how rapidly progressive this is).

Treatment

If there are no symptoms then, unless the PR interval prolongation is extreme, the best policy usually is watchful waiting. It is often helpful to exclude occult episodes of heart block by undertaking a 24-h ECG monitor. If patients with syncope have a long PR interval, then management depends on the clinical situation. In elderly patients with clear-cut Stokes–Adams attacks often a pacemaker is implanted empirically. If the syncope sounds like vasomotor syncope, then prior to implanting a pacemaker one may wish to have more definitive data that heart block is responsible, obtained either from a Holter monitor or reveal device. If there is underlying left ventricular dysfunction, it may be that syncope relates to a ventricular arrhythmia, so ventricular stimulation studies may be needed.

Fig. 55.1 The PR interval is made up of different components, as shown here. In clinical practice, the PR interval can be broken down into the AH interval (atria–His conduction time) and the HV interval (His–ventricular conduction time), which can be invasively measured from appropriately placed electrodes. Prolongation of the PR interval due to prolongation of the HV time is much more likely to progress to complete heart block than that due to prolonged AH conduction. A, atria; AVN, atrioventricular node; BB, bundle branches; BE, bundle electrode; H, bundle of His; HBE, His bundle electrode; HRA, high right atrial electrode; LBB, left bundle branch; P, Purkinje fibres; RBB, right bundle branch; RVA, right ventricular apex electrode; SN, sinus node; V, ventricle.

Fig. 55.2 Long PR interval. It is not easy to see the P wave in those leads usually best suited to examine the P wave (leads II and V1). However, in lead V1 a prominent 'hump', easily confused with a component of the T wave (arrowed) is actually the P wave. This can be confirmed by examining lead V2, where a deflection on the downslope of the T wave is obviously seen to be the P wave. The PR interval is nine little squares, i.e. 360 ms, clearly pathologically prolonged. The ECG otherwise shows small QRS complexes generally, and poor anterior R wave progression. This patient had obesity, normal left ventricular function and isolated conducting tissue disease, which intermittently resulted in high-grade heart block, so requiring a pacemaker.

56 Second degree atrioventricular block

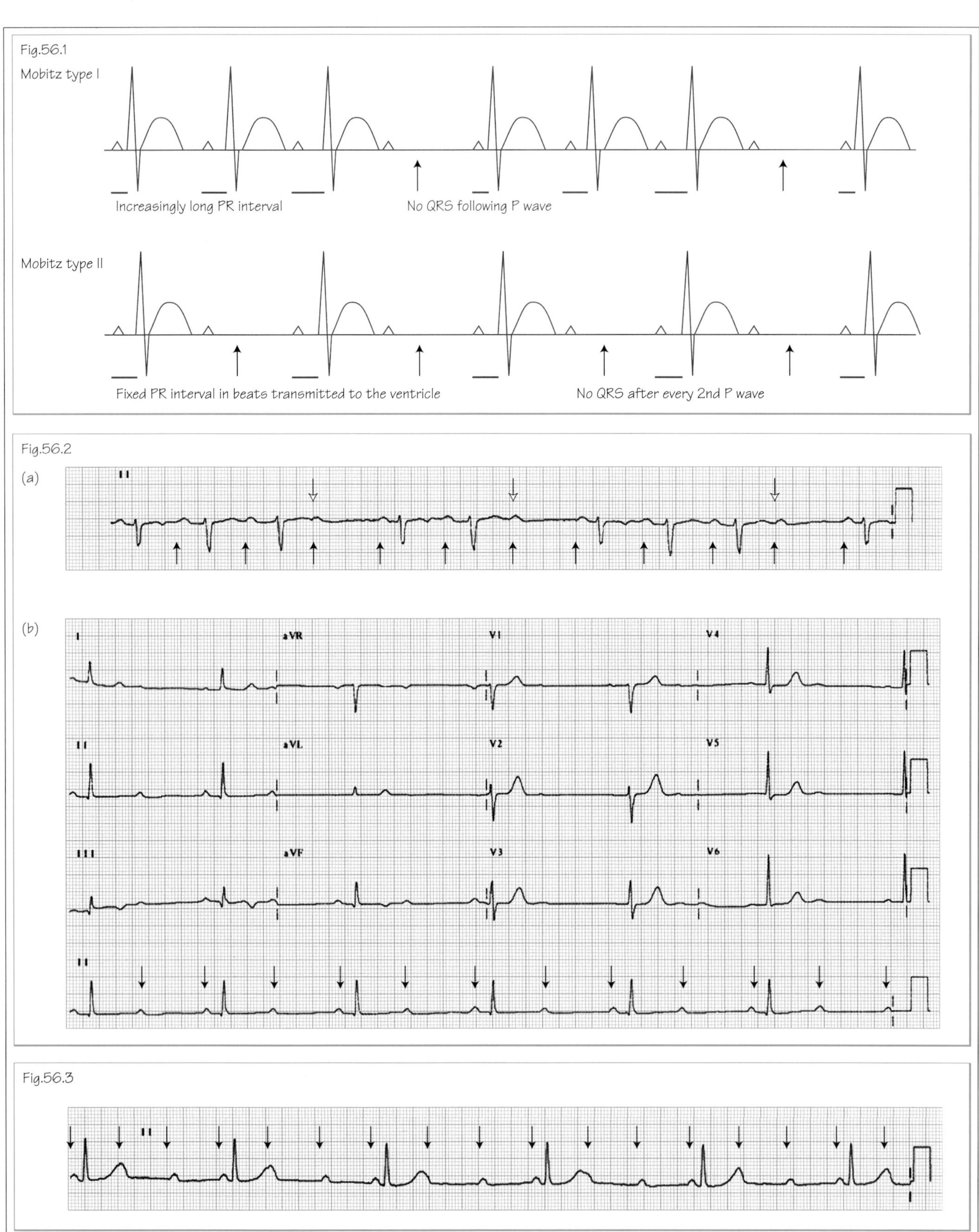

Second degree heart block is a more advanced form of heart block than first degree (long PR interval), and as such is a much more worrying clinical situation. The concern is that second degree heart block will progress suddenly and without warning to third degree heart block, with its attendant risk of asystole and sudden death.

The hallmark of second degree heart block is that not every P wave is transmitted down the conducting system to trigger a QRS complex. Thus there are P waves without any following QRS complexes. There are two forms:

- Type I, also known as Wenckebach, where there is gradual prolongation of each successive PR interval until (usually after 3 or 4 beats), a QRS complex fails to appear. The sequence typically repeats itself, often on multiple occasions. Clear cut type I block is often located in the atrioventricular (AV) node, especially if the QRS complex is narrow, and has a low rate of progression to complete heart block.
- Type II, where after every beat that 'gets through' (i.e. a P wave followed by a QRS complex) there is a fixed number of beats that do not. Most often, every other beat gets through, i.e. there is 2 to 1 (2 : 1) heart block; on occasions every third (3 : 1 block) or, much more rarely, every fourth (4 : 1 block) beat gets through – higher degrees of second degree heart block are rarely found as, if the conducting system is so damaged as to need 5 beats to recover, then usually it is too damaged to conduct at all, and third degree (complete) heart block occurs. The PR interval in those beats transmitted through is usually within the normal range, curiously. Type II block is usually located in the His–Purkinje system and has a high chance of progression to complete block

The only reliable means to ascertain the site of block in type I/II block is by invasive electrophysiological study.

Causes of second degree heart block

The causes are the same as for any conducting tissue disease:

- Isolated (i.e. not involving any other cardiac structures) conducting tissue disease, including infectious causes such as Lyme disease (*Borrelia burghdorferi*).
- Ishaemic heart disease.
- Myocardial disease, such as idiopathic dilated cardiomyopathy. Sarcoidosis has a reputation for causing myocardial disease (which is often rather minor) and more extensive conducting tissue disease.

Consequences

The first consequence is haemodynamic resulting from a decreased cardiac output. This is particularly true in Mobitz type II second degree heart block; in those with left ventricular (LV) disease, chronic heart failure can result, with fluid retention giving rise to peripheral oedema. In many without LV dysfunction, there is a decrease in effort capacity (as the heart is unable to increase its heart rate with exercise), either for rather non-specific reasons or due to breathlessness.

The second consequence results from the progression of the conducting tissue disease, and the development of third degree AV block, and the attendant risk of asystole. The risk is highest in those who have had symptoms of near or actual syncope, as these usually relate to transient episodes of third degree heart block (with symptoms arising from the asystole that commonly accompanies the onset of third degree AV block). However, many patients with acquired second degree heart block regardless of the presence or otherwise of symptoms usually progress in fairly short order to third degree heart block and from there, if untreated, to asystole and death. Accordingly, second degree heart block, unless due to a reversible cause, is an indication for insertion of a permanent pacemaker.

Treatment

Almost always a permanent anti-bradycardic pacemaker is required as soon as practical (see Chapter 59). If there is any recent syncope, the patient should have a temporary pacemaker until the permanent system can be implanted.

Fig. 56.1 Scheme outlining the differences between type I and type II second degree heart block. In type I second degree heart block, there is gradual prolongation of the PR interval over 2–4 beats, and then a P wave occurs which is not transmitted down to the ventricles. Usually, the sequence is repeated many times. In type II heart block, 1 beat is transmitted down for every 2–4 not successfully transmitted. The PR interval of successfully transmitted beats is usually normal, and is the same for each transmitted beat.

Fig. 56.2 (a) Mobitz type I (otherwise known as Wenckebach) second degree heart block. If one looks at the rhythm strip, one can see gradual prolongation of the PR interval over three cardiac cycles, then a non-conducted beat (i.e. one not transmitted to the ventricle). The sequence then repeats itself, though with two beats occurring before the P wave fails to get to the ventricle. (b) Type II Mobitz heart block. Every second P wave is transmitted to the ventricle (see arrows on the rhythm strip showing the P waves). The PR interval in the transmitted beats is normal. The underling ECG is fairly unremarkable aside from mild T wave inversion in the inferior leads – this raises the possibility that the heart block is the result of right coronary artery territory ischaemia.

Fig. 56.3 Mobitz type II heart block showing 3 to 1 (3 : 1) block. The arrows on the rhythm strip show where the P waves are; the P wave rate is fairly unremarkable, but only every third P wave is transmitted to the ventricle. It is relatively easy to miss the 'third' P wave, hidden in the T wave. As the severity of the heart block is greater here than in the ECG in Fig. 56.2b, there is greater concern that this patient will go on to develop third degree heart block, despite the narrow QRS complex on the transmitted beats.

57 Atrioventricular block – third degree (complete) heart block

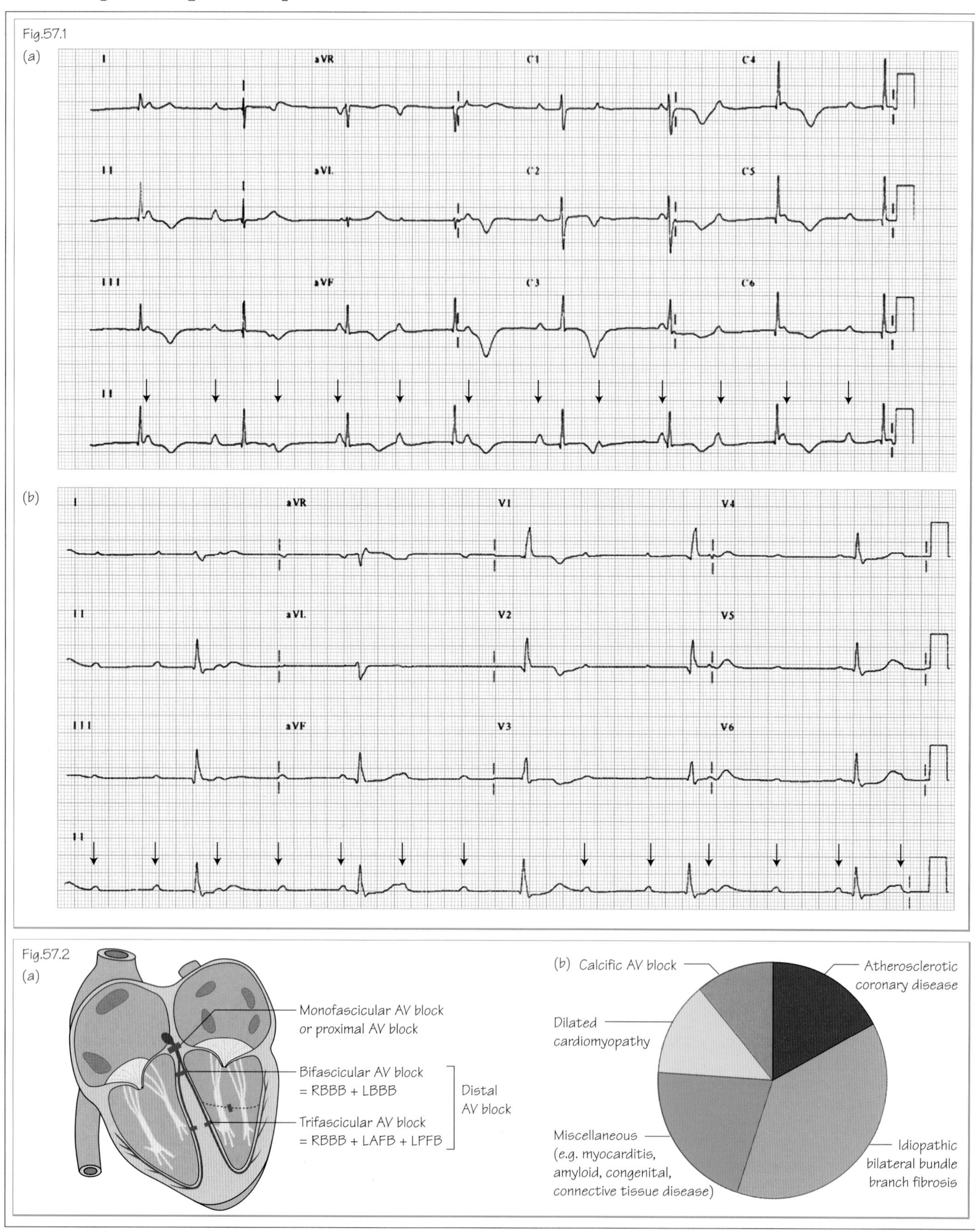

In third degree (complete) heart block (CHB) there is no electrical connection between the atria and the ventricle. It is common and serious – untreated, most patients with acquired CHB die within 2 months, many much earlier. At the moment when the electrical connection between the atria and the ventricle is severed, several events occur:

• Firstly, in many patients, ventricular standstill occurs, causing total loss of cardiac output and syncope. Ventricular asystole typically lasts for seconds rather than minutes. In some patients ventricular activity never resumes and death occurs.

• Secondly, a spontaneous pacemaker starts up in the specialized conducting tissue of the ventricle immediately below the level of the block (Table 57.1). The higher up the block is in the conducting system, the higher the level of the tissue immediately below the block that can act as a pacemaker and the higher is the spontaneous heart rate (Fig. 57.1a,b). Spontaneous ventricular rates in CHB typically vary between 15–40 b/min. The higher the level of block, the more conducting tissue that the impulse can use, so the narrower the QRS complex.

ECG appearance of CHB

• The key ECG finding is atrioventricular (AV) dissociation, i.e. there is no relationship between the P waves and the QRS complex (Figs 57.1a,b & 57.2a,b).

• In atrial fibrillation (AF), P waves are not visible, so one cannot determine the relationship between atrial activity and QRS complexes. Complete heart block is diagnosed in AF by determining the regularity or otherwise of the QRS complexes. In AF with intact conducting tissue, QRSs occur irregularly. In AF with CHB, the QRS complexes occur regularly.

Symptoms in CHB

The symptoms are predictable from knowing the electrical events in CHB. With the onset of CHB, asystole develops and brief syncope results, followed by rapid and full recovery of higher mental faculties as the escape rhythm develops, restoring cardiac output. Though the heart is beating slowly, the cardiac output is rarely depressed enough to cause symptoms at rest. However, the exercise heart rate and cardiac output are greatly depressed, resulting in effort breathlessness, fatigue, possibly angina, and tiredness. Examination shows bradycardia, AV dissociation in the venous pressure and variable intensity of the first heart sound, an ejection flow murmur and sometimes signs of heart failure.

Prognosis

The outlook in the absence of treatment is poor. Increasingly long episodes of asystole followed by increasingly slow escape beats are likely, resulting in further syncope, until finally asystole occurs not followed by a ventricular escape rhythm and death. Occasionally the bradycardia leads to a high-grade ventricular arrhythmia, often a long QT dependent arrhythmia such as torsade-de-pointes. Clearly this is lethal unless terminated quickly.

Treatment

Most acquired CHB requires a permanent pacemaker. Whether a temporary pacemaker ('wire') is needed prior to the permanent pacemaker depends on the stability of the escape rhythm, the safety of temporary wire insertion locally and the delay in permanent pacemaker implantation. Unstable rhythms are those where syncope (i.e. significant asystole) has occurred, where the heart rate is very low (i.e. ≤ 30 b/min) or the QRS complex is broad. Escape beats with a continually changing QRS morphology indicate a very high risk of early asystole. Complete heart block that does not require a temporary or permanent pacemaker needs to have a stable escape rhythm and a reversible cause, e.g. CHB complicating an inferior wall ST segment elevation myocardial infarction (STEMI). Congenital CHB (due to maternal systemic lupus erythematosus [SLE] damaging fetal cardiac conducting tissue *in utero*) is often managed without pacing, though there is accumulating data that permanent pacemakers may prolong life.

Table 57.1 Relative frequency, clinical characteristics and ECG findings in third degree AV block due to conduction block at different sites.

		Escape beat		
Site of block	Relative frequency	Rate	Asystole risk	QRS width
AV node	20%	≥ 45 b/min	No	Narrow
His bundle	20%	≤ 45 b/min	Medium	Broad
Below His	60%	≤ 35 b/min	High	Very broad

AV, atrioventricular.

Fig. 57.1 (a) Congenital complete heart block (CHB), due to maternal systemic lupus erythematosus (SLE). The rhythm strip (bottom) shows no relationship between the P waves (arrowed) and the QRS complexes, i.e. there is atrioventricular (AV) dissociation. A good way to diagnose AV dissociation is to examine the time from the QRS complex to the immediately preceding P wave. If this is variable, and it is highly variable here, AV dissociation is highly likely. Atrioventricular dissociation is then confirmed by finding P waves not followed by any QRS complexes. Atrioventricular dissociation is the hallmark of CHB. The QRS beats are escape beats and the heart rate is 48 b/min. Narrow complex (i.e. QRS duration ≤ 120 ms) beats arise from high up in the conducting system, in or near the AV node. Narrow complex escape beats arising from high up in the conducting tissue, in the setting of congenital heart block, are stable and unlikely to stop. Symptoms are minimized as the heart rate increases with exercise, unlike the 'fixed' heart rate of acquired CHB. Pacing is only infrequently needed. The T waves are abnormal, with antero-lateral deep symmetrical T wave inversion, which is common in CHB, and by itself does not imply additional pathology. (b) Acquired CHB. There is AV dissociation, with no relationship between the P waves (arrowed) and the QRS complexes, which can only be due to CHB. The QRS complex heart rate is about 30 b/min. The QRS complex is broad with a right bundle branch block pattern (suggesting that the escape beat is of left ventricular origin) and an inferiorly directed axis (negative QRS complex in lead I, positive in leads II and III). The slow heart rate implies that the level of the block is relatively low down in the conducting system, confirmed by finding a broad QRS escape beat complex. This form of heart block is unstable (i.e. asystole can occur suddenly).

Fig. 57.2 (a) Site of block. (b) Causes of acquired complete heart block (CHB).

58 Pacemakers – basic principles

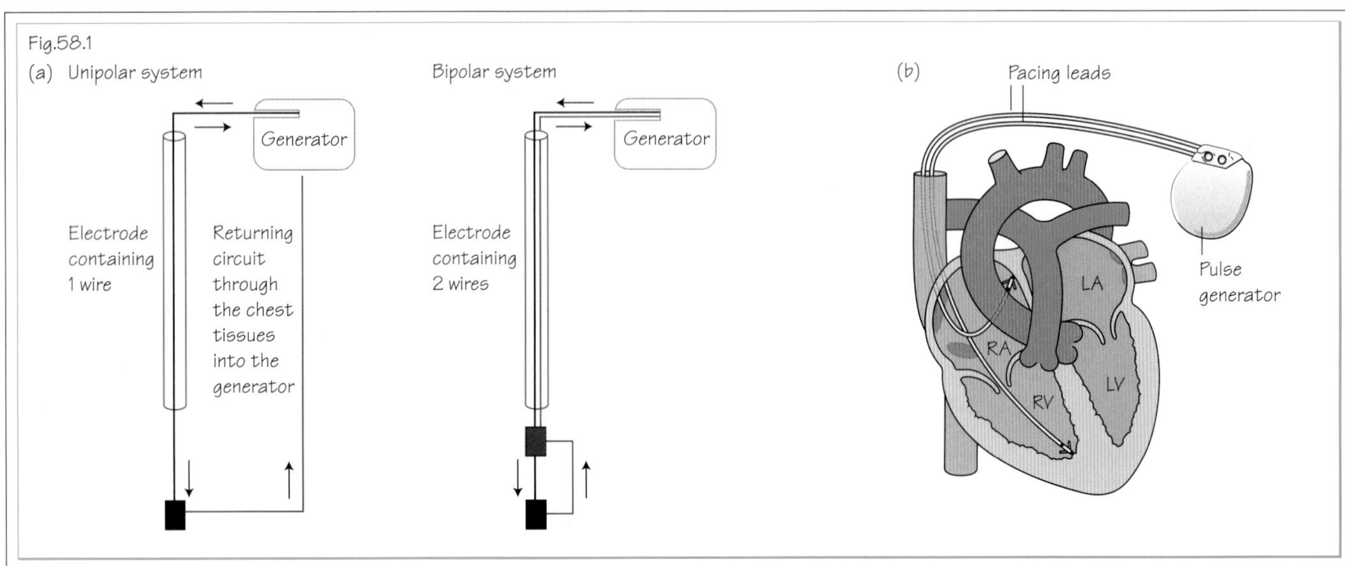

Fig.58.2

(a)

I aVR V1 V4

II aVL V2 V5

III aVF V3 V6

II

(b)

(c)

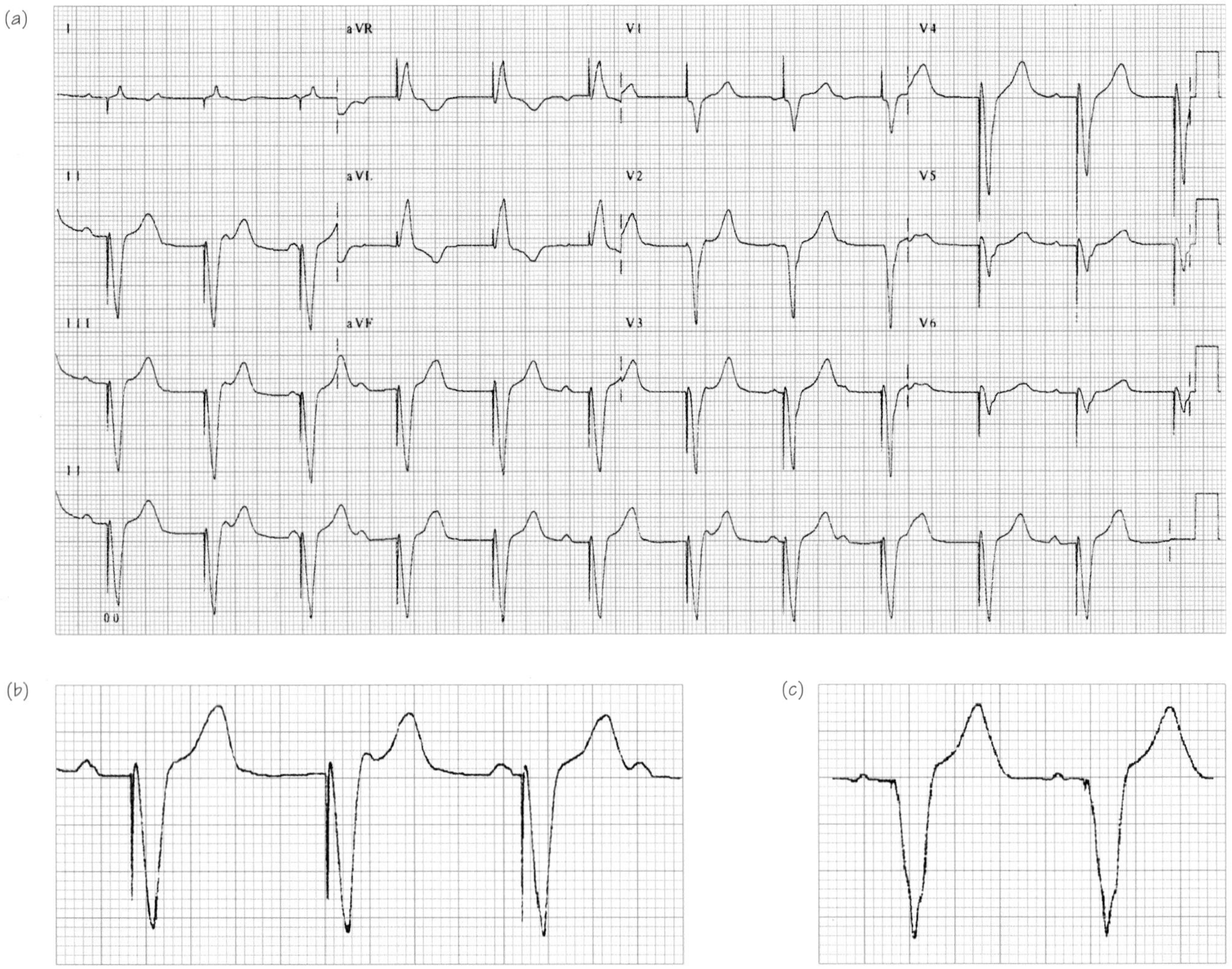

Principle of pacing

Pacemakers treat slow heart rhythms (anti-bradycardia devices), fast heart rhythms (anti-tachycardia devices) and improve ventricular function in heart failure (cardiac resynchronization therapy [CRT]). These functions can be combined. Pacemakers work because:

• Cardiac activity is associated with current flow, which can be detected.

• An intrinsic property of the heart is that an action potential firing in a few cells spreads as a self-propagating wave throughout that chamber. Pacemakers listen out for normal heart activity, and if this does not occur, induce action potentials by passing depolarizing currents into a cardiac chamber (1–5 V, for 1–2 ms) triggering a self-propagating wave so restoring chamber electrical and thus mechanical function.

Pacemaker components

• An **electrode**(s) to pass electricity from spontaneous cardiac activity into the generator, and electricity from the pacemaker into the heart (Fig. 58.1).

• A **generator**, for the power source (lithium battery) and logic circuits that determine the response to cardiac electrical activity, which are: (i) do nothing, e.g. anti-bradycardic devices when normal cardiac activity detected; (ii) pace at a normal heart rate, e.g. anti-bradycardic pacing when no activity is detected or very fast for tachyarrhythmias ('over-drive' pace); (iii) defibrillate (implantable cardioverter defibrillators [ICDs]) when rapid heart rates suggesting ventricular tachycardia (VT)/ ventricular fibrillation (VF) occur. Pacemakers are programmable (Table 58.1); they receive and transmit data/programming instructions through the skin using electromagnetic waves.

Electrode types

• **Unipolar systems** are simple (one electrode/wire) and reliable: current flows from the generator down the electrode, into the heart, and returns through cardiac, thoracic, and chest wall tissues, into the generator via its metal casing. Current flows through poorly conducting non-cardiac tissue, leading to current wastage (shortening battery life, as higher currents are used, so also increasing the 'pacing spike' size) and detection of extraneous extracardiac currents (e.g. pectoral muscle activity), misinterpreted as coming from the heart, inhibiting pacing even if the heartbeat has not occurred. Syncope can result, e.g. when the left arm is used.

• **Bipolar systems** have two wires/electrodes, are complex, expensive, more fragile and likely to fail. Current flows out of the generator, down one wire, into the heart, across a small amount of cardiac tissue and up the other wire. The circuit outside the pacemaker hardware is short, small amounts of electricity are required for cardiac depolarization (prolonging battery life, minimizing the pacing artefact). Extraneous extracardiac electrical activity is not detected and cannot interfere with pacemaker function.

Classification

The international classification system uses five letters: in practice only four are used. First letter is the chamber paced (A = atria, V = ventricle, D = both), second the chamber sensed (O if no sensing function), the third is the response to spontaneous cardiac activity (O = no sensing, T = triggered, D = both). Thus one might have:

• VOO (ventricle paced, no sensing function [a temporary mode used to check pacing threshold]).

• VVI (ventricle paced and sensed, if spontaneous cardiac output detected, then the device is inhibited).

• DDD. Dual chamber pacemaker can trigger (T) ventricular pacing if atrial activity is sensed.

The fourth letter relates to pacing rate adjustment in response to exercise (i.e. rate responsive), designated using the letter 'R'. A common pacemaker is a VVI-R, i.e. a single lead that senses and paces the ventricle, and if the patient exercises, increases the paced heart rate. The fifth letter designates whether anti-tachycardic functions are present.

Generator functions

The generator detects cardiac activity when present and remains silent, and paces when no such activity occurs. Most pacemaker functions can be programmed, by applying a programming head (which emits electromagnetic waves) over the pacemaker, connected to a programmer (a computer that drives the head):

• Pacing mode: most dual chamber systems can be programmed to single chamber mode (e.g. DDD to VVI, useful if the atrial electrode fails).

• Output: the energy delivered to the electrodes can be altered; a lower level conserves power and prolongs battery life, a higher level ensures pacing always occurs when needed. The voltage output is usually set to 50% above the capture threshold. It can be increased if 'exit block' occurs (e.g. due to scar tissue forming around an electrode, raising the capture threshold). The pulse duration can also be altered.

• Sensitivity, the level of current that the generator recognizes or ignores as coming from a cardiac chamber. Currents from pectoral muscle generate 2–3 mV, and from the heart 5–15 mV. For most patients, sensitivity is set at around 4–5 mV, so excluding pectoral muscle/distant chamber activity. If the electrode starts to fail, the amount of electricity passed up the electrode may decrease, leading to failure to sense, and inappropriate pacing. Altering the sensitivity can deal with this problem.

• Refractory period: pacemakers must not misinterpret activity from one chamber as coming from another, e.g. an atrial electrode sensing ventricular activity, labelling it as atrial, and so being inappropriately inhibited. Programming the generator not to detect any electrical activity at certain times of the cardiac cycle (e.g. the atrial electrode, during the time period when normal ventricular activity occurs) can prevent this.

• Rate adaptation: some generators (rate-responsive ones) detect physical activity (using motion detectors, or QT interval sensors), and react by increasing the pacing rate, useful in mimicking the physiological effects of exercise on heart rate

Fig. 58.1 (a) Bipolar and unipolar electrodes. (b) Pacing system (from www.sjm.com/assets/popups/pacemaker.gif).

Fig. 58.2 (a) Paced ECG, VVI pacemaker. P waves occur randomly (examine the rhythm strip), unrelated to the QRS complexes. Pacing spike before each QRS complex, followed by a broad complex beat (electricity transmission from the electrode through the heart is by the slow myocyte-to-myocyte transmission). The QRS complexes for the standard ventricular pacemaker have a left bundle morphology (best shown in lead aVL), indicating the left ventricle is activated last, as the electrode is situated in the right ventricle. (b) Unipolar electrode – large pacing spike. (c) Bipolar electrode, small pacing spike.

59 Anti-bradycardic pacemakers

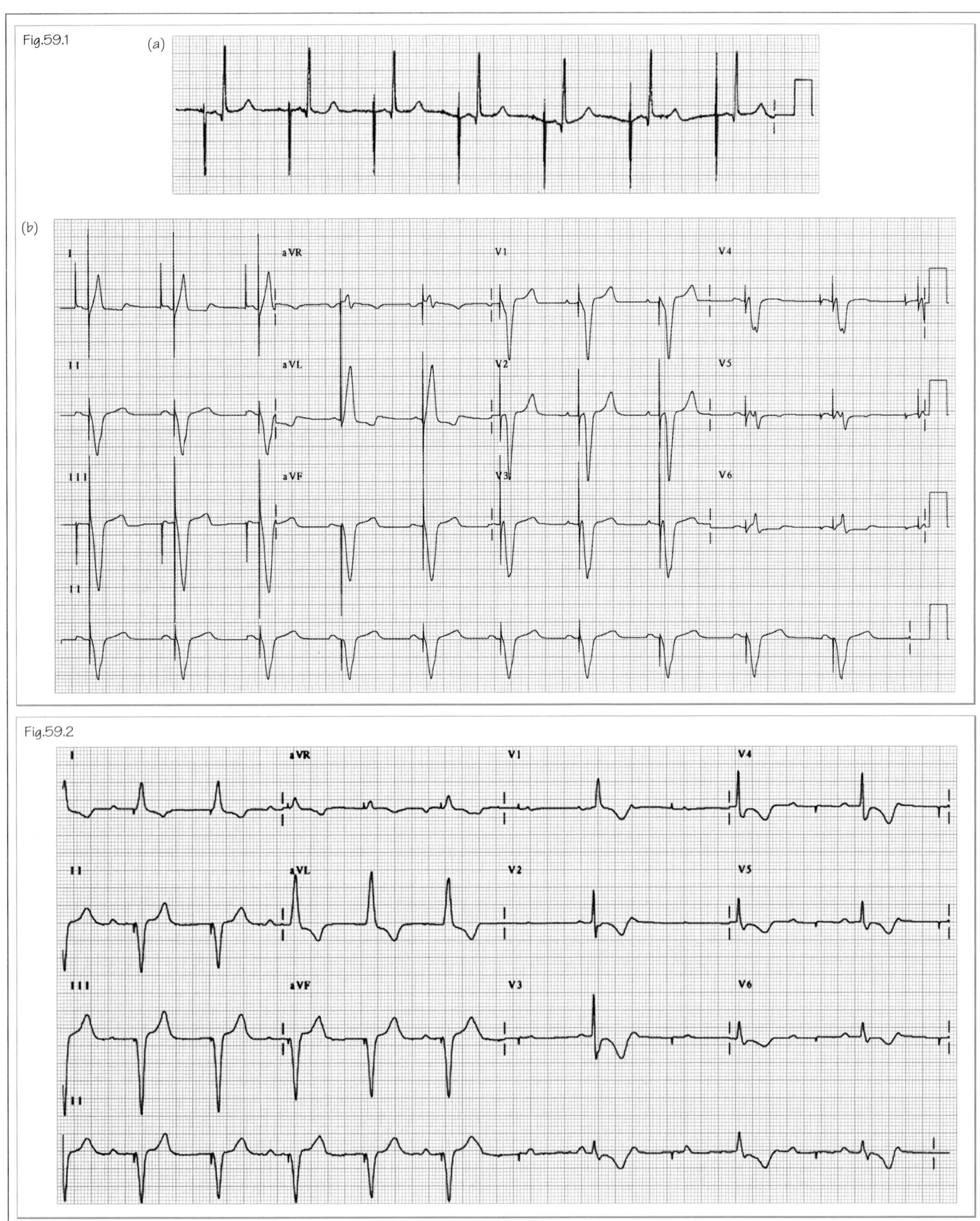

Anti-bradycardia pacemakers comprise the majority of pacemakers (88% of the 35 000 pacemaker device implanted in the UK in 2004). They determine whether normal cardiac electrical activity has occurred; if so, they are silent, if not, then they stimulate the heart to beat. The common indications are: third degree atrioventricular (AV) block (30% of implants), sick sinus syndrome (25%), atrial fibrillation with bradycardia (20%), second degree heart block (15%), others (10%). Except in rare circumstances (see Chapter 60) they do not prevent tachycardias (e.g. in atrial fibrillation [AF] with pauses anti-tachycardic medication is still needed post-pacemaker implantation).

Pacemaker implantation

Pacemakers are implanted under local anaesthetic, in the left upper chest of right-handed individuals. The skin is cut, the cephalic vein identified and opened, the electrode introduced and pushed into the relevant heart chamber, guided into position under X-ray imaging, tested (see below), stitched so it cannot withdraw from the heart, and connected to the generator. The generator is inserted into a pocket made medially in the chest, over pectoral major and under the dermis/subcutaneous fat. The skin wound is sewn up. The procedure takes 30–60 min. The complication rate is low (pneumothorax, haemothorax, pacemaker infection, arrhythmias).

The paced ECG

A paced ECG complex shows two features: (i) A narrow 'pacing spike' (the 'pacing artefact'), which reflects the energy delivered from the generator down the electrode that depolarizes the paced chamber. (ii) The P wave/QRS complex immediately following the pacing artefact. The paced P wave is of normal duration and shape (the atrial electrode is close to the normal sinus node so the spread of depolarization is normal). The paced ventricular complex is always broad (the ventricle is depolarized by slow myocyte-to-myocyte depolarization) and of left bundle morphology (the electrode sits at the apex of the right ventricle [RV], so the left ventricle [LV] is the last to depolarize, as in left bundle branch block [LBBB]).

Determining the pacing threshold

The pacemaker is usually set to AOO or VOO mode (i.e. obligatory pacing without sensing), and the output decreased by a fixed amount every beat – eventually, the pacemaker fails to capture the atria/ventricle (i.e. a pacing spike not followed by a P/QRS complex). The threshold is the pacemaker output that just captures the chamber.

Sensitivity

A pacemaker should detect relevant cardiac activity, then not pace, and ignore non-relevant cardiac electrical activity. For atrial pacemakers the relevant activity is the P wave, for ventricular systems the R wave. The 'sensitivity' is the level above which activity is regarded as being a P wave/QRS complex, below which is ignored, e.g. if the sensitivity is set at 5 mV, R waves ≥ 5 mV inhibit pacemaker ventricular pacing; R waves ≤ 5 mV, lead to ventricular pacing.

Determining whether correct sensing and pacing is present

Normal function leads to: (i) Pacing at an appropriate interval after the last paced/spontaneous beat. (ii) No pacing if P/R waves occur. There are two forms of failure to pace: (i) A spike with no following P wave/QRS complex = 'failure to capture', due to electrode failure (e.g. fracture), 'exit' block (i.e. fibrous tissue around the pacemaker tip that cannot be electrically penetrated) or drugs raising the pacing threshold. (ii) No spike and no paced beat, caused by generator/complete electrode failure or 'over-sensing'/'far-field sensing', i.e. the generator receives an electrical input misinterpreted as being cardiac activity, whereas the electrical activity is either non-relevant (e.g. pectoral muscle activity in unipolar lead systems) or from a distant cardiac chamber (e.g. the atrial electrode senses ventricular activity 'far-field sensing' so believing that the atria have fired when they have not, and so does not fire when it should).

Failure to sense

With correct sensing, if there is an atrial or ventricular beat, there should be no paced beat within the time period determined by the minimum paced rate. If there is, then the pacemaker has failed to sense; there are several causes for this, including various forms of electrode failure, or the 'sensitivity' being set too high (this is a programmable function, and can be adjusted).

Complications of anti-bradycardic pacemakers

- Infection, a feared complication, suspected when anyone with a pacemaker *in situ* presents with an inflammatory illness (some – rarely all – of the following: fever, weight loss, anaemia, raised erythrocyte sedimentation rate [ESR] and C-reactive protein [CRP], positive blood cultures). Treatment is antibiotics, complete pacemaker system removal, and when sterility achieved, new system insertion.
- Lead problems, including fracture and displacement (which prevent pacing/sensing or prematurely deplete the battery).
- Programming problems: inadequate output, incorrect sensitivity, incorrect blanking periods (leading to inappropriate inhibition or pacemaker mediated tachycardia [PMT]).
- Pacemaker mediated tachycardia; in dual chamber pacemakers, the electrodes and generator can act as an accessory pathway, leading to tachyarrhythmias. These can be terminated by: (i) adenosine; (ii) DOO mode (applying an external magnet); (iii) changing the blanking periods; (iv) internal pacemaker algorithms.
- Pacemaker syndrome; patients with VVI pacemakers and intact AV conduction (e.g. sick sinus syndrome) can develop retrograde VA conduction, so that shortly after ventricular systole the atria fire, contracting on a closed AV valve, resulting in atrial distension, brain natriuretic peptide release and reflexes that lower blood pressure, causing faintness/syncope. Lowering the rate at which pacing starts (so less pacing occurs) or upgrading to a DDD system deals with this problem.

Fig. 59.1 (a) AAI pacing. Large pacing spike followed by very small voltage P waves. The clue that atrial pacing occurs is finding a QRS complex ± 200 ms (= PR interval) after every pacing artefact, i.e. the atria must have fired. (b) DDD pacing. Atrial pacing spike (variable amplitude, best seen in lead I), followed by P wave, then ventricular pacing spike followed by a broad QRS complex. Dual chamber pacemaker.

Fig. 59.2 Failure to pace. The first six beats show a pacing spike followed by a paced QRS complex (VVI pacemaker), then the pacing spike occurs (arrowed) but no paced beats follow, 'failure-to-pace'. Fortunately, the underlying heart rhythm, complete heart block, rapidly emerged. The pacemaker output was set too low; the problem resolved when it was increased.

60 Anti-tachycardic and heart failure devices

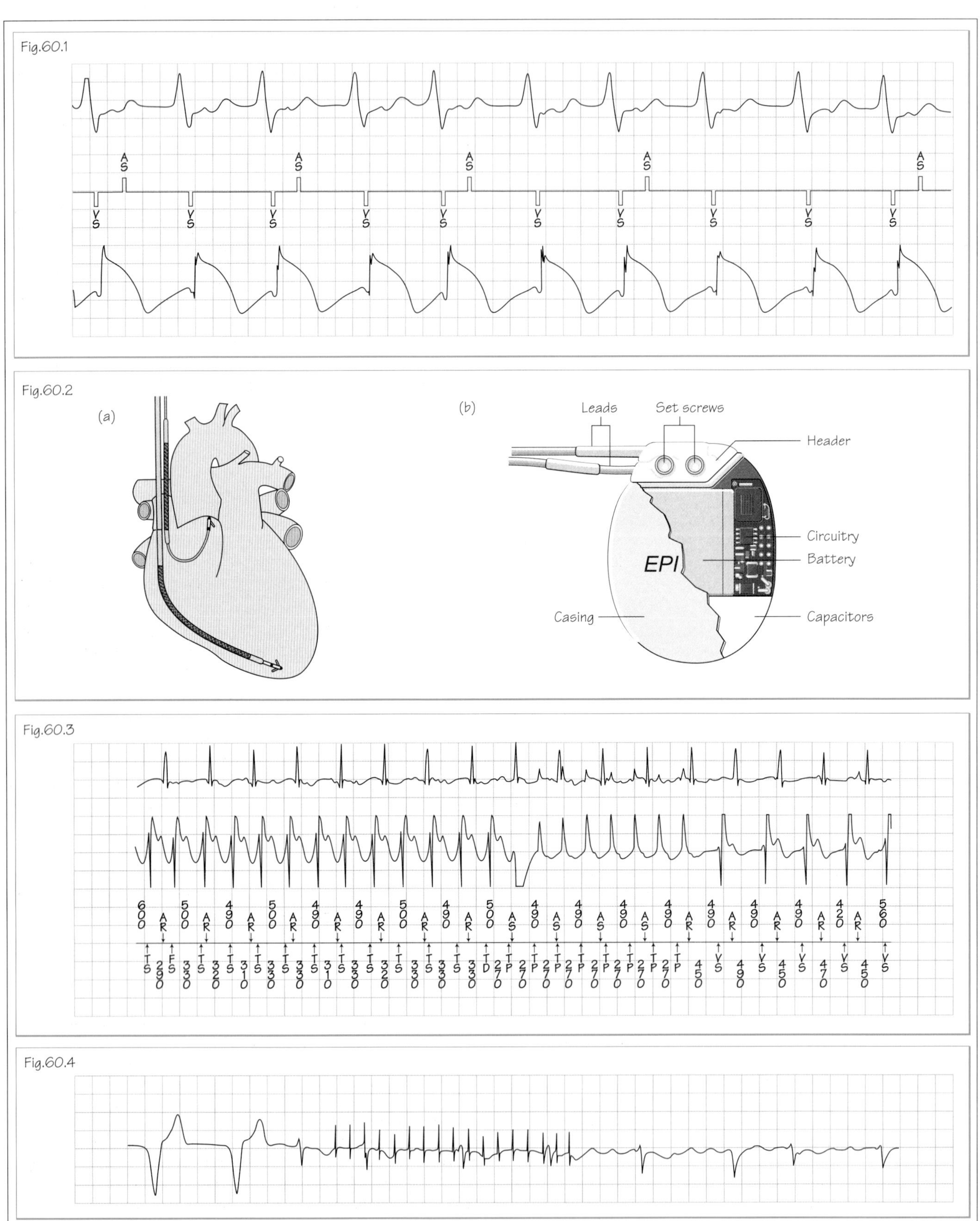

Anti-tachycardia and heart failure devices are commonly implanted; 2700 implantable cardioverter defibrillators (ICDs) were implanted in the UK in 2004, and 1500 cardiac resynchronization therapy (CRT) devices (50% combined ICDs, 50% only pacing). These numbers are increasingly rapidly, by 10% per year (ICDs), 30–50% per year (CRT).

Anti-bradycardia pacing to suppress tachycardias

Occasionally 'standard' anti-bradycardia devices are implanted specifically to suppress tachycardias: (i) AAI pacing to prevent atrial fibrillation (AF) in sick sinus syndrome-induced bradycardia; (ii) long QT dependent torsade-de-pointes (TDP) type ventricular tachycardia (VT). Pacing (DDD) increases heart rate, shortens QT interval and so prevents TDP, especially acutely (e.g. drug toxicity + heart disease + low K^+). Pacing does not terminate TDP once present.

Implantable cardioverter defibrillators

Implantable cardioverter defibrillators (Fig. 60.2b) comprise several functions in one device, i.e. standard anti-bradycardic pacing, VT overdrive pacing and the unique ability to deliver an internal DC shock to the ventricle. For this they possess a battery that stores substantial energy, which can charge the capacitor rapidly. This energy is then delivered between two 'coils', one at the right ventricle (RV) apex another in the supraventricular tachycardia (SVC) (Fig. 60.2a), usually contained in one complex bulky electrode. The generator responses can be fully programmed. The device has a solid-state memory, allowing recording of all events for further analysis (e.g. to determine the appropriateness of shocks). Implantable atrial defibrillators for AF remain experimental and have been superseded by anti-AF ablative treatments.

How devices diagnose ventricular arrhythmias

Devices diagnose ventricular arrhythmias using, mainly, the number of electrical impulses detected by the RV electrode, i.e. the number of R waves. Arrhythmias definitions are programmed and altered according to the clinical situation, e.g. normal heart rhythm 60–150 b/min, slow VT 150–200 b/min, fast VT 200–250 b/min and ventricular fibrillation (VF) ≥ 250 b/min. The device is programmed to treat according to heart rate, e.g. slow VT leads to overdrive pacing, fast VT to overdrive pace three times and if this fails, defibrillation, VF defibrillation immediately. Problems with using heart rate to diagnose VT/VF are: (i) if the heart rate increases from a supraventricular arrhythmia (e.g. AF), VT may be misdiagnosed; (ii) occasionally a prominent T wave is counted as an R wave, leading to double counting, incorrect diagnosis of VT and inappropriate anti-VT therapy. Accordingly, additional diagnostic strategies are used:

- The onset of the arrhythmia (sudden in tachycardia).
- The stability of the arrhythmia (VT is a regular heart rhythm not irregular).
- The morphology of the QRS, i.e. broad complex.

Overdrive pacing to terminate VT

Pacing can be highly successful in terminating monomorphic (not polymorphic) VT. The ventricle is paced just above ('overdrive' pacing) or below ('underdrive' pacing, though this is less successful) the VT rate, to 'capture' the ventricle and break the re-entry circuit. After each VT cycle, those parts of the ventricle that have depolarized, repolarize and become susceptible to further depolarization, either by the re-entrant VT beat returning or, before this occurs, by a wave of depolarization spreading from the RV electrode. If a significant part of the ventricle is susceptible to depolarization, or if the electrical anatomy of the heart is otherwise suitable, an appropriately timed stimulus from the pacing wire can allow a wave of depolarization to spread over the heart that meets and nullifies the depolarization wave from the VT re-entrant circuit. In the electrophysiology (EP) laboratory, single or double appropriately timed ventricular premature contractions (VPCs) are used; outside the EP laboratory, a 'burst' of pacing will often by chance be timed such that the ventricle is captured. Occasionally overdrive pacing results in VT speeding up (i.e. becoming haemodynamically unstable) or VF, in which situation DC shock therapy is delivered. Devices using burst atrial pacing to terminate AF are available (Fig. 60.4).

Cardiac resynchronization therapy

In heart failure, a broad QRS complex is common, the broader the QRS and the quicker the increase the worse the outcome. A broad QRS complex is associated with regional differences in the onset of left ventricular (LV) contraction (dyscoordinate 'asynchronous' contraction). This results in wasted mechanical energy as blood is moved within, rather than out of the ventricle, and a reduced cardiac output. These patients have more mitral regurgitation and reduced diastolic filling time. If LV contraction were to start simultaneously then less blood would be shunted within the ventricle, and more propelled into the aorta. Left ventricular contraction can be synchronized if the LV free wall is paced from an electrode positioned in a coronary sinus branch. Standard pacing electrodes are also placed in the right atrium and RV apex/outflow tract. These three wires are connected to a CRT generator, programmed so that the two ventricular wires are activated simultaneously. These devices relieve symptoms of heart failure, improve prognosis, and lessen the chance of ventricular arrhythmias. Fifty per cent of devices have standby ICDs.

Fig. 60.1 Intracardiac electrogram (bottom) compared to surface ECG (top trace): the intracardiac recording more closely reflects cellular events, and looks remarkably similar to an action potential.

Fig. 60.2 (a) Electrodes from an implantable cardioverter defibrillator (ICD), one positioned to pace/sense the right atrium, one to pace/sense the right ventricle. The shocking circuit is between the two heavily hatched areas on the two electrodes. (b) Components of an ICD.

Fig. 60.3 Implantable cardioverter defibrillator (ICD) – overdrive pacing terminating ventricular tachycardia (VT). Top = atrial electrogram, middle = ventricular electrogram, bottom = timings between P and R waves. Initially VT is present (P waves less frequent than R waves, no relationship between them). Short burst of ventricular pacing (partly seen by the atrial electrode but best seen in the ventricular electrode trace), terminating the arrhythmia. Sinus rhythm is then restored, with each P wave followed by an R wave.

Fig. 60.4 Anti-atrial fibrillation (AF) pacing. Two paced ventricular beats, then a non-paced QRS beat, then a large number of pacing spikes through which non-paced QRS beats can be seen. Following this, AF is seen. This is a system with algorithms for anti-AF pacing. On this occasion, the device failed to terminate AF.

61 External and internal loop recorders

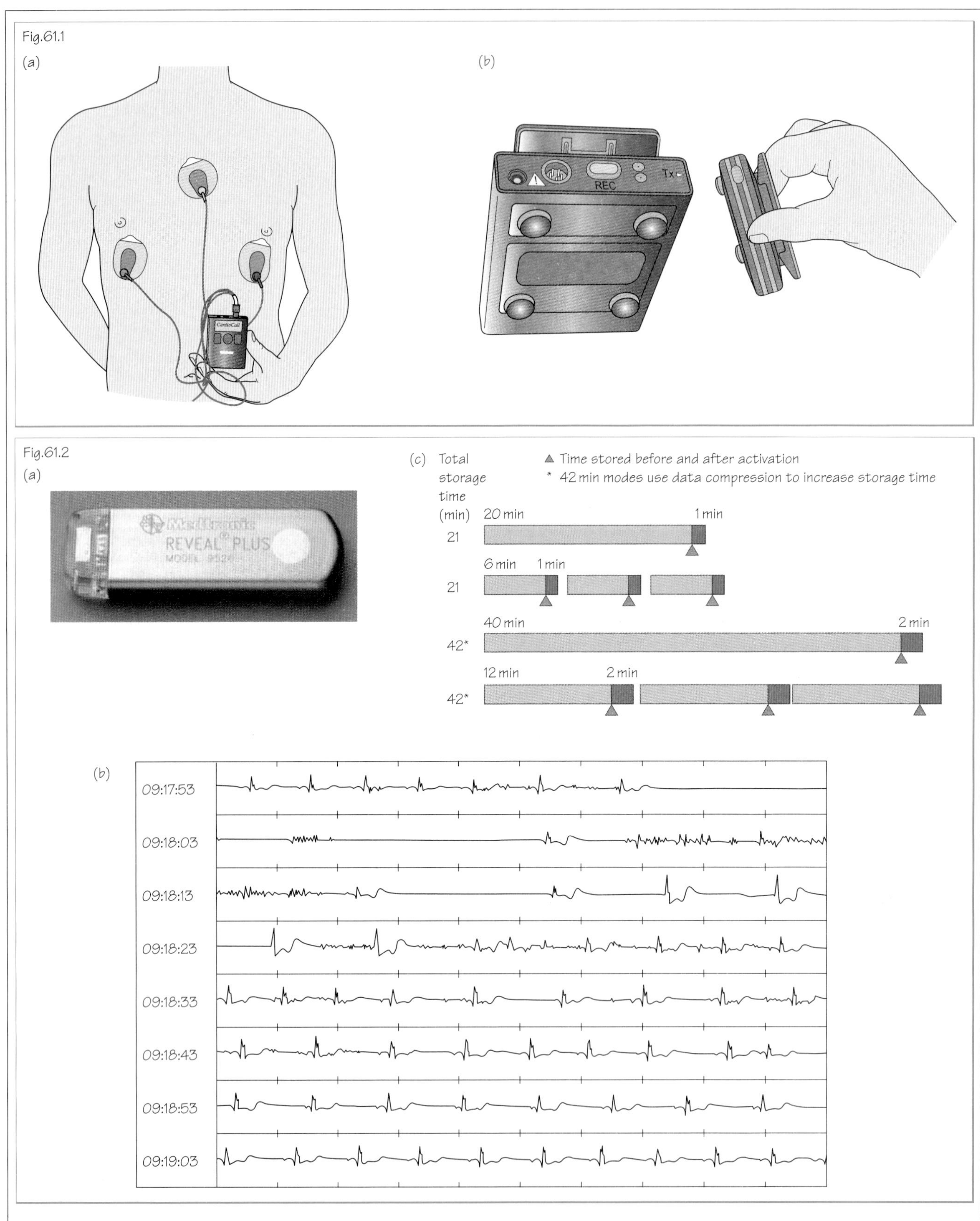

A key aspect in the investigation of symptoms that could be arrhythmic is to obtain an ECG during the event (Table 61.1). An ECG remote to the event along with the clinical history gives clues to the diagnosis, but the 'clincher' is *the ECG during the event*. How best to obtain such an ECG depends on the nature and frequency of symptoms:

• **Palpitations** (breathlessness, etc.): if they last long enough to present to hospital or general practitioner surgery, etc., telling the patient to report to such a facility immediately symptoms start is the best approach. If they do not last this long then a 24-h ECG (see Chapter 63) may be diagnostic. If symptoms occur every few days, a 7-day ECG (known by its commercial name as an 'R' test). If symptoms occur weekly or so an externally applied single channel ECG machine ('Cardiomemo®' device, Fig. 61.1) is the right approach.

• **Syncope**: an ECG is diagnostic if obtained at the moment syncope starts. ECGs recorded *after* the start of the event are usually non-diagnostic, so *the ECG machine must be in place prior to the onset of symptoms*. What sort of device is required depends on symptom frequency, and the probability of a dangerous arrhythmia? Symptoms every few days are diagnosed using 24-h or 7-day ECG recorders, every few weeks by an external loop recorder, less frequent symptoms (especially if possibly reflecting a dangerous arrhythmia) are best diagnosed by an internal loop recorder ('Reveal®' device, Fig. 61.2).

Cardiomemo® device

This externally applied oblong device (12 × 5 × 2 cm) has four electrodes built into the corners of one side. When symptoms occur the device is pushed against the chest wall near the heart, activated and a single channel ECG recorded. This recording does not correspond to any standard ECG lead so though crucially helpful in determining whether an arrhythmia is present, few other conclusions can be drawn. The device stores six recordings of 32 s duration. The data can be downloaded telephonically. The device is most useful for patients who have very symptomatic palpitations of obscure origin. See Fig. 61.1b.

Table 61.1 Diagnostic yield according to investigation in syncope. From http://www.medtronic.com/physician/reveal/syncope_diagnostic_tools.html.

Test/procedure	Yield (%)
ECG	2–11
Holter monitoring	2
External loop recorder	20
Tilt-table test	11–87
EP study without SHD	11
EP study with SHD	49
Neurological testing (CT scan, carotid doppler)	0–4
Reveal® Plus ILR	43–88

CT, computed tomography; EP, electrophysiology; ILR, internal loop recorder; SHR, structural heart disease.

External loop recorders

These comprise a solid-state recording device with memory, usually worn on the belt, or a cord around the neck, attached to the chest by 2–4 electrodes. They continually record an ECG signal into their limited memory. As new ECG signal memory is laid down, data > 10–30 min old is 'wiped' out. When the patient activates the device, the memory is 'frozen'. Up to 10–30 min of memory prior to device activation are available for analysis, a time period that usually captures the onset of symptoms. This data is then downloaded (or transmitted telephonically) to the cardiology department. The advantage of this system is that, *provided the patient activates the device within 10–30 min of symptoms onset*, the ECG at the onset of symptoms is available for analysis, often the time one is crucially interested in. The downside is that if patient fails to activate the device within this time period, the full data may be lost. However, modern machines have overcome even this limitation by automatically storing ECGs when the heart rate falls into a (programmable) bradycardia or tachycardia zone, e.g. below 40 b/min or above 150 b/min, etc. See Fig. 61.1a.

Internal loop recorders

Internal loop recorders (known by the commercial name of a Reveal® device) are the ultimate in loop recorders. They comprise a small implantable device, 6 × 2 × 1 cm. The device has a bipolar electrode at each end. It is implanted subcutaneously in the upper chest wall under local anaesthetic, and secured in position using non-absorbable sutures. The device continuously stores a single channel ECG, but like its external cousin, only has limited memory, so must wipe out the oldest memory in order to store new data (i.e. the data is looped). About 40 min of ECG can be recorded. When a 'wand' is applied by the patient externally and activated, it sends an electromagnetic signal to the device, freezing the currently stored ECG. This data can then be downloaded and analysed later. The device can be programmed to automatically store data if the heart rate drops below or exceeds certain rates (e.g. ≤ 40, ≥ 150, etc.) or if asystole ≥ 3.0–4.5 s occurs. This device is enormously useful in obtaining the ECG in patients who may have dangerous arrhythmias or unpleasant intrusive events, but whose symptoms occur infrequently. These devices show that 20% of patients with intractable epilepsy have a cardiac cause (e.g. prolonged intermittent asystole). The battery within the device lasts 14 months, and devices are explanted either once a definitive diagnosis has been achieved, or when the battery is depleted. See Fig. 61.2.

Fig. 61.1 (a) Attachments for an external loop recorder, similar to a 24-hour Holter monitor. (b) External event monitor, applied to the chest wall during an event to obtain a single channel ECG.

Fig. 61.2 (a) Internal loop recorder, a Reveal® device, which is implanted subcutaneously in the left upper chest. (b) Recording from a Reveal® device, showing profound bradyarrhythmias. Each line is 10s long. The trace shows sinus arrest with ventricular escape beats; the sinus arrest lasts about 30s, during which 8 ventricular beats occur. The longest pause is nearly 10s long, during which syncope cccurred. The patient responded well to DDD pacing. (c) Memory functions of the interval loop recorder: the device can be programmed to whatever memory function is felt most appropriate for the patient. The key advantage of the Reveal® device is that it allows for the analysis of an ECG before an event starts – critical if one wishes to determine whether a brady or tachycardia underlies syncope.

62 Tilt-table test and carotid sinus massage

Fig.62.1

(a)

Type 1 **Mixed**	Heart rate falls at the time of syncope but the ventricular rate does not fall to less than 40 b/min or falls to less than 40 b/min for less than 10 s with or without asystole of less than 3 s. Blood pressure falls before the heart rate falls
Type 2 **Cardioinhibitory**	(a) Cardioinhibition without asystole. Heart rate falls to a ventricular rate less than 40 b/min for less than 10 s but asystole of more than 3 s does not occur. Blood pressure falls before the heart rate falls (b) Cardioinhibition with asystole. Asystole occurs for more than 3 s. Blood pressure falls with or occurs before the heart rate falls
Type 2 **Vasodepressor**	Heart rate does not fall more than 10% from its peak at the time of syncope
	Exception 1 Chronotropic incompetence. No heart rate rise during the tilt testing (i.e. less than 10% from the pre-tilt rate)
	Exception 2 Excessive heart rate rise. An excessive heart rate rise both at the onset of the upright position and throughout its duration before syncope (i.e. greater than 130 b/min)

(b)

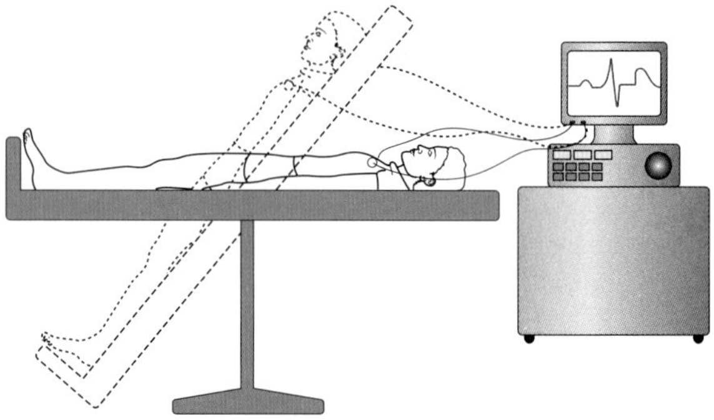

Fig.62.2

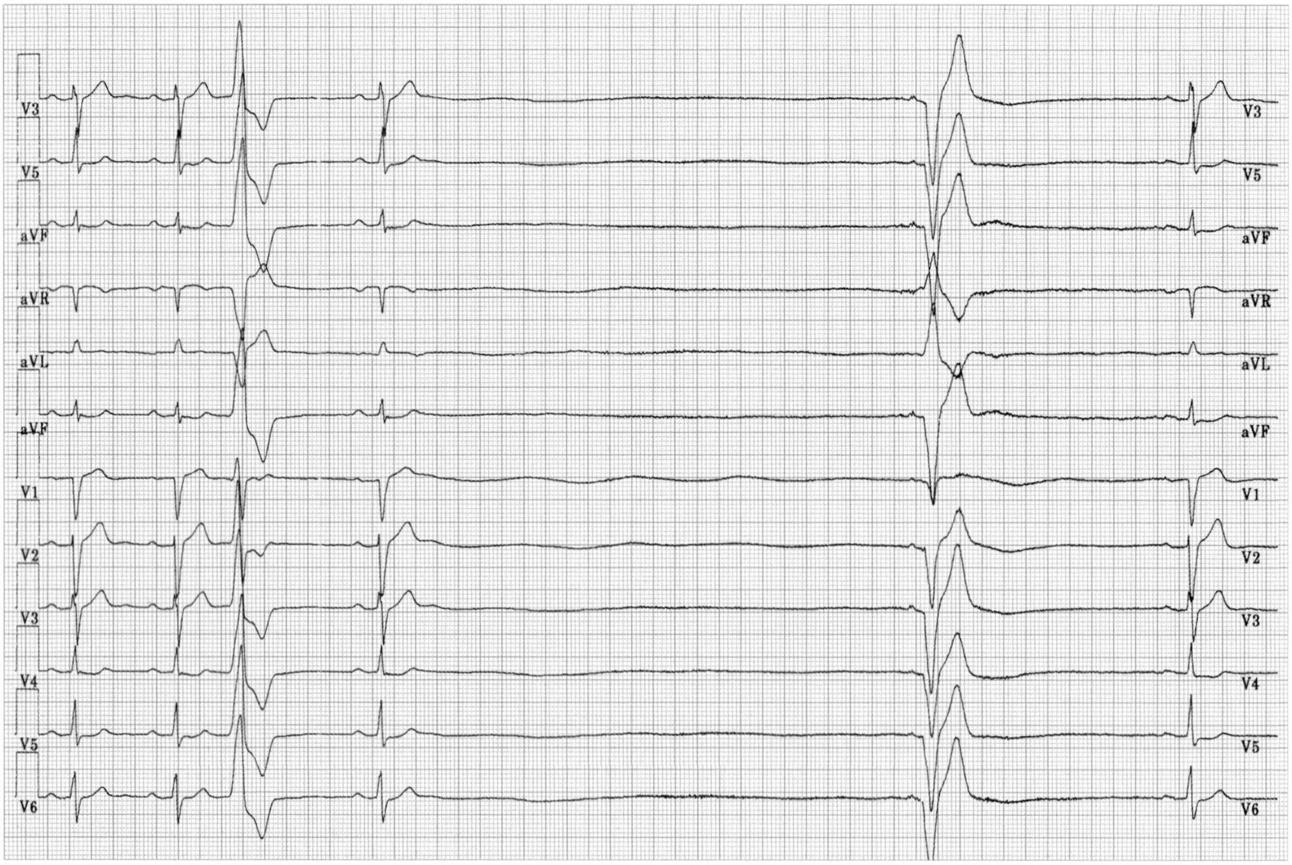

Syncope has many causes (see Chapter 23): in clinical practice the important question is whether an arrhythmia is the cause (which is likely to be dangerous) or whether it is 'reflex', i.e. a transient disruption in 'the control of the circulation' (when the prognosis is usually benign). In determining whether an arrhythmia underlies the event, obtaining an ECG during the episode is diagnostic. This can be difficult; various technologies are helpful (24-h, 7-day recordings, or external or internal loop recordings). If there is a high probability that a 'disorder in the control of the circulation' underlies symptoms, various 'provocative' tests help. These tests are designed to disturb the circulation, and then examine whether the response to this disturbance is normal, or such that could result in syncope. There is some controversy about these tests; some units find them highly reliable and reproducible, other are concerned about poor reproducibility and poor correlation with clinical events.

Tilt-table test

See Fig. 62.1. The principles underlying the tilt-table test are that: (a) Assumption of the upright position in health activates cardiovascular reflexes that result in blood pressure rising, heart rate not changing or increasing slightly. (b) Placing someone passively in the upright position tests the integrity of these homeostatic reflexes. Patients are strapped (to prevent them falling off later) onto a motorized table, initially in the horizontal position, then tilted at 60–80° upright. They are maintained in this position while their heart rate and blood pressure (BP) are measured continuously (beat-to-beat, by a Finapress™ device) for up to 45 min. There are several possible responses:

- **Normal**: no symptoms, rise in BP, unchanged or slightly increased heart rate.
- **Vasodilator syncope**: faintness or actual syncope, fall in BP (usually ≥ 50 mmHg), essentially unchanged heart rate.
- **Bradycardic syncope**: faintness or actual syncope, progressive bradycardia preceding a substantial fall in blood pressure, with heart rate falling to < 20 b/min, and ≥ 4 s of asystole. This form is most likely to have a symptomatic response to permanent pacemaker implantation.
- **Mixed**; with features of vasodilator and bradycardic, neither predominating. Pacing may lessen but not remove symptoms.
- **Neurogenic** (rare, disputed): symptoms (faintness or actual syncope) but no haemodynamic changes.

Patients with postural hypotension (e.g. severe autonomic neuropathy, drugs) have immediate falls in blood pressure on tilting; patients with vasodilator neurocardiogenic syncope have an initially normal response, but after some time, develop a significant BP fall.

The frequency of positive tests can be increased by providing additional stresses to the circulation during the test e.g. by running an isoprenaline infusion, giving glyceryl trinitrate (GTN). Unfortunately this also results in an increase in the number of false positive tests, to 15–20%. The reproducibility of the test (e.g. repeated after several weeks, months) is not high.

Carotid sinus massage

The carotid bulb baroreceptors have an important role in informing the cardiovascular centre in the brain stem of the instantaneous blood pressure, so that appropriate homeostatic changes can be made as necessary. This reflex loop (baroreceptors–brain stem–periphery) can misbehave in patients with *carotid hypersensitivity syndrome*. Here even mild pressure on the neck can lead to inappropriate and profound bradycardia (progressive, with asystole of ≥ 4 s) with BP fall of ≥ 50 mmHg (bradycardic carotid hypersensitivity syndrome), or just a BP fall, with little or no change in heart rate (vasodilator carotid hypersensitivity syndrome). Pacing can substantially lessen the chance of subsequent syncope in those with predominantly bradycardic carotid hypersensitivity syndrome. The test for carotid hypersensitivity syndrome is the *carotid sinus massage (CSM)* test. Here, the patient lies flat on a bed, connected to an ECG machine with continuous printout and a Finapress™ device for beat-to-beat BP measurement. The right side of the neck, at the level of the carotid bulb, is gently massaged for 5–10 seconds, and then after a short delay, the left side similarly massaged. If the test is negative, it is repeated with the patient in 60° head-up tilt. Patients with carotid artery bruits, significant carotid artery disease, or recent strokes, should not have the test. The clinical utility and reproducibility of this test is better than for the tilt-table test, though still not that high.

Fig. 62.1 (a) Classification of tilt-table responses. From Brignole M, Menozzi C, Del Rosso A *et al*. New classification of haemodynamics of vasovagal syncope: Beyond the VASIS classification; analysis of the pre-syncopal phase of the tilt test without and with nitroglycerin challenge. *Europace* 2000; **2**: 66–76. (b) Tilt-table set up; a motorized tilt table is used, if possible all cardioactive medication is stopped for > 5 half lives. The patient should not fast for > 2 h (to avoid the compounding effects of dehydration), and rests quietly for 30–45 min before the test. The test takes place in a quiet darkened room. The motorized table is tilted at 60–80°, until symptoms, hypotension (≥ 50 mmHg change from baseline) or asystole (5 s) occurs. In their absence, the test is discontinued at 45 min. ECG is recorded continuously, blood pressure also preferably, but if not, at least every minute.

Fig. 62.2 Carotid sinus massage: after excluding recent stroke, and carotid artery stenosis (clinically or by carotid Doppler), first the right then the left (shown here) carotid is gently massaged for 5 s. A continuous ECG printout is made, and blood pressure recorded every minute. A pause of 5 s results, then a single beat occurs, probably from a low atrial pacemaker (abnormal P wave shape, short PR interval), resulting in a broad QRS complex (of left bundle branch block morphology), then a further short pause, followed by normal sinus rhythm. This is a fairly strongly positive bradycardic response; the patient responded to dual chamber pacing.

63 Twenty-four hour ECGs

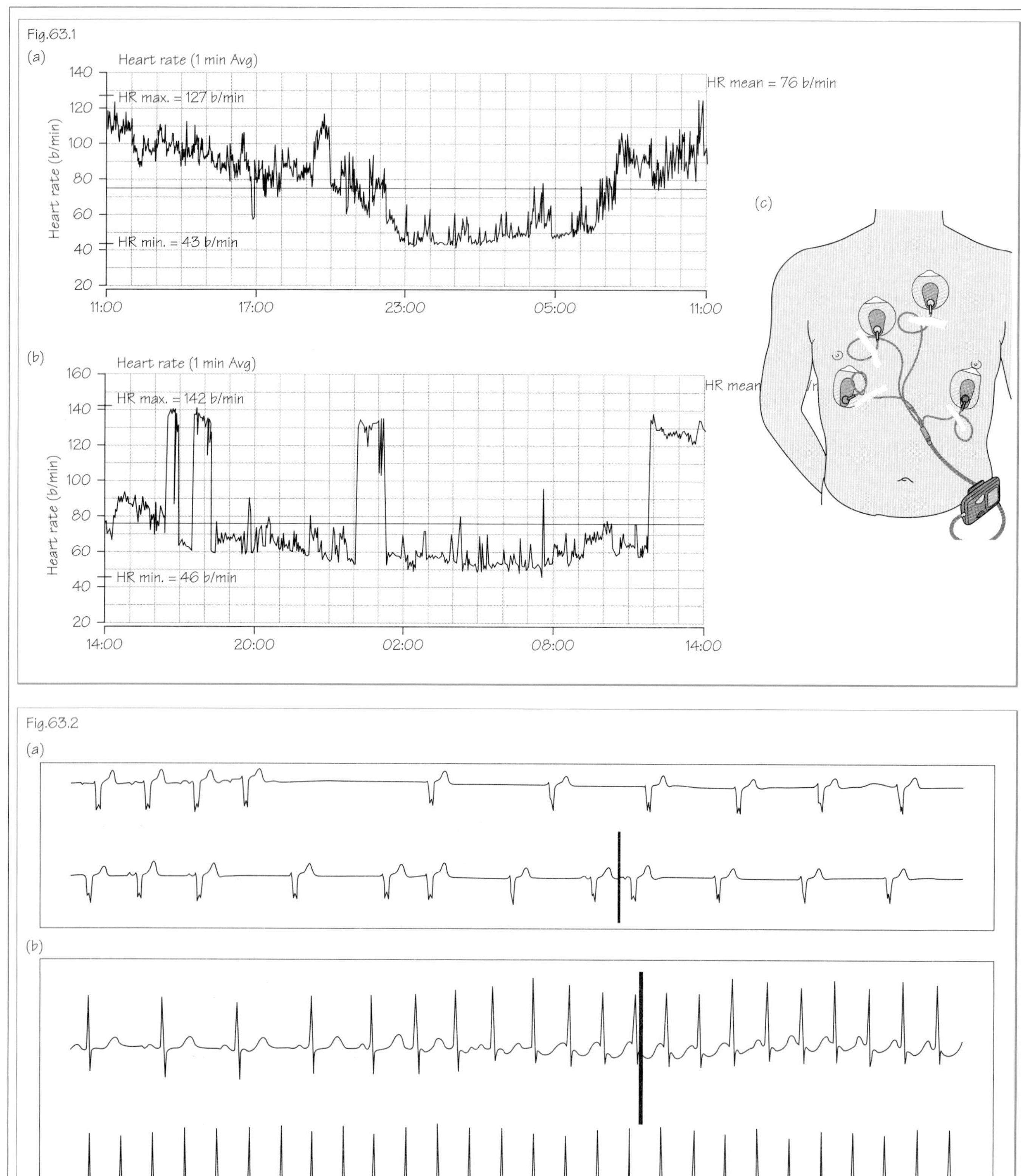

Fig.63.1
(a)
Heart rate (1 min Avg)
HR mean = 76 b/min
HR max. = 127 b/min
HR min. = 43 b/min
Heart rate (b/min)
140
120
100
80
60
40
20
11:00
17:00
23:00
05:00
11:00
(b)
Heart rate (1 min Avg)
HR max. = 142 b/min
HR min. = 46 b/min
Heart rate (b/min)
160
140
120
100
80
60
40
20
14:00
20:00
02:00
08:00
14:00
(c)
Fig.63.2
(a)
(b)

Twenty-four hour ECGs (Holter monitors, after Norman J. Holter) are an indispensable part of modern cardiology practice. Subjects are connected (using 3–5 ECG electrodes attached in a non-standard position called CM5, Fig. 63.1c) for 24 h to a device that records all cardiac electrical activity, the Holter monitor. During this time subjects undertake their usual day-to-day activities. One to three ECG channels are stored in the solid-state memory and analysed after the recording. Patients push a button to mark when symptoms occur. The Holter monitor is useful for determining:

- Heart rhythm, especially to determine whether an arrhythmia underlies symptoms (e.g. palpitations, breathlessness, chest pain, dizzy spells or syncope). *This is the main clinical use of the Holter.*
- Arrhythmia status, a clue to the presence of disease and/or its prognosis:
  (a) Frequent/complex ventricular premature contractions (VPCs) may indicate left ventricular (LV) (rarely right ventricular [RV]) dysfunction, though these can occur in normal hearts (see Chapter 47). Ventricular ectopics are classified according to their frequency and complexity using the Lown grading system (Table 63.1).
  (b) Non-sustained ventricular tachycardia (NSVT) has prognostic significance in post-myocardial infarction (MI) -impaired LV function.
  (c) In extensive conducting tissue disease (e.g. bi- or tri-fascicular block etc.) episodic second/third degree heart block may indicate the need for a permanent pacemaker.
- Heart rate: particularly in atrial fibrillation (AF) to ensure optimal heart rate control, but also in diagnosing 'unfitness' (high resting heart rates/brisk increases with effort), or sick sinus syndrome.
- Heart rate variability (HRV), a surprisingly little used function of the Holter monitor.
- Post-MI risk stratification: by determining average heart rate (the lower the better), occult arrhythmias (especially NSVT) and HRV (the higher the better).
- Ischaemic burden; the amount/duration of ST depression (even if not associated with angina) in ishaemic heart disease (IHD) is a prognostically important and relevant target for intervention.
- QT intervals: the Holter monitor is helpful in this specialized field, giving data on:
  (a) Absolute QT interval data, i.e. is the QT interval prolonged?
  (b) QT interval variability, i.e. how the QT interval changes with heart rate, and how it is affected by the circadian rhythm (normal subjects have longer QT intervals at night than daytime at any given heart rate).

How to read a Holter monitor report

1 Check the patient's name and date of birth! Frequently reports on another patient are inserted into the wrong notes.

2 Look to see what the analysing technician has written on the front page – this gives most of the clues as to what the tape shows!

3 Look at the patient's diary – did symptoms occur and if so when? Look at the printed strips at this time to examine the heart rhythm/rate. *If the patient did not have typical symptoms during the recording, then one cannot conclude what has caused their symptoms.* It is crucial to go to some considerable lengths to obtain an ECG during symptoms and if the 24-h ECG does not allow this, consider other technology, e.g. memo device or loop recorders (see Chapter 61).

4 Look at the heart rhythm on the strips printed out when the patient is free of symptoms – what is the rhythm, and do you agree with the report?

5 Look at the heart rate over the 24 h (graph at the front of the report, Fig. 63.1a), useful in:

(a) Determining the control to arrhythmias, such as AF.

(b) Sudden increases in heart rate often indicate the onset of an arrhythmia (Fig. 63.1b).

(c) A fixed lower limit to the heart rate means either the patient has a pacemaker or an arrhythmia such as atrial flutter (which in many never conducts at less that a 4 to 1 rate, i.e. 75 b/min).

(d) How variable is the heart rate? There are two ways to do this: the first is to eyeball the heart rate graph versus time-of-day; the second is to look at the formal measures of HRV. Reduced HRV means: (i) sinus node disease; (ii) an inactive patient; (iii) a disease process lowering HRV (see Heart rate variability section below).

6 Look at the VPC graph (see the front page of the Holter report): how frequently do they occur and when? Ventricular premature contractions are frequently not of significance, but when very frequent, complex or occurring mainly at high heart rates, this significantly raises the possibility of underlying heart disease (see Chapter 47).

7 Look at the table of arrhythmias, both for tachycardias and bradycardias. Both are usually arbitrarily set (e.g. 140 b/min for tachycardia, ≤ 40 b/min for bradycardias). Confirm from the printouts that you agree that these are arrhythmias.

Variants of normal

What constitutes a pathological arrhythmia is a difficult question? It is important not to rush to conclusions, as normal hearts are not incessantly in sinus rhythm, and may demonstrate:

- Non-sustained ventricular tachycardia.
- Nocturnal atrioventricular (AV) block (e.g. short periods of Wenckebach block).
- Frequent VPCs.

Table 63.1 Lown grading of ventricular premature contractions (VPCs).

Grade	Description
0	None
1	< 30/h
2	≥ 30/h
3	Multiform
4a	2 consecutive
4b	≥ 3 consecutive
5	R-on-T

Fig. 63.1 (a) Tachogram (plot of heart rate against time) from a normal 24-h ECG. A clear diurnal rhythm is shown, with slower heart rates when the subject sleeps. Sudden increases/decreases in heart rate indicating significant (normal) heart rate variability. (b) Tachogram from an individual with supraventricular tachycardia (SVT). The sudden increases in heart rate to about 140 b/min are when an SVT with a rate of 140 b/min occurs. (c) Twenty-four hour ECG in place.

Fig. 63.2 (a) Print out from the time a patient was 'dizzy'. Sinus rhythm gives way to a narrow complex bradycardia without preceding P waves. This is sinus arrest due to sick sinus syndrome, with junctional escape beats. (b) Supraventricular tachycardia (SVT). Sinus rhythm gives way to a narrow complex tachycardia, with increasing ST depression over time. In both traces the bold upright bar is the patient activated marker, indicating symptoms.

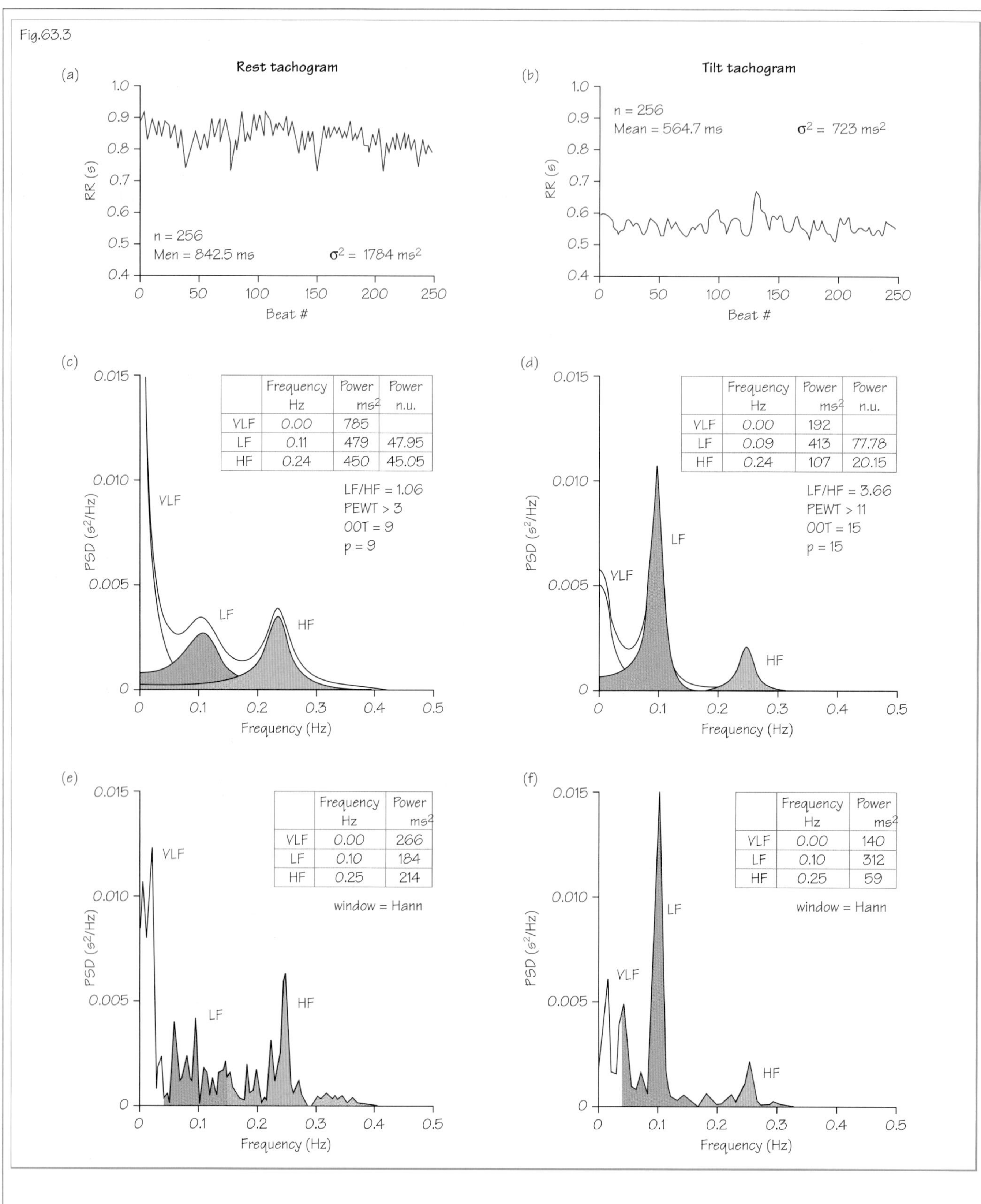
Fig.63.3
(a)
Rest tachogram
RR (s)
n = 256
Men = 842.5 ms
σ2 = 1784 ms2
Beat #
(b)
Tilt tachogram
RR (s)
n = 256
Mean = 564.7 ms
σ2 = 723 ms2
Beat #
(c)
PSD (s2/Hz)
VLF
LF
HF
Frequency (Hz)
	Frequency Hz	Power ms2	Power n.u.
VLF	0.00	785	
LF	0.11	479	47.95
HF	0.24	450	45.05
LF/HF = 1.06
PEWT > 3
OOT = 9
p = 9
(d)
PSD (s2/Hz)
VLF
LF
HF
Frequency (Hz)
	Frequency Hz	Power ms2	Power n.u.
VLF	0.00	192	
LF	0.09	413	77.78
HF	0.24	107	20.15
LF/HF = 3.66
PEWT > 11
OOT = 15
p = 15
(e)
PSD (s2/Hz)
VLF
LF
HF
Frequency (Hz)
	Frequency Hz	Power ms2
VLF	0.00	266
LF	0.10	184
HF	0.25	214
window = Hann
(f)
PSD (s2/Hz)
VLF
LF
HF
Frequency (Hz)
	Frequency Hz	Power ms2
VLF	0.00	140
LF	0.10	312
HF	0.25	59
window = Hann

• Short runs of a supraventricular tachycardia (e.g. 10–12 beats of AF). Given this, be careful before ascribing pathological significance to a 24-h ECG finding.

Indications for prolonged ambulatory ECG recordings

• Evaluation of palpitations and syncope (as above, and see Chapters 22 and 23).
• Guiding anti-arrhythmic therapy in atrial fibrillation (AF). Most patients in AF have a tachycardia at rest and during exercise. This should be controlled, to minimize symptoms and to prevent the development of a 'rate-related' cardiomyopathy (too high a heart rate for too long leads to left ventricular function falling off). The best way to evaluate heart rate in AF is the ambulatory ECG; if it is too high, then bradycardia-inducing therapy is introduced/dose adjusted. Good heart rate control in AF means; night time heart rate ± 50 b/min, any nocturnal pauses = 3–4 seconds, most heart rate during the day ± 60–90 b/min, and only rare episodes of heart rate > 100–110 b/min.
• Assessing arrhythmic risk: in structural heart disease, increasing frequency and complexity of ventricular premature beats VPCs and especially non-sustained ventricular tachycardia (ns VT), increases the risk of future serious arrhythmias (sustained VT/VF). The 24-hour ECG is used to identify patients who benefit from more intense evaluation and treatment.
• Heart rate variability, see below.
• ST depression: modern ambulatory technology allows the detection and analysis of ST depression over 24 hours. This has some uses though, just as in the standard exercise test, be aware that there are many causes of ST depression other than ischaemia. In proven coronary disease, the presence of extensive asymptomatic ST depression ('silent ischaemia') increases the probability of an adverse event.
• QT interval analysis, often used by regulatory authorities to examine the pro-arrhythmic properties of drugs, rarely used in clinical practice.
• T wave alternans (alternate increases and decreases in T wave amplitude in successive QRST complexes) is an interesting research tool; when high it increases the chance of a ventricular arrhythmia occurring.

Heart rate variability

Heart rate variability (HRV) is an important property of the circulation and unexpectedly can (partly) predict outlook.

What is HRV?

If successive RR intervals are measured and plotted against beat number (Fig. 63.3) a pattern emerges. In stable circumstances (e.g. lying flat, standing still) one might expect a flat line, i.e. successive RR intervals not altering, the heart rate fixed. This is not so – successive RR intervals alter markedly; the instantaneous heart rate varies, producing HRV. Why is this? The most likely explanation is the influence of:

• The autonomic nervous system:
(a) The vagus nerve causes a marked perturbation in instantaneous heart rate, i.e. altering successive beats by ≥ 50 ms.
(b) Sympathetic influences change heart rate over a longer time period than the vagus, over several beats rather than one.
(c) The speed at which heart rate changes occurs is measured as a frequency – the vagus nerve influences heart rate at a frequency of 0.25 Hz, the sympathetic nervous system 0.1 Hz, i.e. a full cycle of changes takes the vagus nerve 4 s, the sympathetic system 10 s. Maximum change occurs halfway through the cycle, i.e. 2 s for the vagus, 5 s for the sympathetic system.
• Much HRV, especially those taking a long time to influence the heart (low frequency components) are poorly understood and their origin is speculative.

Determination of HRV

Prerequisites in determining HRV are: (i) sinus rhythm with no/few VPCs; (ii) no sinus node disease. An ECG recording is made (0.2–24.0 h) and a RR interval versus beat number file is obtained using computerized QRS detection. When comparing HRV data, similar length time recordings must be used. There are two main approaches to determine HRV:
• Time domain methods use simple mathematical tools (Appendix, Table 1). Simple statistical methods are most reliable (provided 24-h recordings are employed) and applicable to clinical practice, e.g. SDNN or NN50 count. These methods are easy to obtain, reproducible, reliable and hardly prone to operator error.
• Frequency domain methods (Appendix, Table 2): These all use a basic mathematical principle, that vanability in any system can be broken down into several sine waves of varying amplitude (power) and frequency. The number, frequency and power of these sine wave can be determined, using non-parametric means (fast fourier transform [FFT] – a simple fast, reliable algorithm, Fig. 63.3e,f) or parametric methods, e.g. autoregressive power spectrum analysis, Fig. 63.3c,d, which produces beautiful results, particularly for short-term recordings, e.g. 5–20 min, but is prone to error and requires much greater operator experience for correct interpretation. The frequency domain methods are useful in scientific research, but rarely in clinical practice.

HRV and routlook

Why measure HRV? The main reason is that in many diseases it relates to outlook, and is improved by therapies improving outlook e.g. acute MI depresses HRV, those with the lowest HRV have the worst outcome. Angiotensin receptor inhibitors and beta-blockers increase HRV. Unfit patients have low HRV, heart failure patients have very low HRV, and in both there is a sympathetic predominance.

Fig. 63.3 Heart rate variability lying (left) and tilted (right). (a,b) Heart rate tachogram. Lying shows much high frequency variability (sudden dips up and down) accounted for by vagus outflow, tilted shows little/no high frequency variability, and more lower frequency variability, due to increased sympathetic activity and less vagus outflow (n = number of beats, RR = RR interval, σ^2 = variance of RR intervals). (c,d) power spectral analysis, showing (c) vagal predominance over sympathetic activity when lying, reversed (d) when tilted (PEWT, OOT, n = technical aspects of the model). (e,f) Fast fourier transform (FFT) analysis; similar results to power spectral analysis though less visually appealing. (PSD = power spectral density: the power for each frequency required to produce this variability.)

64 The exercise stress test

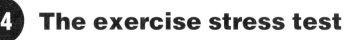

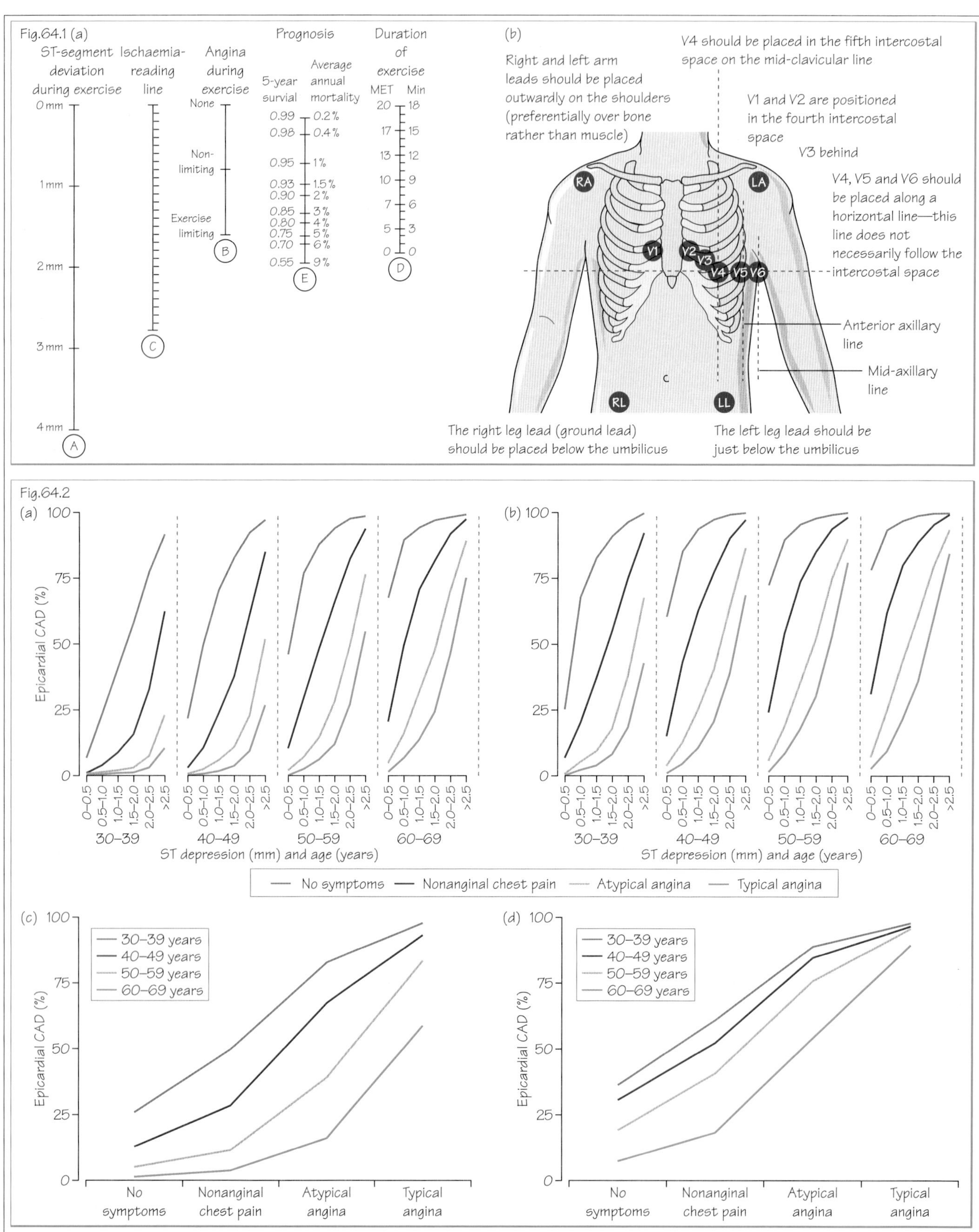

Fig.64.1 (a)
ST-segment deviation during exercise
0 mm
1 mm
2 mm
3 mm
4 mm
A
Ischaemia-reading line
C
Angina during exercise
None
Non-limiting
Exercise limiting
B
Prognosis
5-year survial
Average annual mortality
0.99 0.2%
0.98 0.4%
0.95 1%
0.93 1.5%
0.90 2%
0.85 3%
0.80 4%
0.75 5%
0.70 6%
0.55 9%
E
Duration of exercise
MET Min
20 18
17 15
13 12
10 9
7 6
5 3
0 0
D
(b)
Right and left arm leads should be placed outwardly on the shoulders (preferentially over bone rather than muscle)
V4 should be placed in the fifth intercostal space on the mid-clavicular line
V1 and V2 are positioned in the fourth intercostal space
V3 behind
V4, V5 and V6 should be placed along a horizontal line—this line does not necessarily follow the intercostal space
RA
LA
V1
V2
V3
V4
V5
V6
Anterior axillary line
Mid-axillary line
RL
LL
The right leg lead (ground lead) should be placed below the umbilicus
The left leg lead should be just below the umbilicus
Fig.64.2
(a)
Epicardial CAD (%)
0-0.5 0.5-1.0 1.0-1.5 1.5-2.0 2.0-2.5 >2.5
30–39 40–49 50–59 60–69
ST depression (mm) and age (years)
(b)
No symptoms
Nonanginal chest pain
Atypical angina
Typical angina
(c)
30–39 years
40–49 years
50–59 years
60–69 years
No symptoms
Nonanginal chest pain
Atypical angina
Typical angina
(d)

Probably no test is as used and abused as the exercise stress test (EST). The test has four aims:

• **To diagnose/rule out coronary disease.** Compared to the 'gold' standard (coronary angiography) the EST has a sensitivity of 70% and a specificity of 80% (nuclear myocardial perfusion imaging has a higher sensitivity at = 85%, and specificity at = 90%). The problems therefore in using the EST to diagnose ishaemic heart disease (IHD) are: (i) those with coronary disease may have a normal test; (ii) those without IHD may have an abnormal test, i.e. significant ST depression (due to female sex, left ventricular [LV] hypertrophy, digoxin or idiopathic). Thus, though the diagnostic role of the EST is useful, it does have major limitations.

• **To estimate prognosis**, probably its major function (see below).

• **To objectively measure exercise capacity** (often serially to document changes over time). This is a very helpful function, especially when there is variance between clinical findings and reported exercise capacity. Exercise stress testing combined with gas exchange measurement provides evidence as to the physical fitness of the subject.

• **To provoke arrhythmias**, useful in patients with effort related palpitations, especially in structural heart disease.

Indications

The indications for stress testing reflect the utility of the test, as outlined above. In practice, tests are usually carried out: (a) to determine whether someone with an intermediate probability of coronary disease and symptoms compatible with coronary disease actually has coronary disease (e.g. middle-aged men with a few risk factors, middle-aged women with substantial risk factors); (b) to assess prognosis in those known to have coronary disease, e.g. post-acute coronary syndrome (ACS) risk stratification.

Methods

Most tests are performed using a motorized treadmill, which increases speed and inclination according to the protocol used. A static bicycle ergometer is occasionally used. Blood pressure (BP) is measured every few minutes. A 12-lead ECG is recorded at the start (lying and standing), every minute during the test, and for at least 5 min after the test (or longer until symptoms/ECG changes resolve). Patients exercise:

1 Until symptoms force them to stop. One should carefully ascertain exactly what these symptoms are, because their exact nature impacts on the interpretation of the test, e.g. with similar ST segment depression, typical angina provoked by the test increases the probability of coronary disease compared to either atypical angina or no symptoms.

2 Until pre-specified increases in heart rate have occurred, or excess increases/decreases in BP.

3 If substantial ST depression occurs (usually ≥ 3–4 mm).

4 If significant arrhythmias occur (e.g. atrial fibrillation [AF], supraventricular tachycardias [SVTs], obviously ventricular tachycardia/ventricular fibrillation [VT/VF]).

Interpretation

The interpretation depends on the pre-test probability of disease and the test findings:

• The greater the number of risk factors for coronary disease (especially age, but also male sex in the middle-aged, smoking, diabetes, hypertension, etc.) the greater the probability of coronary disease. The EST can alter this probability, but only rarely does it make coronary disease inevitable or impossible.

• Typical symptoms of myocardial ischaemia provoked by the test, regardless of any other test finding, increase the probability of coronary disease: the further symptoms are from typical angina the less likely is coronary disease.

• Exercise capacity is probably the single most important piece of data to come out of the stress test, and relates reasonably well to prognosis (see Duke score, a nomogram derived from Duke University, North Caroline, USA, Fig. 64.1a), regardless of whether coronary disease is present or not.

• ST depression: the greater the ST depression, the more widespread, and the more downsloping (as opposed to upsloping or planar), the more likely coronary disease is to be present (see Fig. 14.1b). ST depression confined to the inferior leads has the weakest relationship to coronary disease, if this extends laterally, the probability of IHD increases, and if this extends anterolaterally (especially if V3 is involved) the probability becomes quite high. Typical 'ischaemic' changes occurring in the first minute following exercise (Fig. 16.1) increase the probability of IHD further. ST changes on the pre-test ECG lower the significance of any exercise induced ST depression.

Implications

A high-level (i.e. ≥ end of stage III of the Bruce protocol) negative (i.e. no ST changes or symptoms) EST is associated with a very good outlook. In the absence of intrusive symptoms further tests for coronary disease are usually not required. A low-level (i.e. stage I or II) positive test (i.e. ≥ 2 mm ST depression with typical angina symptoms) is associated with a reduced outlook, and normally leads on to coronary angiography. Intermediate tests either lead on to nuclear myocardial perfusion scans (thallium or myoview) (few symptoms) or coronary angiography (the more symptomatic, those with more risk factors or impaired LV function).

Risks and complications

The risk of death is 1 per 10 000 in outpatients, 3 per 10 000 with a recent myocardial infarction (MI). There is a higher risk of inducing MI, arrhythmias (SVT, AF and VT/VF). To minimize risks, it is important to avoid EST in those with symptomatic aortic stenosis, ≤ 2 days from a small MI, ≤ 5–7 days from a larger MI, ACS with ongoing chest pain (i.e. chest pain within 48 h), uncontrolled heart failure, uncontrolled arrhythmias (e.g. AF with a fast heart rate response), febrile patients, gross hypertension (≥ 200/120 mmHg) or in haemodynamic disturbance (e.g. due to pulmonary embolism).

Fig. 64.1 (a) Duke nomogram estimating prognosis in outpatients referred for evaluation of possible coronary artery disease. The ST depression (A) and symptom (B) lines are connected, obtaining a point on the ischaemia reading line (C), which is then connected to the exercise duration (D), to obtain the annual mortality (E). (b) ECG wiring points for treadmill testing.

Fig. 64.2 Presence of epicardial coronary artery disease (CAD) related to age and sex (a) women, (b) men, (c) symptoms and (d) ECG changes.

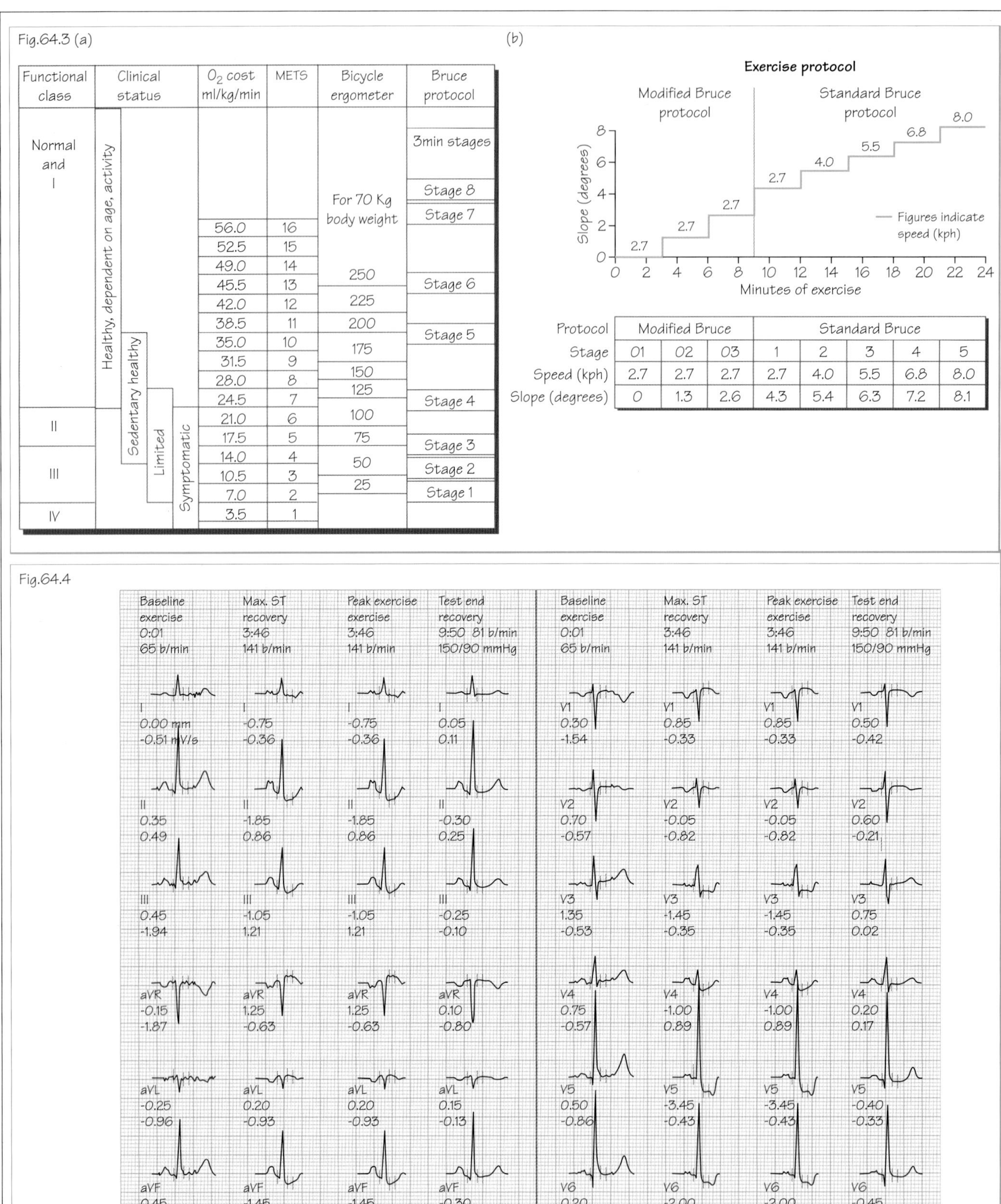

Protocol	Modified Bruce			Standard Bruce				
Stage	01	02	03	1	2	3	4	5
Speed (kph)	2.7	2.7	2.7	2.7	4.0	5.5	6.8	8.0
Slope (degrees)	0	1.3	2.6	4.3	5.4	6.3	7.2	8.1

How to analyse an exercise ECG

1 Check the patient's name, date of birth, and date of the test and ascertain the indication.

2 Determine exercise capacity? Exercise duration is powerfully related to longevity.

3 Why did exercise stop?

- Angina – increases the probability of IHD.
- Breathlessness: associated with a worse outcome, not necessarily due to a cardiac event.
- Fatigue, a non-specific finding, due to joint/musculoskeletal illness, deconditioning or poor motivation.
- 'Dizziness' is organic when associated with a BP fall (≥ 30 mmHg from the resting value).
- Arrhythmias.
- ST changes.

4 What was the heart rate response? Increases quicker than normal usually indicates physical unfitness, slower may indicate physical fitness, sinus node disease or drugs, e.g. beta-blockers/rate slowing Ca^{2+} channel blockers.

5 Blood pressure response? Excessive increases usually mean undertreated hypertension, a flat response either pre-test anxiety (the usual cause), or LV dysfunction, a fall may indicate severe multivessel coronary artery disease (CAD) or severe LV dysfunction.

6 What was the heart rate–BP double product at peak effort (= heart rate × systolic BP); symptoms/ECG changes occurring at lower double products are of greater diagnostic and prognostic importance.

7 What does the resting ECG show? Is it normal, or is there evidence of old infarction (Q waves/loss of R wave height)? Are there T wave changes (flattening/inversion); these render effort-induced ST depression of much less diagnostic significance. Left bundle branch block renders the ECG uninterpretable. Right bundle branch block normally results in repolarization (ST/T wave) changes in the right-sided chest leads during exercise.

8 What is the ST segment response to effort? Nothing (CAD less likely). ST depression: the greater, the higher the chance of CAD. Upsloping depression is the least likely to indicate CAD, planar or downsloping (most likely to be CAD). ST elevation may indicate an MI!

9 ST changes post-exercise. ST depression/biphasic T waves in the first 1–2 min after exercise ('post-exercise ischaemic changes') increase the probability of CAD.

The EST should be reported as lowering (or increasing) the probability of CAD by a little (or a lot). Rarely does it allow conclusive diagnosis/exclusion of CAD.

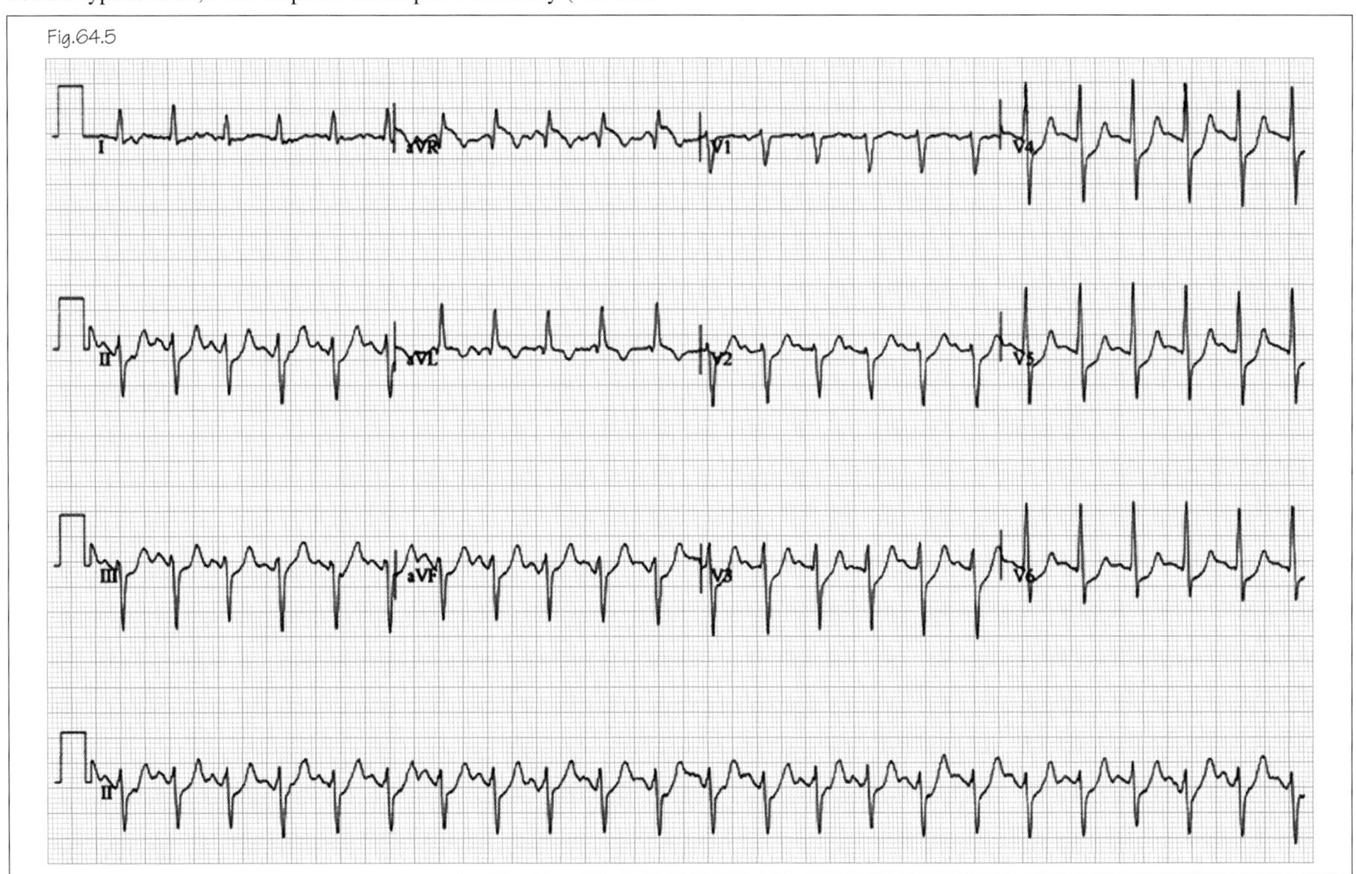

Fig. 64.3 (a) Exercise protocols, and equivalent clinical states and metabolic expenditure. (b) Bruce protocol exercise test.

Fig. 64.4 Exercise stress test, undertaken for chest pain. Effort ceased at 3 min 45 s due to ST changes, no chest pain, peak heart rate 141 b/min, systolic blood pressure 180 mmHg (unremarkable). Resting ECG normal, with exercise highly significant downsloping ST depression anteriorly (I, aVL, V3–6). Interpretation depends on demographics/symptoms – an elderly male with typical angina, coronary artery disease (CAD) highly likely, a young female with atypical symptoms (see Fig. 64.2) CAD possible, but much less likely. The patient was a young female with atypical symptoms and had a normal coronary angiogram.

Fig. 64.5 Exercise stress testing for angina in a middle-aged male. Exercise lasted 4 min 23 s, stopped due to chest pain (typical angina), peak heart rate 137 b/min, peak systolic blood pressure (not shown) 140 mmHg. Resting ECG (not shown) normal. Peak ECG, widespread upsloping ST depression, up to 4 mm in lead V4. Angiography showed a tight left main stem stenosis, with a blocked right coronary artery, normal left ventricular function. Coronary artery bypass graft undertaken successfully.

65 Invasive electrophysiological studies

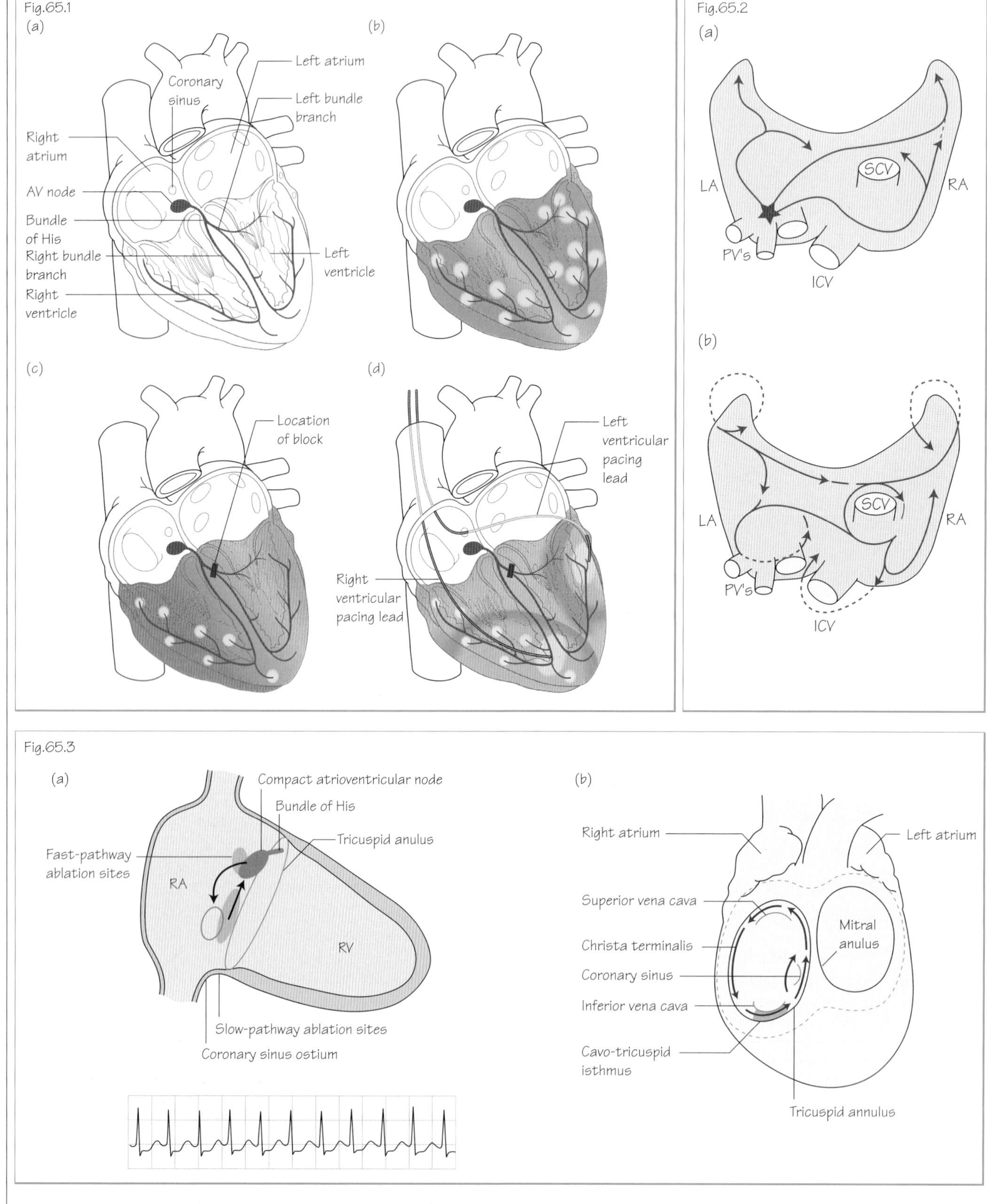

Fig.65.1
(a)
Coronary sinus
Left atrium
Left bundle branch
Right atrium
AV node
Bundle of His
Right bundle branch
Right ventricle
Left ventricle
(b)
(c)
Location of block
(d)
Left ventricular pacing lead
Right ventricular pacing lead
Fig.65.2
(a)
LA
SCV
RA
PV's
ICV
(b)
LA
SCV
RA
PV's
ICV
Fig.65.3
(a)
Compact atrioventricular node
Bundle of His
Tricuspid anulus
Fast-pathway ablation sites
RA
RV
Slow-pathway ablation sites
Coronary sinus ostium
(b)
Right atrium
Left atrium
Superior vena cava
Christa terminalis
Mitral anulus
Coronary sinus
Inferior vena cava
Cavo-tricuspid isthmus
Tricuspid annulus

Specialist electrophysiological (EP) investigations have a small but important role in evaluating arrhythmias. They are expensive and are restricted to a few specialized centres; despite their lack of availability it is crucial to refer patients who may benefit.

Standard EP setup

Electrophysiological studies take place in the catheterization laboratory, with the patient draped, sedated, lying on the X-ray table. Catheters are introduced via the right femoral (subclavian) vein, and placed in the: (i) high right atrium; (ii) alongside the atrioventricular (AV) node/bundle of His; (iii) right ventricle (RV) apex (sometimes RV outflow tract); (iv) coronary sinus. A roving catheter may also be used. Electricity detected by these catheters passes to an ECG machine, which records the signals and prints out high speed/gain paper traces. Electrophysiological catheters detect electricity from multiple sites in and around their tip. The aim is to introduce sufficient catheters to accurately determine when different parts of the heart are activated, both in normal sinus rhythm and during an arrhythmia. Many abnormal pathways that sustain arrhythmias generate electricity during sinus rhythm and can be mapped.

Studies to evaluate supraventricular tachyarrhythmias

• Atrioventricular nodal re-entrant tachycardia (AVNRT), due to additional pathway(s) in/around the AV node, can be demonstrated at EP study (Fig. 65.3). Atrial extrasystoles are introduced: the time taken for these to reach the bundle of His measured and plotted against extrasystoles prematurity. Extrasystoles close to the normal sinus rhythm interval are conducted quickly to the bundle of His. As the coupling period is shortened, there is a marginal increase in the A_{ES}–H_{ES} time. In those with no additional pathways, when the effective refractory period (ERP) is reached conduction ceases. In those with an additional pathway, at short coupling intervals, there is a sudden jump increase in the A_{ES}–H_{ES} time, i.e. an additional pathway that repolarizes rapidly (i.e. has a short ERP) but conducts slowly has become active. Slow pathway modification can ablate this pathway: a catheter is placed on the pathway, radiofrequency ablating energy passed down the catheter, coagulating and destroying the pathway.

• Atrioventricular re-entrant tachycardia (AVRT) with a visible accessory pathway (Wolff–Parkinson–White syndrome). Electrophysiological studies: (i) diagnose the condition; (ii) localize the pathway (from delta wave polarity and using steerable catheters placed where pathway potentials arise or earliest ventricular activation occurs); (iii) determine the risk of sudden cardiac death, high in those with pathways capable of conducting high atrial rates; pacing the atria very fast/inducing atrial fibrillation (AF) determines pathway-conducting ability. 'Slick' pathways are ablated.

• Atrioventricular re-entrant tachycardia with a 'concealed' pathway (no delta wave); responsible for three-quarters of AVRT. Pathways can be identified and ablated.

• Atrial fibrillation: EP work here involves treatment. (i) Paroxysmal AF often occurs from extrasystoles arising in the origin of the pulmonary veins, which can be electrically isolated from the rest of the left atrium by osteal circumferential 'burns', using specialized ablating catheters. (ii) Atrioventricular node ablation for heart rate control in drug-refractory cases. (iii) Percutaneous 'MAZE' procedures that electrically isolate parts of the left and right atrium rendering them unable to support a re-entrant arrhythmia (e.g. macro re-entrant AF).

• Atrial flutter: like AF, the main EP role is treatment. The flutter circuit (Fig. 65.3b) can be easily 'burnt' using modern EP tools.

Studies to evaluate ventricular tachyarrhythmias

Electrophysiological studies determine: (i) whether symptoms are due to ventricular tachycardia (VT); (ii) how high is the risk of VT (impaired left ventricle function post-myocardial infarction [MI]). If VT can be induced, this suggests it is relevant. Ventricular tachycardia induction is attempted using a ventricular stimulation study (ventricular tachycardia study [VTS]). One to three extrasystoles are introduced close to the refractory period, first in sinus rhythm, then with pacing at RR intervals of 600, 500 and finally 400 ms (Wellens protocol). The earlier in the protocol sustained monomorphic VT occurs, the more likely VT is to be clinically relevant. Polymorphic VT and ventricular fibrillation (VF), especially at intense stimulation levels, are a non-clinically relevant response of the heart to extreme stimulation. Ventricular tachycardia study is most useful in ischaemic heart disease post-MI; its utility is low in other forms of structural heart disease and absent in genetic pro-arrhythmic conditions. In some patients with VT, catheter ablation of the circuit is possible. This requires knowledge of the earliest site of ventricular activation, ascertained by: (i) inducing VT, and moving the catheter around until the earliest site of activation is detected (activation sequence mapping), then searching for the 'slow common diastolic pathway' which can be quite remote from the exit site; (ii) pacing the heart from different sites (using a steerable catheter), until the site is found where the resulting 12-lead ECG is exactly the same as during spontaneous VT (pace map). Catheter ablation of VT is greatly aided by complex mapping systems, which plot the catheter position along with electrical data. LV dysfunction promotes VT; in these patients with a low ejection fraction and a broad QRS, delayed contraction of the LV free wall (diagnosed echocardiographically) may reduce cardiac output. In these patients, cardiac resynchronization therapy, CRT (Fig. 65.1) can improve cardiac output.

Studies to evaluate bradyarrhythmias

It is rare to carry out EP studies to study bradycardias. In suspected sinus node disease, the sinus node recovery time (SNRT) has some utility: the atria are briefly paced, the time taken for a normal sinus node beat to occur measured (SNRT). In long PR interval, the mechanism is sometimes ascertained (by measuring the atrial–His conduction time (AH) and His–ventricular conduction time (HV) intervals, using the standard EP setup), as infra-hissian is more likely than supra-hissian block to proceed to complete heart block.

Fig. 65.1 The normal conducting tissue of the heart (a), which nearly simultaneously activates all parts of the ventricle (b). (c) A patient with heart failure, where there is conduction block of a component of the conducting tissue supplying the left ventricle, resulting in delayed activation and so contraction of the LV free wall, dysynchrony, and reduced cardiac output. (d) Pacing leads are implanted to, amongst other sites, the LV free wall, allowing this to be activated simultaneously with the rest of the ventricle, so improving cardiac output.

Fig. 65.2 Mechanism of atrial fibrillation (AF). Some AF originates from electrophysiologically active foci in pulmonary veins – isolating these by radiofrequency burns from the rest of the atrium can prevent AF. Some AF is due to re-entry within the atria – these patients may respond to the percutaneous MAZE procedure.

Fig. 65.3 (a) Sites for ablating atrioventricular nodal re-entrant tachycardia (AVNRT). (b) Mechanism of atrial flutter – a 'burn' across the cavo-tricuspid isthmus prevents the flutter circuit.

Case studies and answers

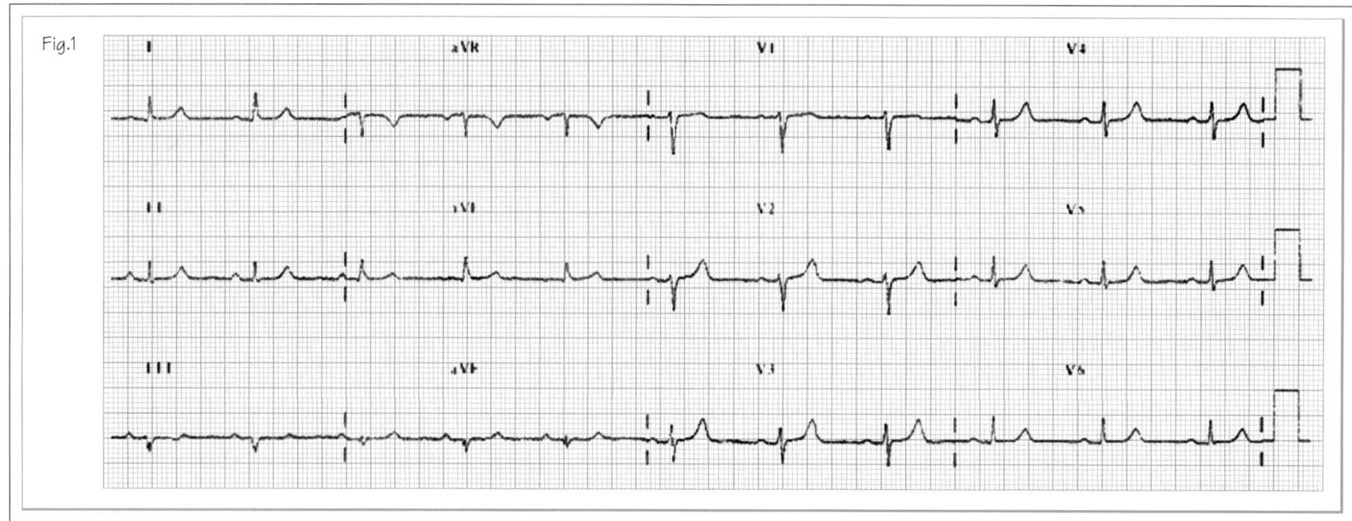

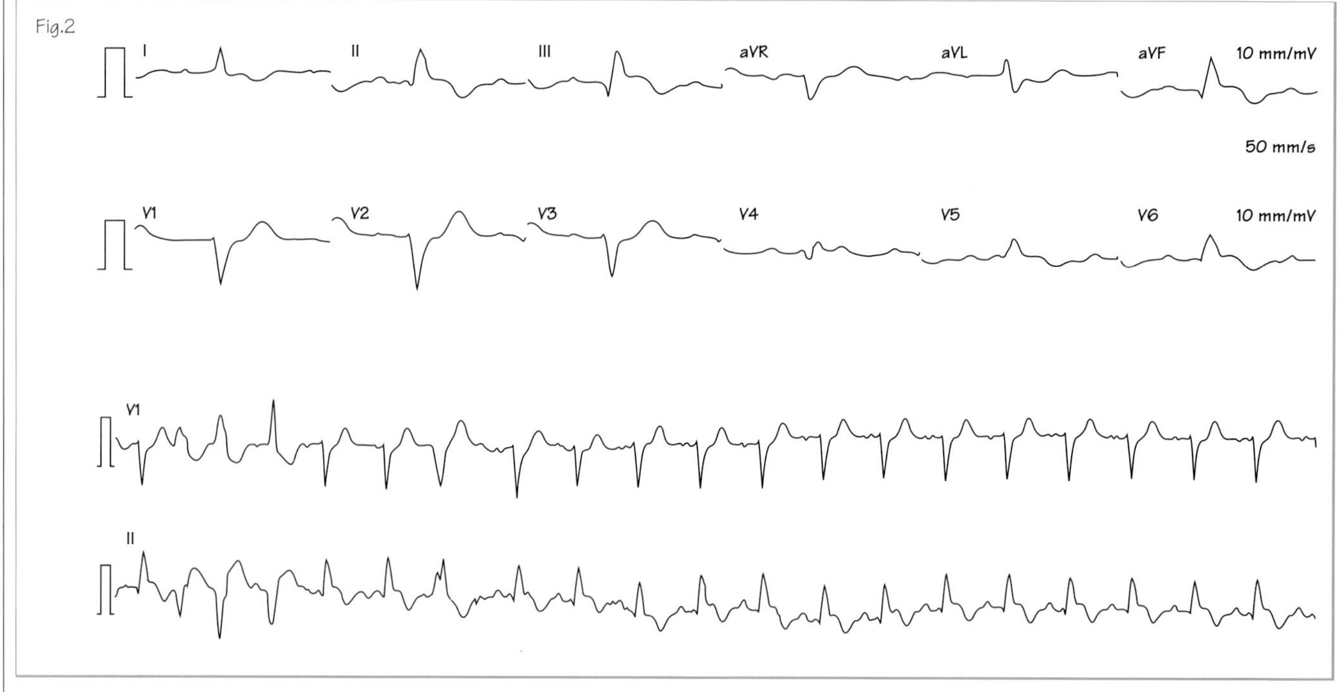

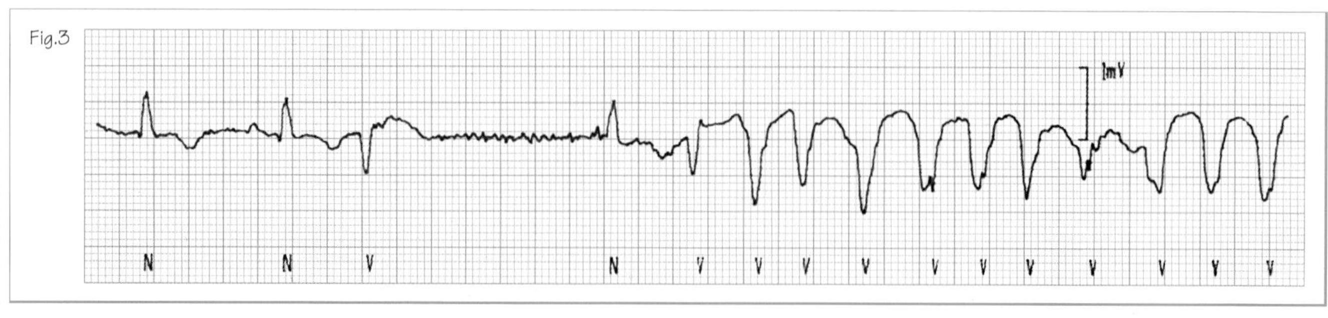

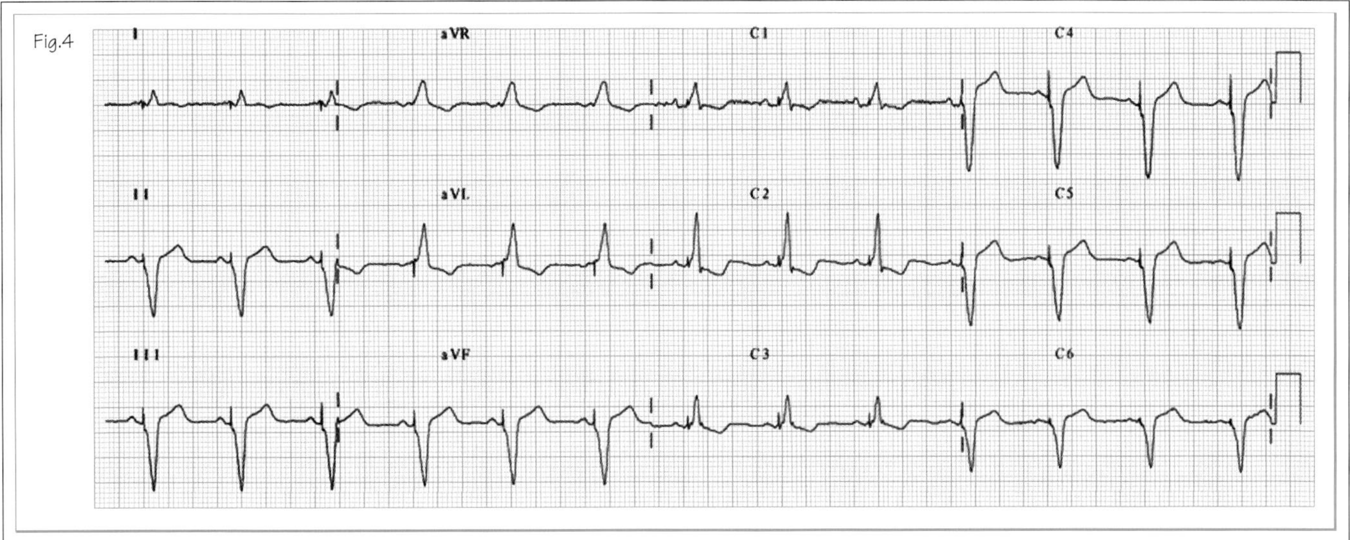

Case 1

Your opinion is requested on the pre-operative risk assessment of a moderately obese 79-year-old female due to undergo hip replacement surgery. She has treated hypertension, no prior cardiac illness, can walk a hundred yards before stopping with hip discomfort. Exam shows sinus rhythm, rate 80, blood pressure 138/82, no signs of heart failure, no murmers. Figure 1 shows her ECG.

1 *What does it show and does it help pre-operative risk assessment? What, if any, further investigations are appropriate?*

She undergoes successful hip replacement surgery. Eight months later she presents acutely with severe chest pain, radiating down both arms, with associated sweating. Exam shows her to be in pain, otherwise unremarkable.

2 *What does the ECG (Fig. 2) show, and how should she be treated?*

Two days after admission, she develops fast regular palpitations, with a blood pressure of 85/55. This ECG (Fig. 3) records the onset of her arrhythmia.

3 *What does it show, and what is the mechanism for her arrhythmia?*

Case 2

The ECG shown in Fig. 4 is taken from a 55-year-old man, known to have heart failure, who presents with increasing breathlessness.

1 *What does it show, and what is the mechanism?*

Answers

Case 1

1 The only abnormality is rather small QRS complexes; this could reflect myocyte loss, but a cardiac ultrasound was normal, the R waves therefore relate to her obesity, and the ECG was normal. Operative risk depends on the nature of the planned surgery, and seven risk factors (age > 70 years, current angina, previous myocardial infarction, chronic heart failure, prior cerebrovascular event, diabetes mellitus and chronic renal failure). The resting ECG does not, in most cases, add data beyond these variables. No further evaluation is required, and the patient underwent uneventful surgery.

2 The ECG is taken at standard sensitivity (10 mm/mV) but twice normal speed (50 mm/s), accounting for the apparent QRS broadening. Sinus rhythm, normal P wave, PR interval, ST elevation II, III, aVF, V4–6. The diagnosis is an infero-lateral ST segment elevation myocardial infarction (STEMI). Thrombolysis or primary percutaneous coronary intervention (PCI) is the treatment. The rhythm strip shows ventricular ectopics of different shapes initially, then sinus rhythm.

3 The strip starts with two supraventricular beats (the second one clearly sinus, with a preceding P wave, the first of less certain aetiology). There is then a ventricular ectopic, and a considerable pause, followed by one sinus beat, then a run of a broad complex tachycardia, clearly ventricular tachycardia. The mechanism of the ventricular tachycardia (VT) is pause-dependent QT lengthening. The VT was sustained and required DC cardioversion.

See Chapter 50 for further details.

Case 2

1 Regular unremarkable P waves. Broad QRS complex, preceded by a pacing spike (best seen in leads V3–6). This is a ventricular paced rhythm; as there is a P waves before each QRS complex, this is a dual chamber pacemaker, tracking the atria, pacing the ventricle. The QRS is dominant (i.e. large R wave) in lead V1 giving the appearance of right bundle branch block, due to late right ventricle activation. 'Normal' ventricular pacing activates the right ventricle first, then the left ventricle (as the pacing wire is sited in the right ventricle apex), giving an appearance similar to *left* bundle branch block. The pattern here indicates that the left ventricle (LV) is activated first, either as the ventricular pacing wire has been placed by mistake in the LV (i.e. going from the superior vena cava/right atrium, via a patent foramen ovale, into the left atrium and ventricle) or, much more likely, if the patient has a *multisite ventricular pacemaker* pacing the LV free wall, resynchronizing dyscoordinate LV contraction.

See Chapter 65, Fig. 65.1 for further details.

Fig.5

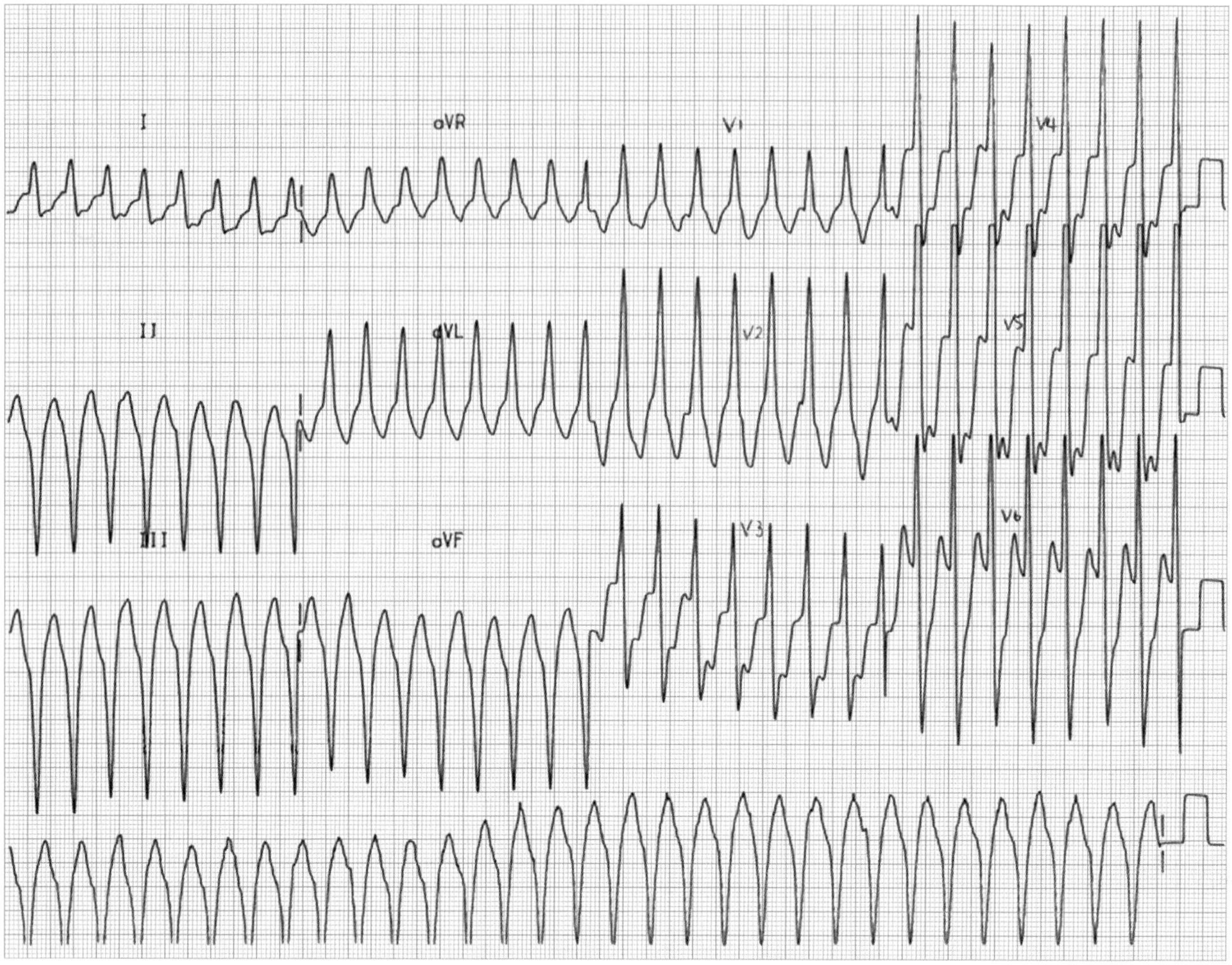

I aVR V1 V4

II aVL V2 V5

III aVF V3 V6

Fig.6

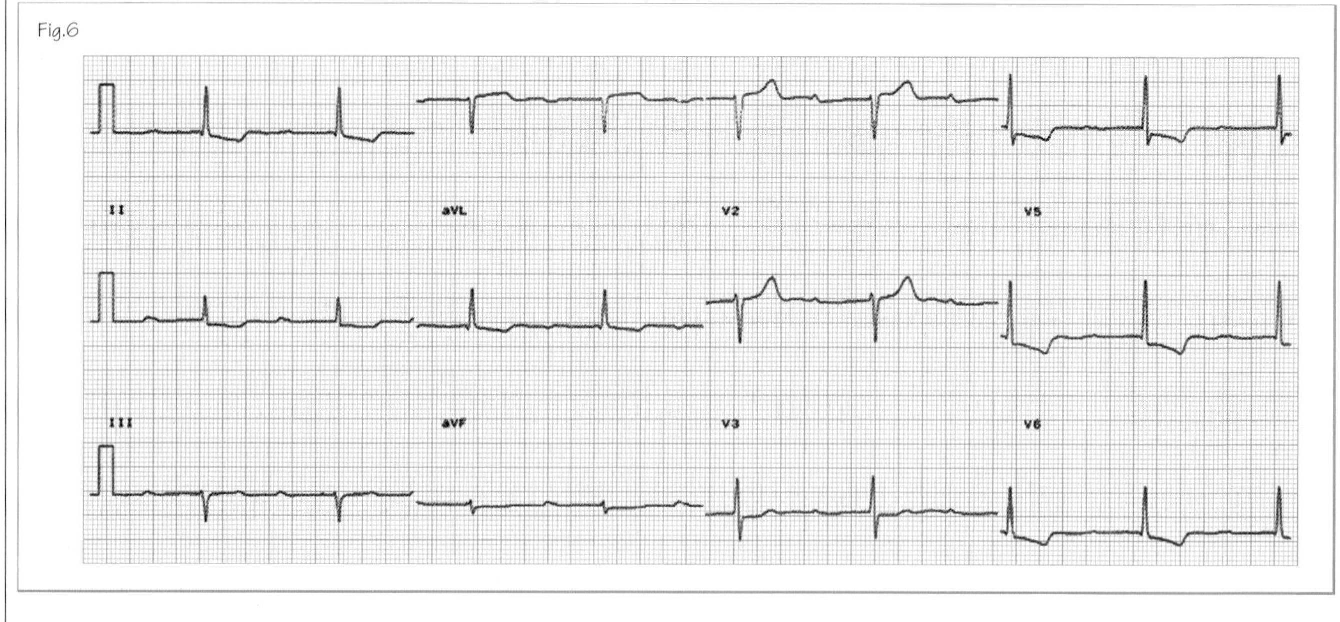

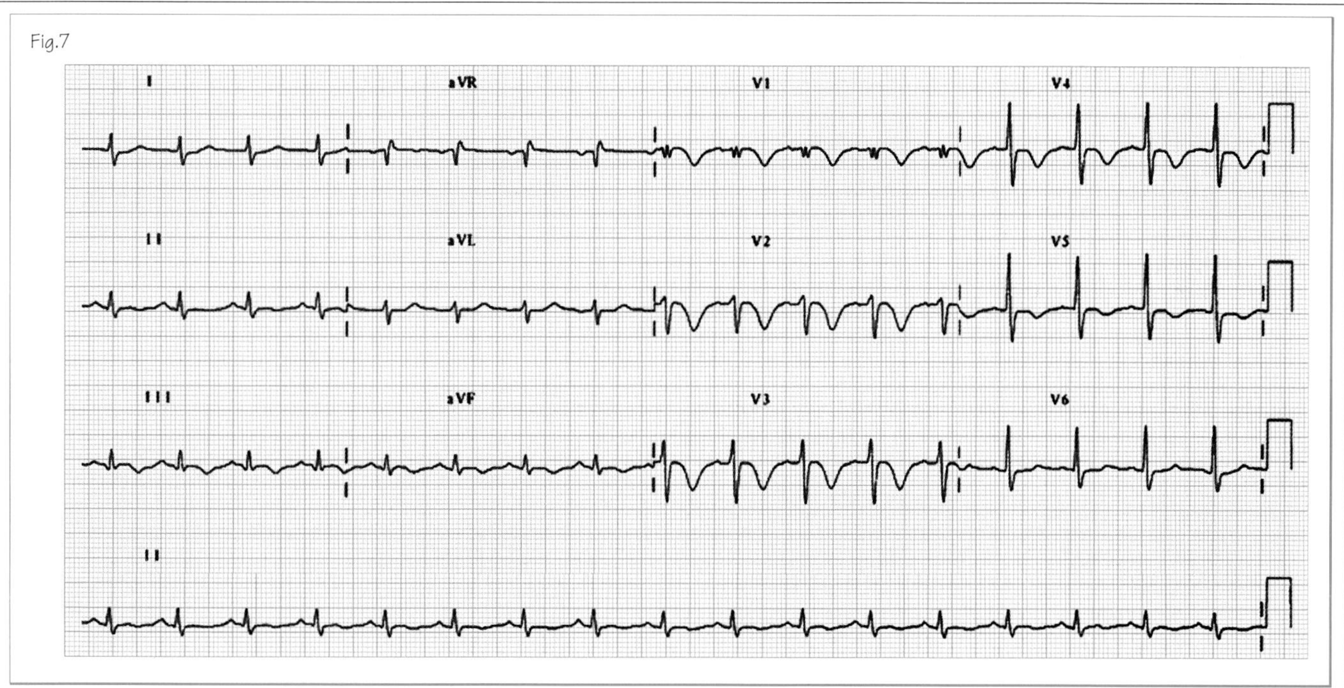

Case 3

A 67-year-old man with a remote myocardial infarction develops fast regular palpitations, with light-headedness. In hospital he is fully conscious, has slightly cool skin, O_2 saturation 97% on air, heart rate 160 b/min, blood pressure 85/50, venous pressure raised, no pedal oedema, an irregular variation in the first heart sound.

1 *What does the ECG show (Fig. 5) and what is the treatment?*

Case 4

An 85-year-old hypertensive man, presents with a blackout. While standing in the kitchen, without warning, he fell to the ground, unconscious. He was described as 'looking dead'. Moments later he recovered fully. Examination shows bilateral black eyes, normal cardiovascular exam. His ECG is shown in Fig. 6.

1 *What does this ECG show? What is the treatment?*

Case 5

A 35-year-old man returns from a holiday in Greece, presents with brief syncope, followed by intermittent breathlessness and anxiety. He looks pale, O_2 saturation 93% on air, heart rate 120 b/min, blood pressure 90/55, venous pressure + 6 cm, loud first heart sound, no murmurs, clear chest.

1 *What does the ECG (Fig. 7) show? What should be done?*

Answers

Case 3

1 This ECG shows ventricular tachycardia (VT). Why? There is a broad complex tachycardia; an experienced observer will instantly recognize VT. Ninety per cent of broad complex tachycardias in those with previous myocardial infarction (MI) are VT, so chance alone says this is VT. In supraventricular tachycardia with aberrancy, the complexes look like right or left bundle branch block (RBBB or LBBB), not the case here. With its dominant R wave in lead V1, this appears most like RBBB, but in fact doesn't look at all like the staggered M of typical RBBB. The straight up-down pattern is highly suggestive of VT. What clinches the diagnosis is the independent (i.e. varying relationship to each QRS complex) atrial activity seen in leads II and V1 as occasional irregularities in the baseline. The right-bundle pattern – superior axis (+ve QRS in lead I, –ve in II, III) suggests the VT originates in the inferior wall of the left ventricle. Though with only mild haemodynamic compromise, one could try intravenous drugs; DC cardioversion under general anaesthesia is a safe reliable treatment. In the longer run, exclusion of another MI, assessment of left ventricular function and coronary anatomy are needed, and probably revascularization and implantable cardioverter defibrillator (ICD) implantation.

See Chapter 49 for further details.

Case 4

1 The P wave is broad (lead II), suggesting left atrial enlargement. The PR interval is 520 ms (normal < 200 ms). The QRS duration and axis are normal. The R waves are unremarkable. The lateral T waves are inverted. The interpretation is: (a) extensive conducting system disease of the AV node or, more likely, the infra-Hissian system, causing an episode of complete heart block and so a Stokes–Adams attack; (b) lateral lead T waves changes could reflect ishaemic heart disease as the T waves changes spread to lead V3, or, despite the normal R waves, hypertensive heart disease (not aortic stenosis, as no murmer) – left ventricular hypertrophy with unremarkable R waves is not rare in the elderly. Digoxin causes a long PR interval (rarely this long) and lateral T changes. Provided there is no acute coronary syndrome, the right treatment is a permanent pacemaker.

See Chapter 55 for further details.

Case 5

1 Sinus tachycardia, 103 b/min, normal P waves, PR interval. QRS axis shifted to the right (+ 107°), impressive T wave inversion septally (V1→3), and more laterally, mildly so inferiorly. The differential diagnosis includes an acute coronary syndrome (ACS) (and myocarditis), but the sinus tachycardia, right axis QRS deviation and V1→3 T wave inversion are together so highly suggestive of a large pulmonary embolism as to be almost diagnostic. A cardiac ultrasound will support the diagnosis (and decrease that of an ACS). A computed tomography (CT) pulmonary angiogram will confirm the diagnosis. Intravenous heparin/thrombolytic therapy may be required.

See Chapter 20 for further details.

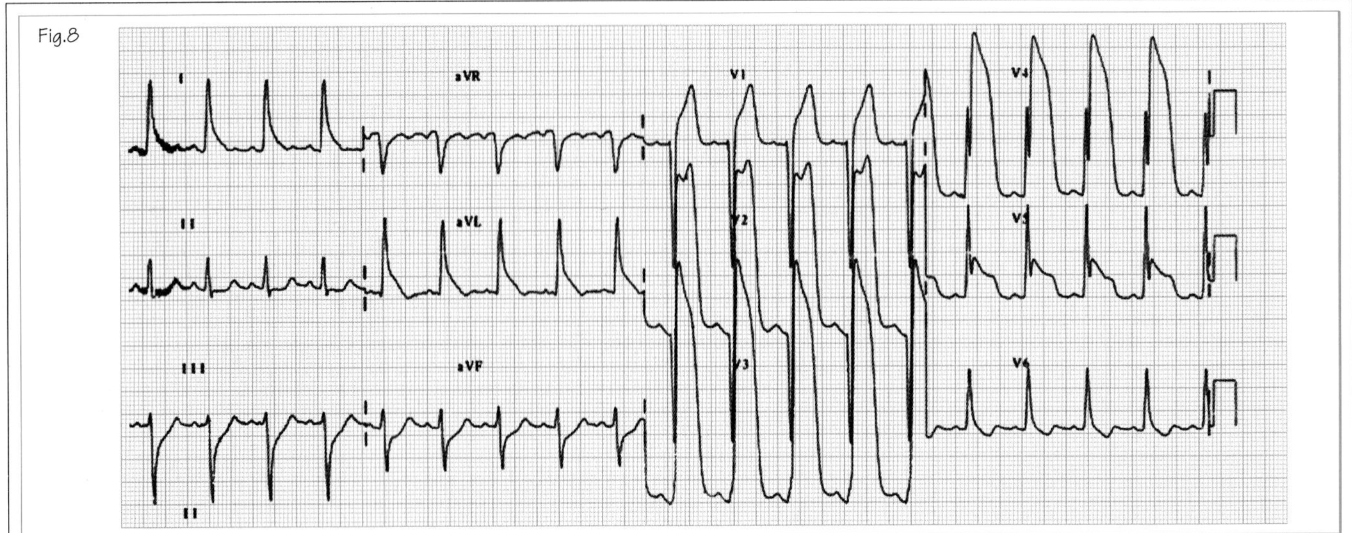
Fig.8
I
aVR
V1
V4
II
aVL
V2
V5
III
aVF
V3
V6
II

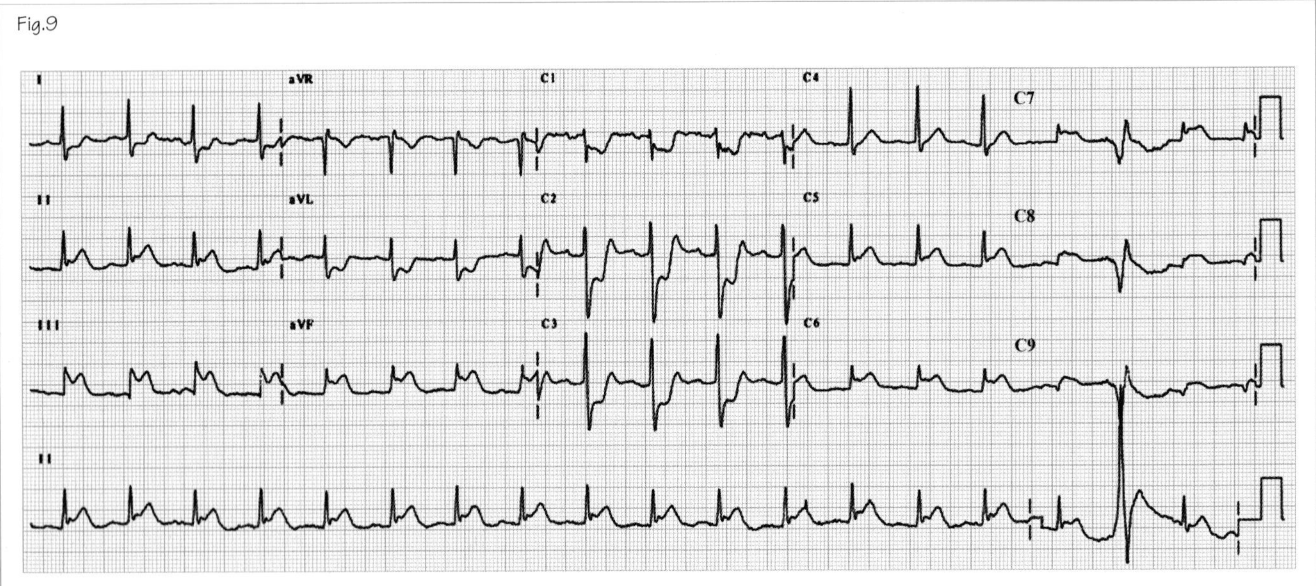
Fig.9
I
aVR
C1
C4
C7
II
aVL
C2
C5
C8
III
aVF
C3
C6
C9
II

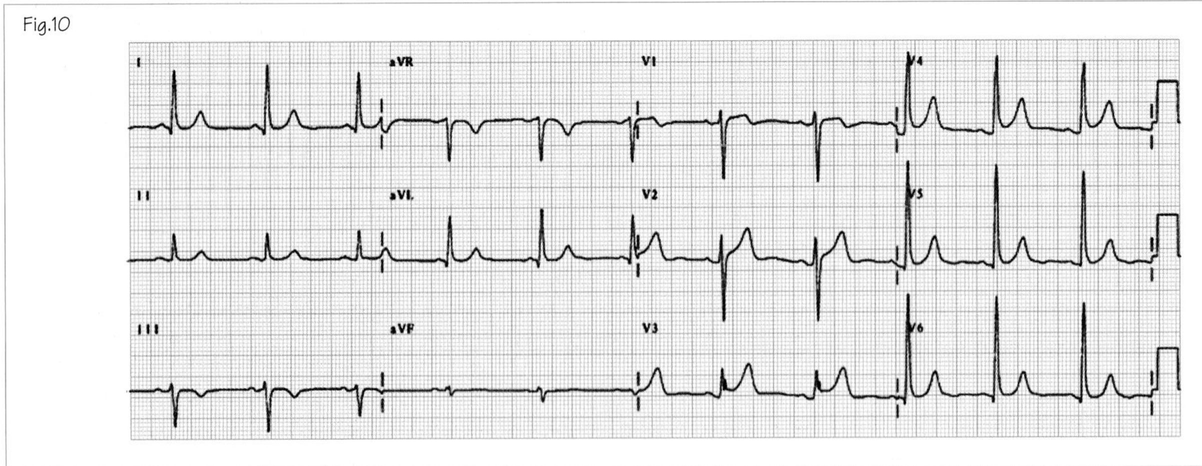
Fig.10
I
aVR
V1
V4
II
aVL
V2
V5
III
aVF
V3
V6

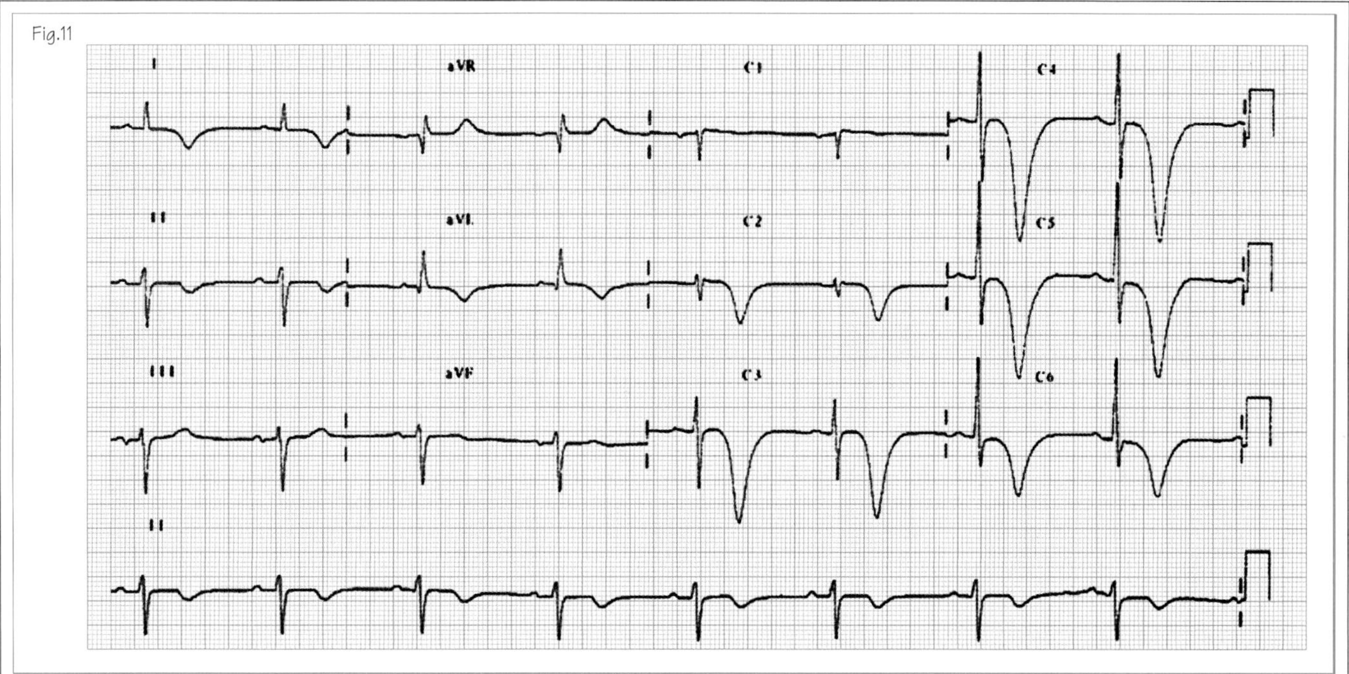

Case 6

A 55-year-old man presents with severe retrosternal chest pain, sweating, nausea, vomiting, and severe breathlessness. He looks grey and ashen and is clammy, heart rate 105 b/min, blood pressure 130/85, jugular venous pressure not raised, moderately loud S3, some bibasilar crepitations. His ECG is shown in Fig. 8.

1 *What does this ECG show? How will you measure the response to treatment?*

Case 7

A 72-year-old man presents with mild chest pain, retrosternal, no sweating. Examination unremarkable except soft third heart sound (Fig. 9).

1 *What does this ECG show, and what is the extent of the problem?*

Case 8

A 34-year-old woman presents with central chest pain, worse on deep inspiration, and on lying back, relieved by sitting forward.

1 *What is the diagnosis from the ECG shown in Fig. 10?*

Case 9

A 75-year-old insulin-requiring diabetic presents with 45 minutes of retrosternal chest pain, having had several much shorter episodes over the previous 2 weeks. His ECG is shown in Fig. 11.

1 *What does his ECG show, and how does this guide treatment?*

Answers

Case 6

1 Sinus tachycardia, normal P waves, PR interval. R waves difficult to see, as there is such impressive ST elevation, maximum 52 mm, affecting leads I, aVL, V1–5, ST depression elsewhere. The appearances are those of a massive anterol-ateral ST segment elevation myocardial infarction (STEMI); massive as: (a) many (seven here) leads show ST elevation and; (b) the amount of ST elevation, which relates to the extent of damage, is gross. Immediate effective reperfusion is needed, preferably primary percutaneous coronary intervention (PCI); its effectiveness can be ascertained by measuring the speed and amount of resolution of the ST elevation, and the subsequent absence of loss of R wave height/Q waves.

See Chapter 31 for further details.

Case 7

1 Sinus rhythm, normal P wave, PR interval, R wave. ST elevation leads II, III, aVF, V5–9, ST depression in leads I, aVL and posteriorly in V1–3. The appearances are those of an infero (II, III, aVF), postero (ST depression V1–3), lateral (V5–9) ST segment elevation myocardial infarction (STEMI), most likely due to circumflex occlusion, given the posterior and lateral involvement. The occluded artery is likely to be a large one, given the extent of the ECG changes. Posterior infarction leads to ST depression in leads V1–3, and ST elevation in leads V7–9; leads not routinely used, though they should be whenever posterior infarction is suspected.

See Chapter 31 for further details.

Case 8

1 This woman has pleuritic position dependent central chest pain, i.e. pericarditis clinically. The ECG shows ST elevation in leads V2–5, saddle-shaped in the mid-chest leads. These findings are by themselves non-diagnostic (and indeed could be physiological); what clinches the diagnosis, however, is finding PR interval depression in leads V3/4 – a rare but relatively sensitive finding for pericarditis. Pericarditis has many possible causes; in a young woman, without a preceding respiratory tract infection (i.e. suggesting that a respiratory virus is an unlikely cause) a possible cause that may need exclusion is systemic lupus erythematosus (SLE).

See Chapter 13 for further details.

Case 9

1 Sinus rhythm, normal P waves, PR interval. QRS left axis deviation (+ve in lead I, –ve in II, III), otherwise unremarkable, deep symmetrical pan-anterior T waves inversion in leads I, aVL, V2–6. The history is highly suggestive of an acute coronary syndrome – the ECG is almost diagnostic of a lesion in the proximal part of the left anterior descending coronary artery, suggesting really quite a dangerous situation. The cause of the left axis deviation is uncertain; the good R waves suggest that little or no myocardial necrosis has as yet occurred. Measuring troponin, while useful, does not alter therapy. Such patients require intense anti-platelet therapy, often including heparin, as a prelude to angiography and revascularization.

See Chapter 16 for further details.

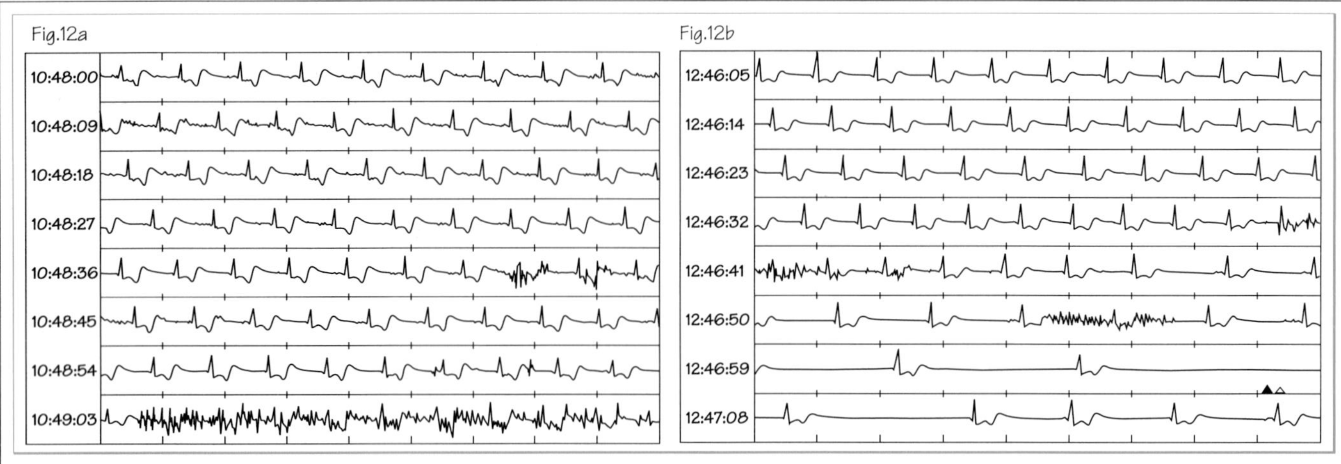
Fig.12a
10:48:00
10:48:09
10:48:18
10:48:27
10:48:36
10:48:45
10:48:54
10:49:03
Fig.12b
12:46:05
12:46:14
12:46:23
12:46:32
12:46:41
12:46:50
12:46:59
12:47:08

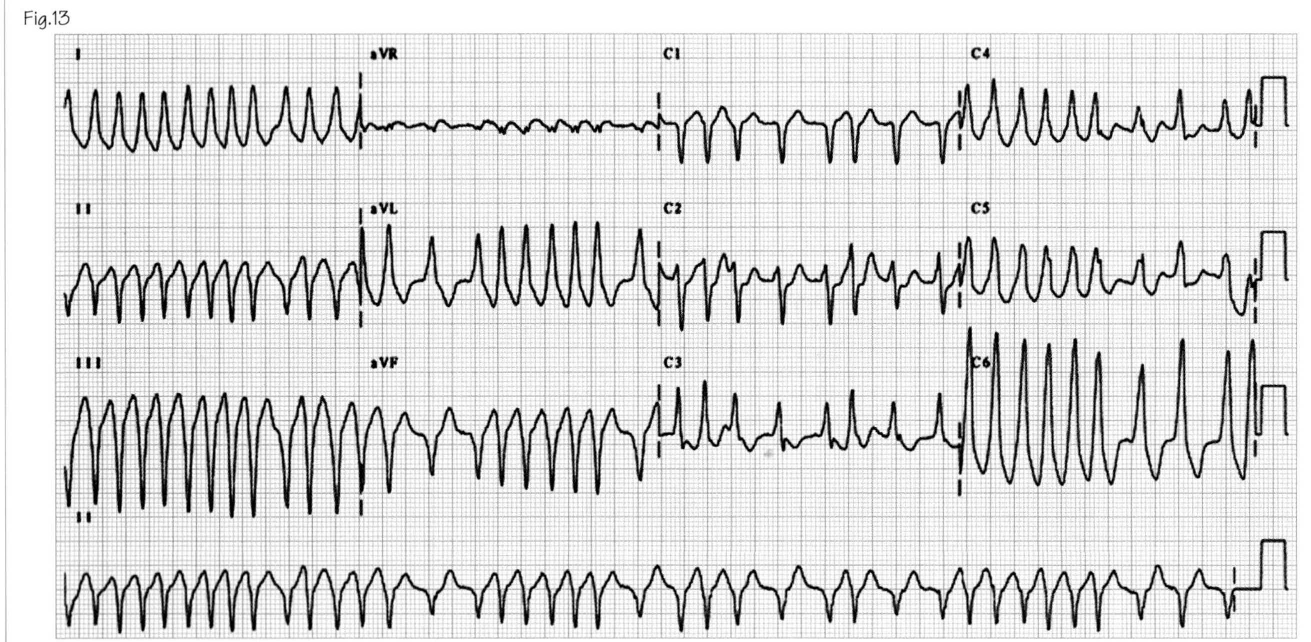
Fig.13
I
aVR
C1
C4
II
aVL
C2
C5
III
aVF
C3
C6
II

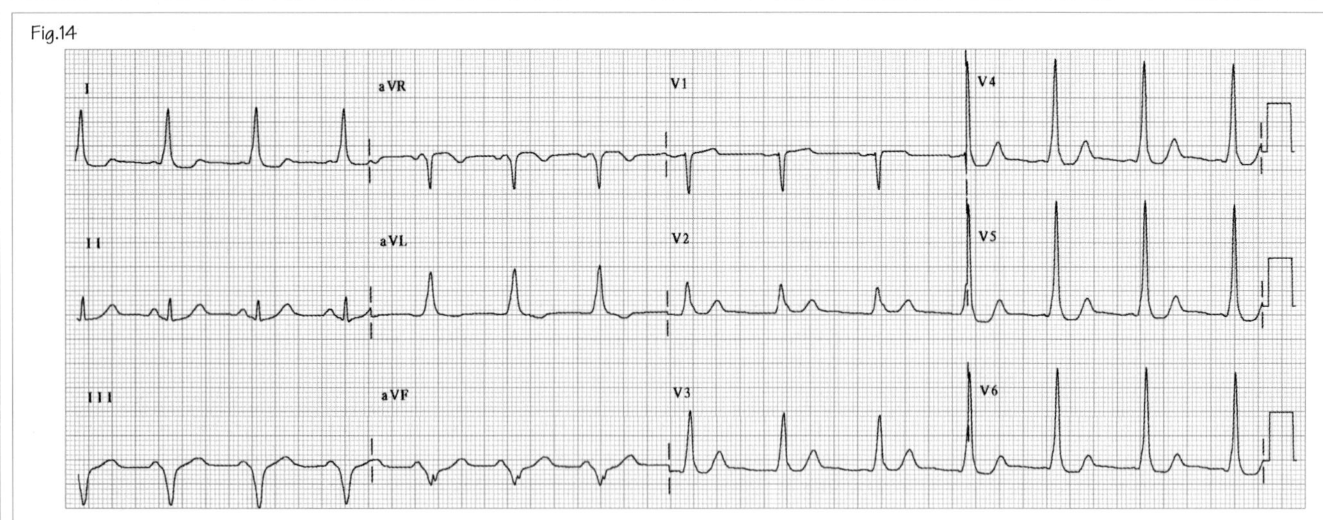
Fig.14
I
aVR
V1
V4
II
aVL
V2
V5
III
aVF
V3
V6

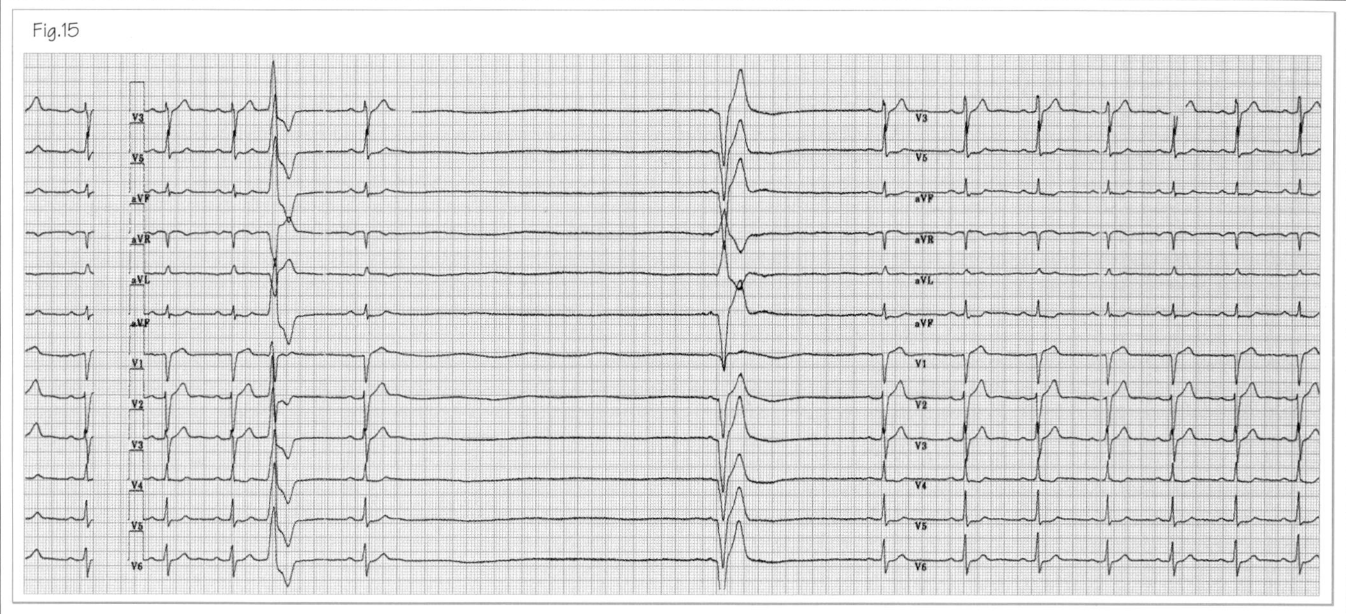

Case 10

A 42-year-old man present with 20–30 episodes of syncope, occurring over 5 years, in the standing position. A brief warning of near fainting and nausea precedes each episode, followed by loss of consciousness, falling to the ground, unconsciousness for 1–2 minutes, then rapid restoration of all faculties. Injury does not occur. Examination, 12-lead ECG, 24-hour ECG and tilt-table test were normal. A Reveal® device was implanted, and these recordings (Fig. 12a,b) made during syncope.

1 *What do they show and what are the implications for treatment?*

Case 11

A 38-year-old woman presents with faintness accompanied by rapid irregular palpitations. Examination shows her to look pale, variable heart rate around 170–200 b/min, blood pressure 90/60, normal heart sounds. Her ECG is shown in Fig. 13.

1 *What does her ECG show and what immediate treatment should be given?*

She has now received treatment (Fig. 14).

2 *What abnormality is shown and where is it located? What is the most appropriate treatment?*

Case 12

A 78-year-old man presents with syncope. He has had three episodes over 2 years, from the standing position, none while exercising. Stereotyped with a brief warning leading to loss of consciousness, falling, brief unconsciousness, rapid restoration of all faculties, bruises but no more severe injury. Normal exam, 12-lead ECG (Fig. 15).

1 *What tests (if any) are appropriate? What is this test, what does it show and how should the patient be managed?*

Answers

Case 10

1 A Reveal® device is an implantable ECG recorder, allowing capture of an ECG during syncope. The first trace (Fig. 12a) shows sinus rhythm early, later (bottom line) there is substantial muscle artefact (high-frequency small voltage waves), while the heart rhythm remains sinus. The second trace (Fig. 12b) shows sinus rhythm giving way to a severe nodal bradycardia, with pauses of 5 s. The demographics and history are highly suggestive of vasomotor syncope, probably neurocardiogenic, though the diagnosis was not supported by the tilt-table test (not infrequently the case). The traces shows that the first syncopal episode is not due to bradycardia (it is vasodilator – or non-bradycardic – in origin); the second shows a moderately profound reflex bradycardia, which by itself or in association with vasodilatation underlies syncope. So, the patient has a mixed bradycardic-vasodilator form of neurocardiogenic syncope. Pacing may lessen the frequency of syncope, and perhaps severity, but episodes (due to vasodilatation) will still occur, so pacing will not remove symptoms.

See Chapter 23 for further details.

Case 11

1 An irregular tachycardia, diagnostic of atrial fibrillation (AF). The QRS complexes in the lateral leads (I, aVL, V4–6) are broad with a slurred upstroke, suggestive of a delta wave. This is '*pre-excited*' *AF* (AF with Wolff–Parkinson–White [WPW] syndrome); most impulses reaching the ventricles via the accessory pathway. The minimum RR interval is 200 ms. Intravenous flecainide can be used, or DC cardioversion.

2 Wolff–Parkinson–White (WPW) syndrome, with delta waves in I, aVL the chest leads (not V1). There is a *pseudo infarction pattern* in the inferior leads (i.e. the Q waves reflect the abnormal ventricular activation pattern, not an old myocardial infarction). Right ventricular postero-septal accessory pathway (see Chapter 12). Catheter ablation is appropriate, given (i) atrial fibrillation (AF); (ii) heart rate during AF.

See Chapter 65 for further details.

Case 12

1 The normal exam and 12-lead ECG, absent antecedent cardiac history, suggests that episodic ventricular tachycardia or complete heart block are unlikely; the demographics suggest vasomotor syncope. The elderly can break bones (dangerous in the elderly) during syncope, so measures to prevent this are appropriate. Pacing may benefit those with bradycardic neurocardiogenic syncope (his tilt-test was negative) and bradycardic carotid hypersensitivity syndrome. This is a carotid sinus massage test, of the left carotid, while lying. A substantial bradycardia is induced; dual chamber pacing abolished syncope.

See Chapter 62 for further details.

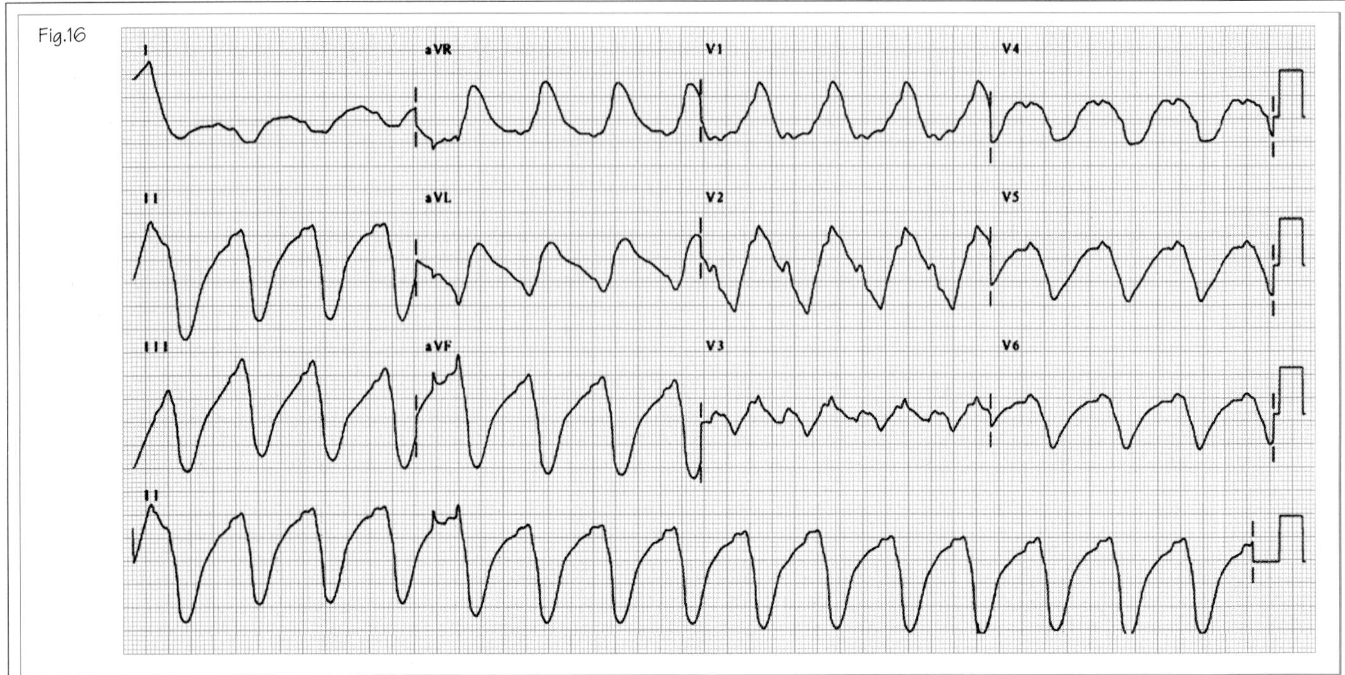
Fig.16
I
aVR
V1
V4
II
aVL
V2
V5
III
aVF
V3
V6
II

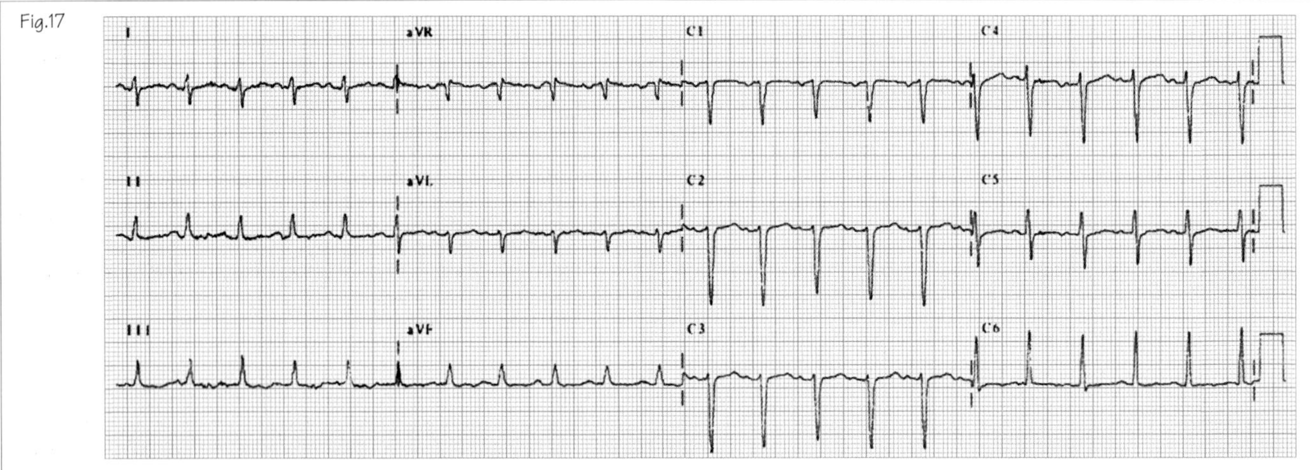
Fig.17
I
aVR
C1
C4
II
aVL
C2
C5
III
aVF
C3
C6

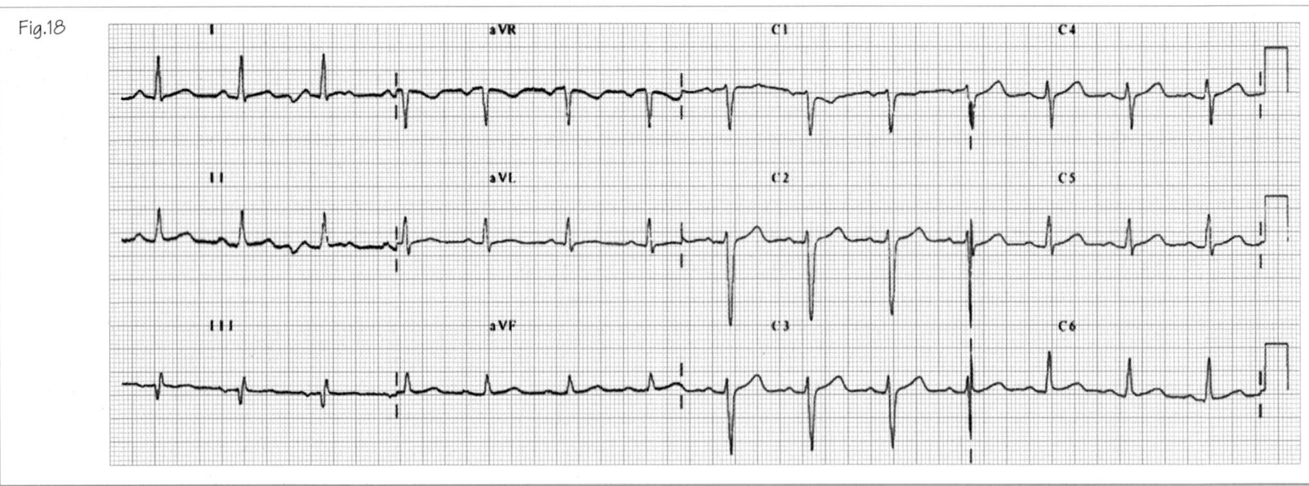
Fig.18
I
aVR
C1
C4
II
aVL
C2
C5
III
aVF
C3
C6

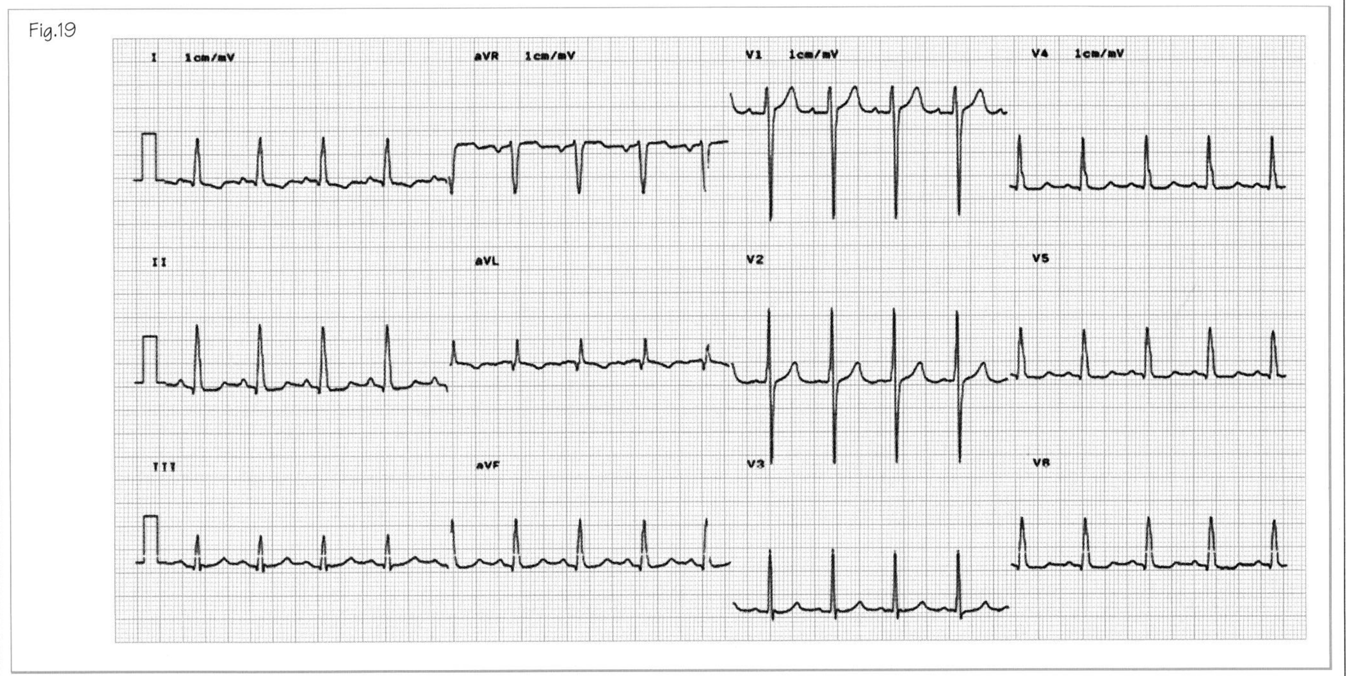

Case 13

A 78-year-old man with a long history of ischaemic heart disease, with previous myocardial infarcts, known poor left ventricular function and coronary surgery, presents with a week's history of diarrhoea, leading to dizziness on standing. He has noticed that for 2 days his urine output has been very poor.

1 *What does his ECG (Fig. 16) show, what is the likely cause, and what is the immediate treatment?*

Case 14

A 36-year-old homosexual man presents with a 2-month history of increasing breathlessness, initially on effort, then waking him up in the middle of the night, relieved by sitting forward. Examination shows a heart rate of 110 b/min, blood pressure 130/80, jugular venous pressure +8 cm, modest clinical cardiomegaly, third heart sound though no murmurs, some bibasal crepitations. His ECG is shown in Fig. 17.

1 *What does his ECG show, and is the cause identifiable?*

He receives treatment, and several months later his ECG is recorded again (Fig. 18).

2 *What does it now show?*

Case 15

A 49-year-old man presents with a 6-month history of increasingly severe effort breathlessness, with vague effort related chest tightness. Examination was normal.

1 *What does his ECG (Fig. 19) show, and can one use it to estimate ejection fraction?*

Answers

Case 13

1 This is a very bizarre ECG – there is a very broad complex rhythm, and it is difficult to distinguish the QRS from the T wave. To ascertain whether this is sinus, or an arrhythmia, the relationship between the P waves and the QRS complexes should be determined, not easy in this ECG. However, in lead V1, a P wave can be seen in the valley between two complexes. This is sinus rhythm with an extraordinarily broad QRST complex. His diarrhoea and postural dizziness suggests that he has become dehydrated, and this, when severe, can lead to renal failure, as evidenced by his low urine output. A complication of renal failure is hyperkalaemia, and his potassium was 9 mmol/l. The treatment required is intravenous calcium, followed by insulin/dextrose, aggressive fluid resuscitation and dialysis.

See Chapter 37 for further details.

Case 14

1 His symptoms and physical findings suggest heart failure, due to a left ventricular problem – this might be due to any one of the large number of causes of a dilated cardiomyopathy, though his sexual orientation places him at risk of human immunodeficiency virus (HIV) infection. His ECG shows sinus rhythm, with evidence of left atrial enlargement (negative P wave in lead V1), rather small QRS complexes, with poor anterior R wave progression, and very widespread ST/T wave flattening throughout the ECG. This ECG cannot diagnose the cause of his heart failure, all one can say is that it is very abnormal, and is likely to reflect a diffuse process affecting the whole heart (rather than coronary disease). A cardiac ultrasound showed globally very poor left ventricular function, his HIV test was positive, and he received anti-retroviral treatment.

2 His subsequent ECG (Fig. 18) is now virtually normal; there is still some poor anterior R wave progression, but the repolarization abnormalities have returned back to normal.

See Chapters 15 and 21 for further details.

Case 15

1 The ECG shows sinus rhythm, normal P waves, PR interval, normal QRS axis, very slight QRS broadening, deep S waves anteroseptally, and, the major abnormality, widespread repolarization (ST/T wave) changes. This ECG cannot reliably estimate ejection fraction – the worse the ejection fraction, generally speaking, the broader the QRS complex, the longer the QT interval, and, in coronary disease, evidence of old infarction (small R waves, Q waves, small QRS complexes). These are all generalizations, and there are many exceptions. This patient had an ejection fraction of 29% due to an idiopathic dilated cardiomyopathy.

See Chapter 21 for further details.

Fig.20

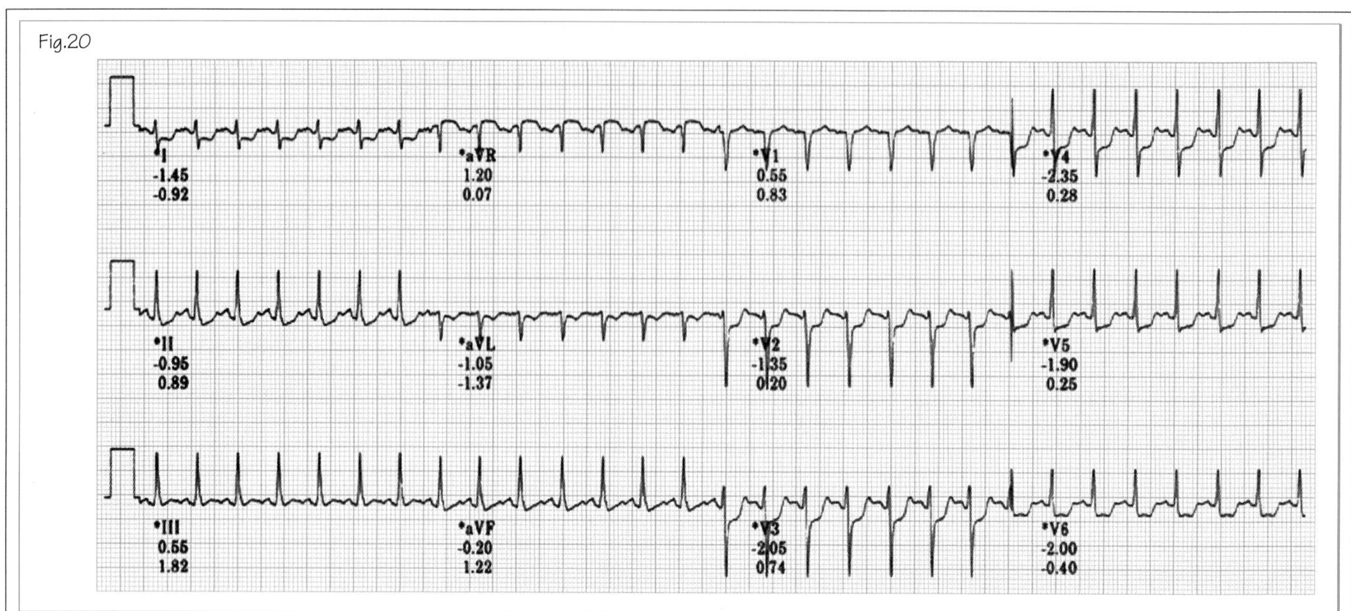
•I
-1.45
-0.92
•aVR
1.20
0.07
•V1
0.55
0.83
•V4
-2.35
0.28
•II
-0.95
0.89
•aVL
-1.05
-1.37
•V2
-1.35
0.20
•V5
-1.90
0.25
•III
0.55
1.82
•aVF
-0.20
1.22
•V3
-2.05
0.74
•V6
-2.00
-0.40

Fig.21

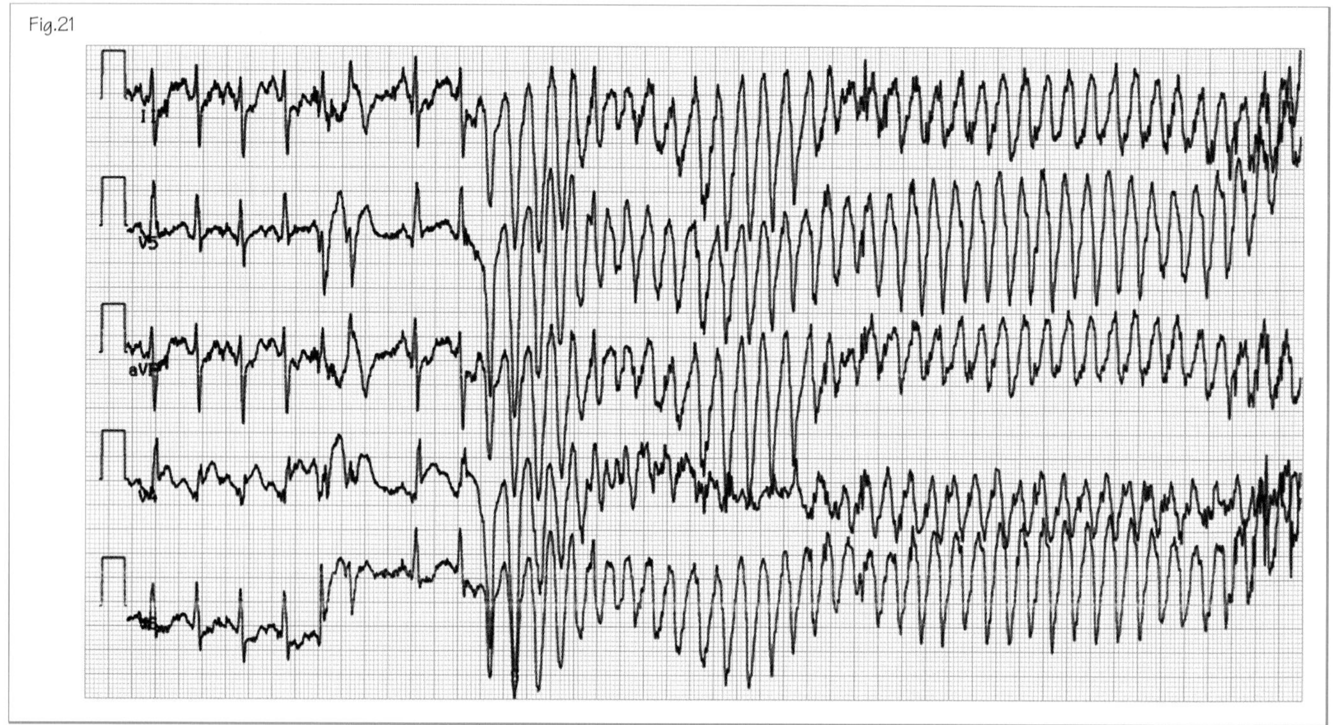
I
V5

Case 16

A 55-year-old male, without major risk factors for coronary artery disease presents with a 12-month history of burning left upper chest discomfort often but not always related to effort. He underwent exercise stress testing (Bruce protocol). The ECG shown in Fig. 20 was recorded at 4.5 mins, when chest pain necessitated discontinuation of the test.

1 *What is his pre-test likelihood for coronary disease?*

2 *What is shown, and what is the interpretation?*

Case 17

A 70-year-old, diabetic man presents with a 6-month history of retrosternal chest heaviness provoked by walking 800 yards, relieved by 1-minute rest, never occurring at rest. Physical examination was normal.

1 *What is the pre-test likelihood for coronary disease?*

Exercise stress testing provoked mild chest discomfort from early stage III. In late III the ECG in Fig. 21 was recorded.

2 *What does it show? What is the management?*

Answers

Case 16

1 The pre-test probability of obstructive coronary artery disease (see Fig. 19.3a in Chapter 19) in this man with atypical angina is 45%, so the test helps diagnostically and prognostically.

2 The ECG shows sinus tachycardia, 171 b/min, widespread anterior ST depression, 2.5 mm in V4, likely to reflect genuine myocardial ischaemia, as the ST depression is planar (not upsloping), severe (> 2 mm), widespread and affects the anterior leads. These factors increase the post-test probability of coronary artery disease to 85–90%. The Duke treadmill score is helpful prognostically (see Chapter 19: = exercise time (mins) – (5× ST-segment deviation, in mm) – 4 if angina occurs and 8 if angina is the reason for stopping the test) and is –17, giving a 5-year mortality of 75%. It is likely severe coronary artery disease is present, and that revascularization improves outcome, i.e. early coronary angiography is indicated.

See Chapters 19 and 64 for further details.

Case 17

1 The pre-test probability of coronary artery disease in this man with typical angina is 98%, i.e. the stress test is not for diagnosis but to ascertain prognosis.

2 The first four beats show sinus rhythm; with ST depression in leads II & aVF (1st and 3rd leads down), ST elevation in lead V4 (4th lead down). Two ventricular ectopics then occur, then two sinus beats, then a broad complex tachyarrhythmia, initially waxing and waning, becoming more, though not absolutely, monomorphic. The ST changes suggest ischaemia, the arrhythmia is ventricular tachycardia, initially polymorphic (?torsade-de-pointes) then possibly monomorphic. If the arrhythmia does not settle spontaneously with rest (the case here), treatment depends on the haemodynamic state, likely to be poor, necessitating immediate DC cardioversion, then anti-platelet therapy and, if ST elevation persists, immediate reperfusion therapy. This exercise stress testing is associated with a very poor prognosis on medical therapy, so early angiography is mandated. A blocked right coronary artery with a tight left main stem stenosis was found; a coronary artery bypass graft was undertaken successfully.

See Chapter 50 for further details.

Appendix

Table 1 Time domain methods for HRH.

Statistical measures		
SDNN	ms	Standard deviation of all NN intervals
SDANN	ms	Standard deviation of the averages of NN intervals in all 5-min segments of the entire recording
RMSSD*	ms	The square root of the mean of the sum of the squares of differences between adjacent NN intervals
SDNN index	ms	Mean of the standard deviations of all NN intervals for all 5-min segments of the entire recording
SDSD	ms	Standard deviation of differences between adjacent NN intervals
NN50 count*		Number of pairs of adjacent NN intervals differing by more than 50 ms in the entire recording; three variants are possible counting all such NN intervals pairs or only pairs in which the first or the second interval is longer
pNN50*	%	NN50 count divided by the total number of all NN intervals
Geometric measures		
HRV triangular index†		Total number of all NN intervals divided by the height of the histogram of all NN intervals measured on a discrete scale with bins of 7.8125 ms (1/128 s)
TINN†	ms	Baseline width of the minimum square difference triangular interpolation of the highest peak of the histogram of all NN intervals
Differential index	ms	Difference between the widths of the histogram of differences between adjacent NN intervals measured at selected hights (e.g. at the levels of 1000 and 10 000 samples)
Logarithmic index		Coefficient of the negative exponential curve $k \bullet e^{-t}$, which is the best approximation of the histogram of absolute differences between adjacent NN intervals

* These measurements of short-term variation estimate high-frequency variations in heart rate and thus are highly correlated.
† These measures express overall HRV measured over 24 hours and are more influenced by the lower than higher frequencies.

Table 2 Frequency domain methods for heart rate variability (HRV). From http://circ.ahajournals.org/cgi/content/full/93/5/1043.

Variable	Units	Description	Frequency range
Analysis of short-term recordings (5 min)			
5-min total power	ms^2	The variance of NN intervals over the temporal segment	0.4 Hz
VLF	ms^2	Power in VLF range	0.04 Hz
LF*	ms^2	Power in LF range	0.04–0.15 Hz
LF norm	nu	LF power in normalized units LF/(total power – VLF) × 100	
HF†	ms^2	Power in HF range	0.15–0.4 Hz
HF norm	nu	HF power in normalized units HF/(total power – VLF) × 100	
LF/HF		Ratio LF [ms^2]/HF[ms^2]	
Analysis of entire 24 hours			
Total power	ms^2	Variance of all NN intervals	0.4 Hz
ULF¶	ms^2	Power in the ULF range	0.003 Hz
VLF‡	ms^2	Power in the VLF range	0.003–0.04 Hz
LF	ms^2	Power in the LF range	0.04–0.15 Hz
HF	ms^2	Power in the HF range	0.15–0.4 Hz
α		Slope of the linear interpolation of the spectrum in a log–log scale	0.04 Hz

* This frequency is held to reflect the impact of the sympathetic nervous system on the heart.
† This frequency is held to reflect the impact of the vagus (and baroreflex) on the heart.
¶ The origin of the ultra low frequency component of heart rate variability is unknown, though is only expressed in 24 hour recordings.
‡ The very low frequency component of heart rate variablility is largely of uncertain origin, but may reflect the impact of thermoregulation on the circulatory system.

Index

Note: page numbers in *italics* refer to figures, those in **bold** refer to tables

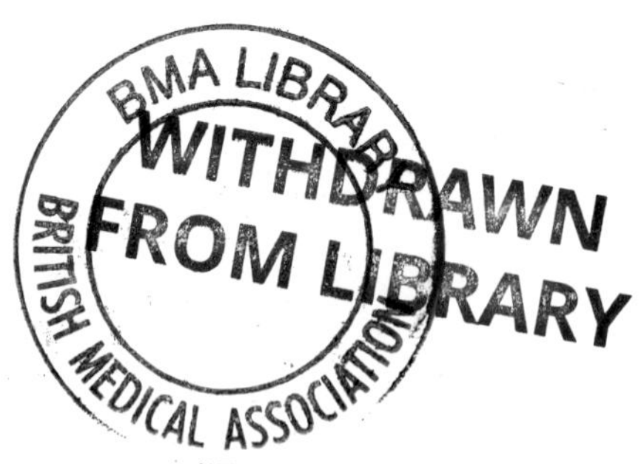